Handbook of Peritoneal Dialysis

Disclaimer:

The field of medicine is vast, complicated, and changing rapidly. The author assumes full and sole responsibility for the accuracy of the information presented in this book but human error or changes in medical information may have occurred. No information in this book can substitute for the caregiver performing due diligence to verify the accuracy of this medical information. Again, the information presented is solely from the author and does not represent the opinion of any past or present hospital, university, or employer.

This edition of the *Handbook of Peritoneal Dialysis* has been enhanced by the expert graphic designs of Mariana Ruiz Villarreal at mrv_taur@gmx.net

Any comments, suggestions, or corrections are welcomed at
guestnest5@yahoo.com

Copyright © 2014 Steven Guest, MD
All rights reserved.

ISBN: 1483932729
ISBN 13: 9781483932729

Handbook of Peritoneal Dialysis

SECOND EDITION

☙

Steven Guest, MD

This book is dedicated to:
Karl Nolph
Jack Moncrief
Zybut Twardowski
Dimitrios Oreopoulos

Preface:

THE ORIGINAL *HANDBOOK OF Peritoneal Dialysis* was published in 2010 and provided extensive clinical information relating to care of the patient on peritoneal dialysis (PD). The book was subsequently translated into Japanese and Mandarin editions and has been available on online bookstores around the world. This second edition is notable for updated and expanded chapters, enhanced graphics, and updated references.

As this book hopes to emphasize, PD remains the most innately physiologic, gentle, continuous, and cost-effective form of dialysis therapy based not on extracorporeal blood circulation but the natural filtering capabilities of the peritoneal membrane. While many countries such as the USA and Japan have been slow to widely adopt this therapy, other countries have reached different conclusions and believe that modern PD, with its novel solutions, newer cycler technologies, reduced complication rates, and recent survival data make this the preferred dialysis modality. These countries believe that PD offers a more rational approach to offering dialysis therapy in the broader context of overall health care expenditures.

It is inevitable that the model of in-center dialysis will need to be altered. Continuing to build brick and mortar dialysis facilities, in an attempt to keep pace with an epidemic of end-stage renal disease, is simply not sustainable and represents a cost to national health care payers that threatens their viability. It is clear that the USA will be moving towards a policy of establishing the home as the point-of-care for dialysis services driven by reimbursement changes to dialysis providers that favor home dialysis with PD. Dialysis providers, physicians, and nurses that anticipate and prepare for these changes will be well positioned to embrace them, develop successful practices that are economically viable, and thrive.

Perhaps this book can serve as a resource for expanding the clinical application of PD. It is evident that caring for satisfied PD patients, who cherish their ability to have care at home, be independent, work, and travel can be rewarding professional experiences.

Table of Contents:

Chapter 1: Brief History of Peritoneal Dialysis 1

Chapter 2: Peritoneal Membrane Physiology 13

Chapter 3: Peritoneal Permeability Tests 23

Chapter 4: Kinetic Modeling / Adequacy of Dialysis. 33

Chapter 5: Residual Kidney Function in PD. 43

Chapter 6: Peritoneal Dialysis Solutions 53

Chapter 7: Catheters and Placement Techniques. 65

Chapter 8: Catheter Dysfunction 83

Chapter 9: PD in Acute Kidney Injury or the Late-Referred ESRD Patient. 93

Chapter 10: Prescribing Chronic PD Therapy. 105

Chapter 11: Infectious Complications. 117

Chapter 12: Non-Infectious Complications. 145

Chapter 13: Volume Management in PD Therapy 175

Chapter 14: PD in the Diabetic Patient 185

Chapter 15: PD in the Obese Patient 203

Chapter 16: Nutritional and Metabolic Issues in PD. 211

Chapter 17: Survival in the PD Population. 231

Chapter 18: Setting Up a PD Program / Infrastructure. 239

Chapter 19: PD in Special Situations 249

Chapter 1:
Brief History of Peritoneal Dialysis

THE LONG HISTORY OF discovery that resulted in the understanding that the peritoneal cavity could be used as a renal replacement therapy is a fascinating compilation of personal dedication, fortuitous clinical observation, and the courage and sacrifice of early practitioners and patients. Descriptions of the peritoneal cavity date to ancient Egyptian hieroglyphics and early Greek descriptions of abdominal injuries, in gladiators, described the peritoneum as "peritonaion"- the roots *peri* meaning "around" and *ton* meaning "to stretch".

More detailed discussions of peritoneal anatomy and pathology were noted in the 1770's in reports of the clinical presentations leading to ascites. Early practitioners such as Christopher Warrick and Stephen Hales wrote of draining ascites with a "leather pipe" and suggested that two trochars could be used to allow for in and out lavage of the ascitic fluid.

Friedrich Daniel von Recklinghausen, in 1862, published the first descriptions of the peritoneal membrane's cellular components. This was followed in 1877 by G. Wegner, a German investigator, who described the concept of peritoneal ultrafiltration. Working with an animal model, he infused hypertonic solutions made of salts and glycerin and noted increased volume of the drained peritoneal fluid. He described metabolic transport processes occurring across the peritoneal membrane that could be altered by changes in the infused concentrated sugar solution. In 1884, work done in the laboratories of two Englishmen, Ernest Henry Starling and Alfred Herbert Tubby, noted that the movement of peritoneal fluid could be bi-directional, as infused hypertonic solutions could lead to an increase in intraperitoneal volume whereas hypotonic solutions resulted in a reduced intraperitoneal volume. They concluded that the bi-directional transport of fluid and solute was between the peritoneal cavity and the blood compartment and was affected by the number of blood vessels in the membrane.

D.Engel working in Prague in 1918 demonstrated that larger molecules such as proteins could transport from the blood compartment into the peritoneal cavity. The following year M. Rosenberg noted that urea from the blood reached equilibrium with peritoneal fluid and concluded that urea could be removed from the body by removing peritoneal fluid. Working with a dog model in 1923, J. Putnam, a neurologist and pathologist by training, concluded that the peritoneum was a "dialyzing membrane" where the rate of diffusion of a solute was dependent on its molecular weight and that solutes could reach a state of osmotic equilibrium between the peritoneal fluid and the plasma. He published the seminal paper "The Living Peritoneum as a Dialyzing Membrane" in the *American Journal of Physiology*. He then returned to neurological interests and was a co-discoverer of phenytoin.

The first attempt at PD in humans was based on this early work. Later in 1923, Georg Ganter, working at the University of Wurzburg, had been creating a model of obstructive uropathy in guinea pigs by ligation of the ureters. He then injected saline into the peritoneal cavity and, after several hours, removed the saline (probably the first description of intermittent PD). He noted that the drained saline had near complete equilibrium of nitrogen compared to the plasma. While doing this research, a patient was presented to him- a young woman with obstructive uropathy secondary to uterine cancer. He determined that the patient would soon die unless a similar procedure could be attempted. He prepared glass bottles to hold the infused solution. The bottles were boiled to make them sterile and then filled with 1.5 liters of a physiological salt solution. A rubber tube was used to infuse the fluid through a needle that had been introduced into the woman's peritoneal cavity. He infused from 1 to 3 liters each time and continued to do so until the blood chemistry became more normal and the uremic woman seemed to improve and was sent home. She died at home and he apparently concluded that the infusions should have been continued. Ganter's work created a foundation of knowledge for the future of PD- that peritoneal access would be required, sterile solutions would be needed, the risk of infection would plague the procedure, that ultrafiltration could be modified by changes in glucose concentration, and that solute removal was determined by the time and volume of the dwell.

Improved access to the peritoneal cavity was needed and in the 1920's, Stephen Rosenak and P. Sewon developed a metal trochar for instillation of fluid into the peritoneal cavity. This was followed by additional clinical activity at the Wisconsin General Hospital. In 1936 a patient presented who was diagnosed with obstructive uropathy. A group of physicians headed by Drs. Wear, Sisk and Tinkle employed peritoneal dialysis acutely and continued the procedure until the obstruction resolved. This demonstrated conclusively that patients could be treated with longer term PD. After World War I, German investigators employed what they termed "internal dialysis" to attempt to treat a variety of acute renal failure cases. Most patients apparently died from the other co-morbidities making any generalized successes of PD still unproven.

Repeated attempts were made to employ materials such as porcelain, glass and metal that could be sterilized for the dialysis procedure. Dr P. Kop, an associate of Willem Kolff's, was working on the concept of hemodialysis using synthetic dialyzing membranes that could be exposed to the blood. Dr. Kop moved to the field of peritoneal dialysis and devised a gravity driven system using large porcelain containers to infuse peritoneal dialysate down latex rubber tubing to a glass catheter that had been placed in the abdomen. They treated twenty one patients many of whom survived.

In 1945, physicians Howard Frank, Arnold Seligman and Jacob Fine used a double catheter for infusion and drainage and successfully treated a patient with acute kidney injury due to a sulfa drug overdose.

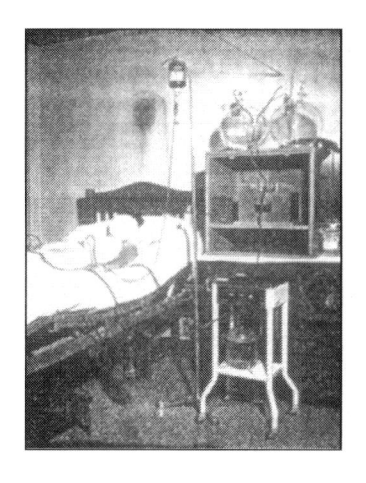

Acute renal failure from sulfa drug exposure successfully treated in Boston with a dual catheter system and gravity driven dialysis

During World War II frustrations mounted as thousands of soldiers died of acute kidney injury and in 1946 a major publication appeared in the Annals of Surgery describing successful peritoneal irrigation prolonging survival in patients. These investigators used large 5 gallon containers with dual abdominal trochars for continuous irrigation of the peritoneal cavity. The implications were that this procedure could be used to treat wounded soldiers with acute kidney injury in the battlefield.

As described, access to the peritoneal cavity remained a barrier and the most common approach employed metal trochars left in place for hours at a time. Further advances in peritoneal access were required and in 1952, Arthur Grollman at Southwestern Medical School in Dallas described use of a polyethylene tube. The tube was attached to a one liter container at one end. The intraperitoneal portion contained many small holes allowing for better infusion and distribution of fluid throughout the abdomen. The tube was more flexible and could be left in place for longer periods of time. He recommended that the infused fluid dwell for 30 minutes and then be drained back into the attached container.

Paul Doolan at the Naval Hospital in San Francisco in 1959 developed a modification of the polyethylene catheter that allowed for longer term implantation. The catheter was flexible and had additional grooves and side holes for better drainage. Dr. Richard Ruben, a physician at the same hospital who had just finished a tour of duty, treated a patient with peritoneal dialysis using this "Doolan" catheter. Her condition improved dramatically but then deteriorated again when the procedure was held. They repeated dialysis and again she improved- but again deteriorated when it was stopped. It was decided to allow the patient to go home for the week but return for dialysis on the weekend. This continued for 7 months.

Dr. Morton Maxwell, in that same year, while working at the Wadsworth Veterans Administration Hospital in Los Angeles, felt that emerging technologies in hemodialysis would be too cumbersome for clinicians so he designed a peritoneal dialysis system to treat acute kidney injury that would be easy to set up, use, and then take down. He approached a local manufacturer of intravenous solutions and requested a peritoneal dialysis solution in a customized glass container that was attached to the infusing tubing and the polyethylene abdominal catheter. Using these components, clinicians could use the "Maxwell Technique" which involved the simple installation of 2 liters of his peritoneal solution into the peritoneal cavity with a dwell time of 30 minutes and followed by a drain back into the original container that was lowered to the floor.

Later in 1959, a thesis was published in Holland by a young doctor named Fred S.T. Boen. Dr. Boen was born in Jakarta Indonesia in 1927 and attended the University of Indonesia and then transferred his studies to the University of Amsterdam. In 1957 he began working on his MD thesis for his supervisor Professor Borst. The subject of his thesis was "Peritoneal Dialysis" and was published in *Medicine* in 1961. The tenants of the thesis were that peritoneal dialysis was a simple procedure that avoided abrupt changes in blood volume, allowed for tailoring of the procedure by changing the dialysate to allow for better control of fluid and electrolyte balance, and could be performed long term as a permanent replacement for the kidneys. Dr. Boen wrote extensively of the past milestones in the understanding of peritoneal anatomy and physiology and detailed diffusion curves and peritoneal clearances for a variety of blood constituents. He described the influence of glucose on ultrafiltration when added to the irrigation fluid and modeled the correction of metabolic acidosis with addition of bicarbonate to the fluid. He also included meticulous flowcharts and other clinical details of patients presenting with acute kidney injury whom received peritoneal dialysis.

After reading Dr. Boen's thesis, Dr. Belding Scribner wrote to this young physician and invited him to come to the Northwest Kidney Center in Seattle to continue his research. Boen accepted the offer and moved to Seattle in 1962 with the intent on automating the procedure. There he developed a "fluid factory" where dialysate was prepared in large 20 to 40 liter bottles and then autoclaved.

Boen devised a latex catheter that could be capped off to allow for intermittent access to the peritoneal cavity. This capped catheter was termed the "Boen Button". He emphasized that the catheter lumen should be of sufficient size with adequate side holes to allow for proper hydraulic flow. He designed a sump drainage container that would hold a larger volume of solution. He recognized that a completely closed system would limit the risk of infection. He therefore designed larger infusion bottles to allow for repeated infusions without the need to re-connect additional bottles. The larger drainage container could accommodate repeated drains and he designed a monitor on the drainage side for measuring fluid removed from the patient. He automated the entire system so that it could operate overnight without requiring the presence of a physician. The Boen system allowed for discharge from the hospital and patients received peritoneal dialysis in their homes.

As clinical experience accumulated, Dr. Boen was concerned about peritonitis. He believed infection originated from the abdominal catheter as the rest of his system was a closed system. Therefore, he abandoned the permanently placed Boen Button and reverted to an earlier catheter that was placed for use and removed at the end of the procedure. With this new catheter patients could still remain at home but a physician was required to travel to the patient's home, place the catheter, set up the dialysis system and return the next day to remove the catheter.

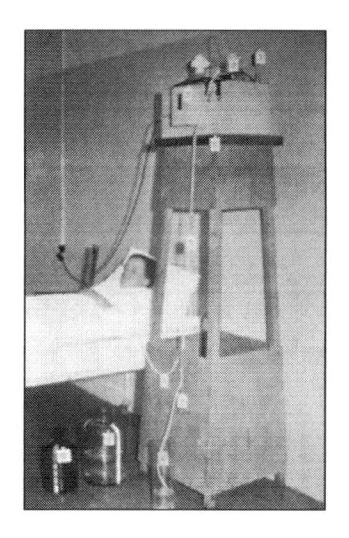

Boen used a gravity driven system with a single catheter- infusion followed by a dwell and then drain to the floor container

Dr. Boen, in the 1960's, wrote the first and only book (at the time) of peritoneal dialysis called *Peritoneal Dialysis in Clinical Medicine*.

Dr. Fred S.T. Boen is truly one of the founding fathers in the field of peritoneal dialysis.

Dr. Henry Tenckhoff at the University of Washington in 1963 began collaborating with Boen's team. It was his opinion that the system was still too cumbersome for wide application and was especially concerned about the difficulties in transporting 40 liter sterile bottles of dialysate to the patient's home. He devised a home-based reverse osmosis water purification system that prepared sterile water that was later mixed with a dialysate concentrate. He added a controller unit that could cycle fluid in and out of the abdominal cavity and be operated by the patient at home.

The procedure required repeated abdominal puncture and in a shocking publication Dr. Tenckhoff described a patient surviving over three years due to 380 catheter placements in the home. Obviously a more satisfactory catheter system was still needed. Tenckhoff addressed this by modifying a catheter that had been originally designed

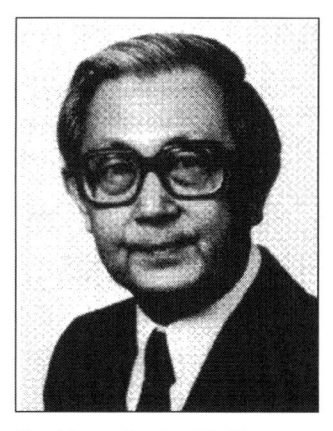

Fred Boen in the 1970's

by Dr. Russell Palmer and Wayne Quinton. The catheter was made of siliconized rubber and he modified it to be shorter and have a straight intra-abdominal segment or a pig-tailed segment. He added Dacron cuffs to allow for tissue ingrowth to seal the skin and peritoneal insertion sites. He stylized an internal metal trochar that would allow placement of the catheter more easily.

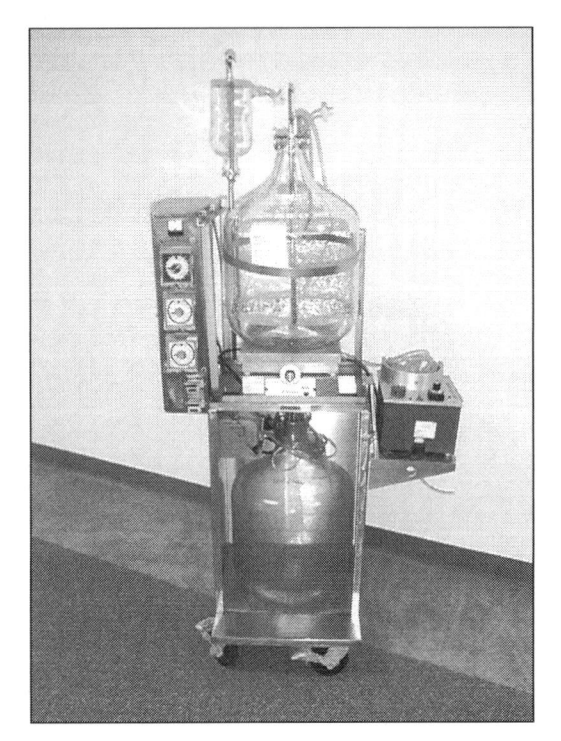

Norman Lasker, who was Acting Director of the Renal Division at the Seton Hall College of Medicine in New Jersey, visited the Seattle group to learn more about this new peritoneal dialysis system but returned somewhat concerned that these automated systems would be too difficult to manage at his location. He began collaborating with others to design a simpler device that used only 2 liter glass bottles, a drainage bag, a device to warm the solutions and to measure the volume of infused dialysate. He soon began treating patients in their homes with his new automated cycler device.

Dimitrios Oreopoulos who had trained in Belfast Ireland

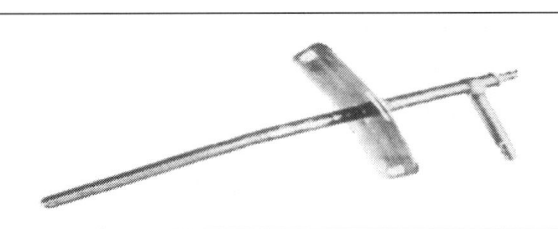

Boen's portable cycler device utilizing glass bottles, control devices on a metal frame with wheels

Metal trochar to instill dialysate

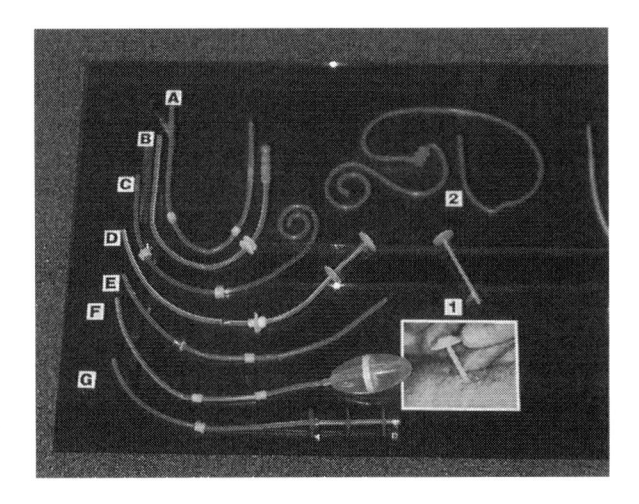

Various catheters, including the Deane's prosthesis (#1) used to seal the entry sinus track to facilitate replacement of the trochar for the next treatment and the Palmer catheter (#2) first describing a coiled configuration

accepted a position at the Toronto Western Hospital and was in charge of a 4 bed intermittent PD program. To allow for patients to move out of his inpatient unit he ordered several Lasker cyclers. His program was successful and eventually expanded to 70 patients making it the largest intermittent peritoneal dialysis program in the world.

Dr. Jack Moncrief established his medical practice in Austin Texas as the Director of Dialysis and Transplantation at the Austin Diagnostic Clinic. He developed an in-center hemodialysis program and in 1975 admitted a patient that would change his entire life. Patient Peter Pilcher had a fistula placed to begin hemodialysis but then thrombosed this and seven subsequent access creations. Dr. Moncrief recommended that the patient move to Dallas where an intermittent PD program had been established. The patient refused and Dr. Moncrief could not accept that his patient would die under these circumstances. He quickly collaborated with Robert Popovich, who had been a biomedical engineer with the Seattle group before moving to Austin to join the Chemical Engineering Department at the University of Texas. Moncrief and Popovich devised a 2 liter bottle system that used simple tubing to connect to a Tenckhoff catheter. Popovich modeled urea transport and determined that 5 exchanges of 2 liters would allow for stable blood chemistries. The fluid would therefore be left in the abdomen for 4 hour dwells and then drained.

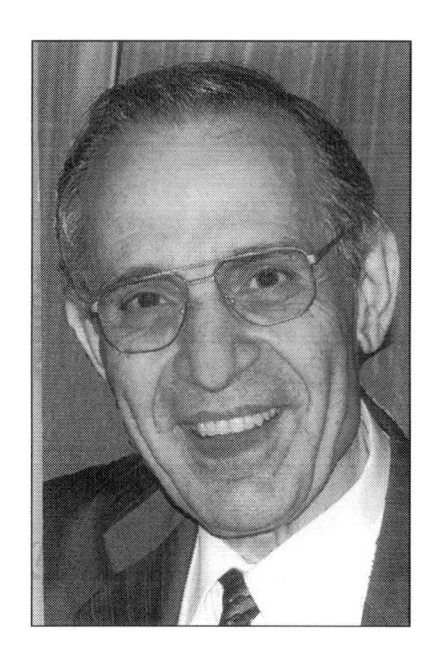

Drawings of schema to construct a PD system in the patient's home

Dr. Dimitrios G. Oreopoulos worked at the Department of Medicine, Toronto Western Hospital and the University of Toronto, Toronto, Ontario, Canada

They originally called this process "equilibrium peritoneal dialysis" and it was taught to patient Pilcher, who performed it at home successfully until he received a transplant. Soon thereafter Moncrief and Popovich formally applied for an NIH grant to allow them to continue to prescribe and research this technique. They received a contract to study the procedure on 4 additional patients. They submitted an abstract describing the procedure to an ASAIO meeting but it was not accepted for presentation.

They began discussing this new "equilibrium dialysis" with Dr. Karl Nolph of the University of Missouri. Dr. Nolph had learned of the work done in Austin and had a long-standing interest in urea kinetics and was asked by the NIH to establish a second center to study this procedure. Dr. Nolph's initial observations were that 2 liter exchanges 4 times a day would be adequate, in most patients, and this became the typical regimen. At an earlier dinner meeting, while discussing how to introduce the procedure into the University of Missouri, Moncrief, Popovich, and Nolph agreed to change the name of the procedure to "Continuous Ambulatory Peritoneal Dialysis" (CAPD) and re-submitted an abstract, this time to the American Society of Nephrology. On this submission, it was accepted and presented at the 1977 November meeting.

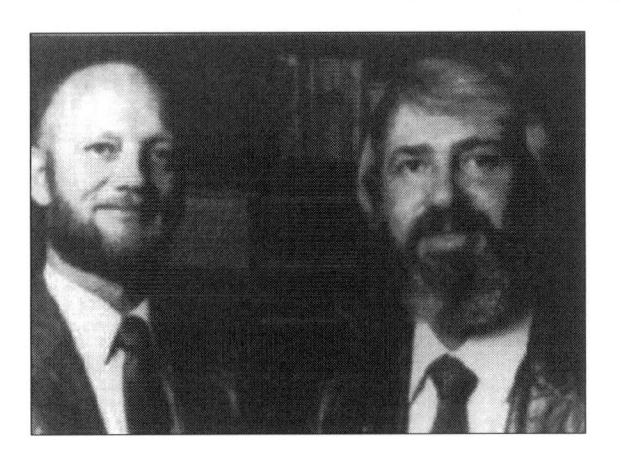

Jack Moncrief (left) Robert Popovich (right)

In 1978, the Toronto group, again, made a major contribution by publishing a paper describing their modification of the CAPD procedure. They had been using predominantly intermittent cycler therapy until one of their renal fellows, Dr. Jack Rubin, returned from a research sabbatical at the University of Missouri's PD unit. He had been involved with this emerging CAPD program and discussed this with Dr. Oreopoulos. Dr. Oreopoulos then tried the CAPD procedure on a patient doing poorly on his cycler therapy and noted that the patient significantly improved. This convinced him to start a Toronto CAPD program but altered the procedure by changing from glass dialysate containers to plastic polyvinylchloride (PVC) bags, which were available in Canada but not the USA. With these plastic PD bags he noted greater ease in transporting solutions, significantly reduced peritonitis rates, and overall improved

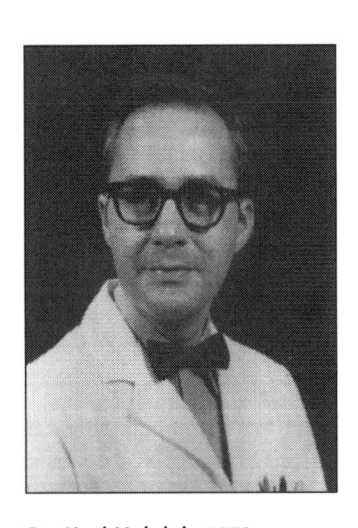

Dr. Karl Nolph in 1972
University of Missouri

Dr. Karl Nolph and his wife Georgia attending a conference in France in 1980

patient acceptance. The plastic bags allowed for the fluid to be infused by gravity, then, when empty, could be rolled up and remain connected. Later, the bags could be unrolled to allow for gravity drainage of the fluid. The drained bag was then removed and a fresh bag was connected. Working with his local Baxter Healthcare representative they modified how new bags would be attached to the tubing by designing a spike at one end of the tubing. This spike was inserted into a receptacle fashioned into the plastic bags and this allowed for an easier, more secure and sterile way to connect the tubing to the plastic bags.

Back in the USA, the Food and Drug Administration, in 1978, gave approval for the CAPD procedure and in 1979 Baxter introduced to the market the first CAPD system that included solution bags, tubing with a spike at one end, a titanium luer lock to connect to the patient's catheter, and an antiseptic solution to clean the spike/bag connection. Three types of dialysis solutions were available based on varying dextrose concentrations.

Upon learning of this new spiking mechanism and subsequent reduction in peritonitis rates, Moncrief and Popovich again made a contribution by inventing an ultraviolet exposure system at the spike site to attempt to further reduce the chances of infection.

Dr. Umberto Buoncristiani in Italy soon invented the so-called Y system where an empty drain bag was connected to the tubing on one end, the patient could be connected at the tubing that formed the base of the Y and then the remaining tubing used to spike a solution bag. This configuration allowed for flushing of new solution and dwelled dialysate away from the patient into the drain bag first, to wash away any contaminating bacteria, before any fresh dialysate was infused. This flush-before-fill technique dramatically reduced overall peritonitis rates. The Y-set was later

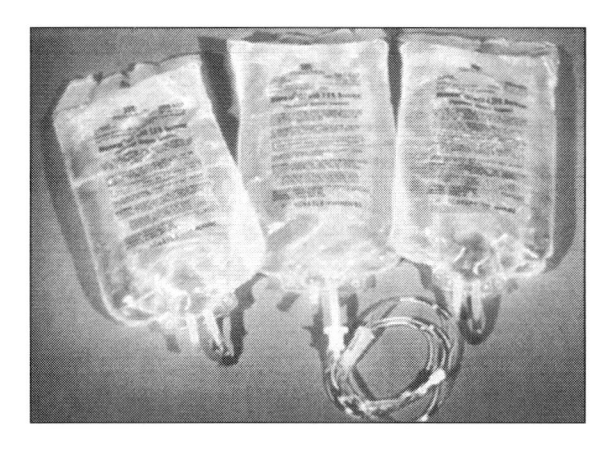

Plastic dialysate bags first used by Oreopoulos in Toronto

modified into a double bag system that allowed for only one required connection, to the patient, further reducing peritonitis risk.

In 1981, Drs. Jose Diaz-Buxo and D. Nakayawa both independently published reports describing a hybrid technique that used a cycler device to repeatedly infuse and drain dialysate during the night followed by a long 1 to 2 liter dwell of fluid during the day. They termed this procedure "Continuous Cyclic Peritoneal Dialysis" (CCPD). This allowed for fluid to be in contact with the peritoneum for 24 hours, similar to CAPD, but with reduced number of required connections.

In the USA, governmental discussions on how to reimburse providers for these procedures soon followed and in 1983 an amendment to Medicare legislation allowed for PD to be compensated at a similar rate as in-center hemodialysis. As word spread of this new form of dialysis, large symposiums were held to present clinical experiences and research. The first international symposium was held in Mexico followed by other large meetings in Buenos Aires, Berlin, Melbourne, Washington, Paris and Austin. Dr. Nolph was contacted by the NIH and asked to organize a national conference on PD that would be yearly. The first such meeting was called "The First National CAPD Conference" and the name was later changed to the "Annual Dialysis Conference" which is still in existence today, sponsored by the University of Missouri. Presentations from this yearly meeting are separately published as *Advances in Peritoneal Dialysis*.

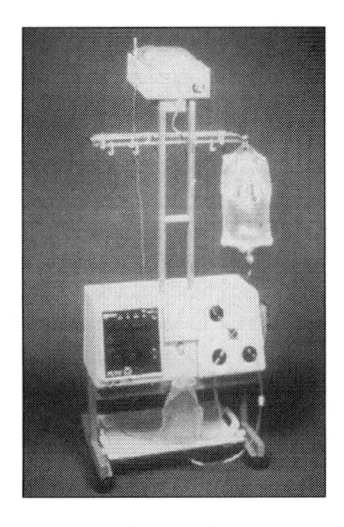

Gravity driven cycler machines used in the 1980's and early 1990's

Jack Maher and Jim Winchester proposed and established the International Society of Peritoneal Dialysis (ISPD) in 1984 and in 1988 the official publication of the ISPD became the journal *Peritoneal Dialysis International* (PDI). The journal was derived from the *Peritoneal Dialysis Bulletin*, started in 1980 by Dr. Oreopoulos as a means to keep in contact with the over 800 visitors that had come to Toronto to view their PD unit. The interest in this publication continued to grow with submissions coming in from around the world. The free publication soon had a circulation of over 13,000 made possible by the "no strings attached" financial support from Baxter. Dr. Oreopoulos served as the editor of the publication for 23 years. Under his leadership the impact of PDI continued to grow and remains the primary publication for clinical and research publications in this discipline. The PD community grieved the death of Dr. Oreopoulos, at age 76, in April 2012.

As CAPD became more common in the USA, a national CAPD Registry was started. Data was initially collected from 15 centers but by 1988 the final report included data on over 26 thousand patients from 498 centers. The usefulness of this registry in understanding trends and outcome measures in CAPD was followed by the establishment of the US Renal Data System (USRDS) to better follow all patients with ESRD.

The popularity of PD continued to grow world-wide as a cost effective option for dialysis. As the field of PD continues to innovate and excite, with the advent of newer solutions, improved connectology, and smaller cyclers, it is important to remember the historical context in which these changes are occurring. The courage and persistence of many physicians, nurses, scientists and policy makers allowed this field to mature to the point that now over 11% of the world's dialysis population are alive on peritoneal dialysis.

Author's Note;
THE AUTHOR WISHES TO thank John A. Sweeny for providing several images. Mr. Sweeny is retired Technical Training Manager, Global Technical Services, Largo, Florida and past curator of Baxter's History of Dialysis Museum.

In addition to Dr Oreopoulos, the PD community has recently mourned the loss of Dr. Popovich.

References:

Bliss S, Kastler AO, Nadler SB. Peritoneal lavage. Effective elimination of nitrogenous wastes in the absence of kidney function. Proc Soc Exp Biol and Med 1931;29:1078-1079.

Boen ST. Peritoneal dialysis: a clinical study of factors governing its effectiveness. Kidney Int 2008;73:S5-17.

Boen ST. Kinetics of peritoneal dialysis. A comparison with the artificial kidney. Medicine 1961:4:243-287.

Fine JH, Frank HA, Seligman AM. The treatment of acute renal failure by peritoneal irrigation. Ann Surg 1946;124:857-875.

Guest S, Divino Filho J, Krediet RT. Celebrating the 50th anniversary of the thesis on peritoneal dialysis by Dr. Fred S.T. Boen. Perit Dial Int 2009;29:601-604.

Lasker N, Shalhoub R, Habibe O, Passarotti C. The management of end-stage kidney disease with intermittent peritoneal dialysis. Ann Intern Med 1965;62:1147-1169.

Maxwell MH, Rockney RE, Kleman CR, Twiss MR. Peritoneal dialysis. JAMA 1959;170:917-924.

Moncrief JW, Popovich RP, Nolph KD. The history and current status of continuous ambulatory peritoneal dialysis. Am J Kidney Dis 1990;16:579-584.

Nolph KD, Khanna R. Dimitrios Oreopoulos: fondly remembered and greatly missed. Perit Dial Int 2012;32:373-374.

Oreopoulos DG, Robson M, Izatt S, et al. A simple and safe technique for continuous ambulatory peritoneal dialysis (CAPD). Trans Am Soc Artif Intern Organs 1978;24:484-489.

Oreopoulos DG. Peritoneal Dialysis International: its origins and impact. Semin Dial 2004;17:346-348.

Oreopoulos DG, Thodis E. The history of peritoneal dialysis: early years at the Toronto Western Hospital. Dial Transplant 2010;August:338-342.

Popovich RP, Moncrief JW, Nolph KD, Ghods AJ, Twardowski Z, Pyle WK. Continuous ambulatory peritoneal dialysis. Ann Intern Med 1978;88:449-456.

Putnam TJ. The living peritoneum as a dialyzing membrane. Am J Physiol 1923;63:543-565.

Tenckhoff H, Shillipetar G, Boen ST. One year's experience with home peritoneal dialysis. Tran Am Soc Artif Int Organs 1965;11:11-14.

Teschner M, Heidland A, Klassen A, et al. Georg Ganter- a pioneer of peritoneal dialysis and his tragic academic demise at the hand of the Nazi regime. J Nephrol 2004;17:457-460.

Nolph KD. 1975 to 1984- an important decade for peritoneal dialysis: memories with personal anecdotes. Perit Dial Int 2002;22:608-613.

Twardowski ZJ. History of peritoneal access development. Int J Artif Organs 2006;29:2-40.

Chapter 2:
Peritoneal Membrane Physiology

IN PD, THE INNATE peritoneal membrane serves as a dialyzing membrane that enables solutes to diffuse from the capillary blood compartment to the dialysate-filled peritoneal cavity. The membrane has a large effective surface area, estimated to be 1 to 2 square meters. The total membrane area includes the visceral peritoneum (60%), peritoneum covering the mesentery and omental surfaces (30%), and the parietal peritoneum (10%).

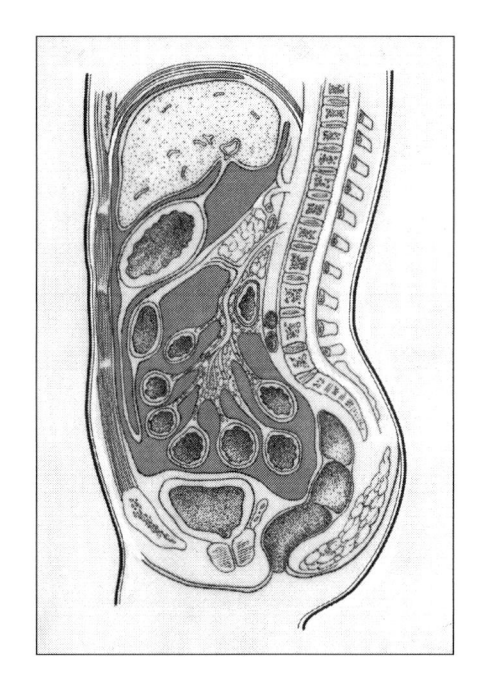

Although the parietal peritoneum consists of only 10% of the total peritoneal membrane area, there is evidence to support the belief that this parietal anatomy constitutes the main anatomic location for the dialysis process. Imaging studies performed after the infusion of radio-isotope tracers or contrast material have demonstrated that dialysate collects largely in the dependent pelvic region and into the lateral abdominal paracolic "gutters" and maintains contact most significantly with the parietal surfaces. Scant tracer

The large visceral and parietal peritoneal membrane surface area participates in solute transport during peritoneal dialysis

activity or contrast is visualized in the central abdomen in the vicinity of the visceral peritoneum. Most convincing of all studies were those performed by Rubin and colleagues in 1986 in which mongrel dogs were anesthetized, given peritoneal access catheters and underwent urea and glucose clearance studies. The dogs were then subjected to complete evisceration of intestines and omentum. Clearance measurements did not appreciably change after the evisceration, strongly suggesting that the visceral peritoneum contributes relatively little to the dialysis process.

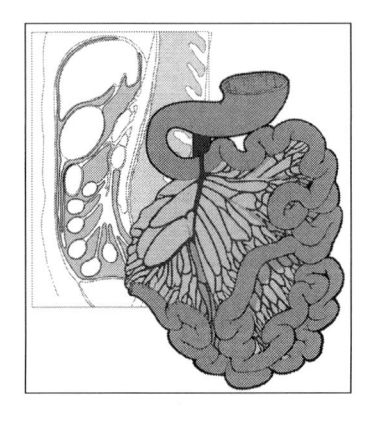

Extensive peritoneal blood supply allows for solute delivery to capillary bed for diffusion and convection

The peritoneal membrane has an extensive blood supply, with the visceral peritoneum supplied by the mesenteric arteries that drain ultimately into the portal circulation, and the parietal peritoneum supplied by the smaller epigastric, intercostals, and lumbar arteries that drain directly into the inferior vena cava. The estimated total peritoneal blood flow is 50 to 100 mL per minute.

The Peritoneum as a Dialyzing Membrane

Three major peritoneal components could potentially filter toxins from the blood compartment into the peritoneal space:

1. Mesothelial cell layer
2. Interstitial space
3. Capillary endothelium

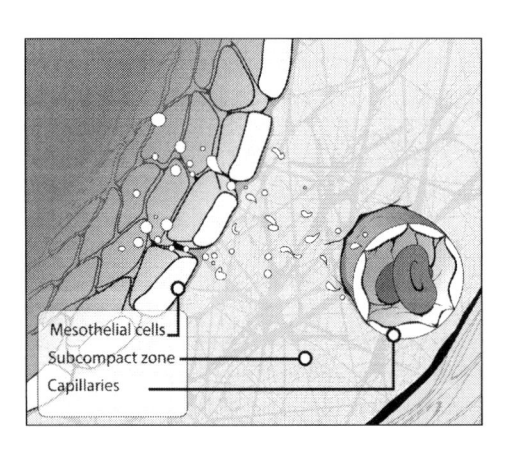

The mesothelial layer and interstitial space are felt to offer only minor resistance to the flow of toxins. The primary filter determining solute transport appears within

The three main determinants of the peritoneal membrane- the mesothelial cell layer, the underlying interstitial tissue, termed the subcompact zone, and the peritoneal capillary bed

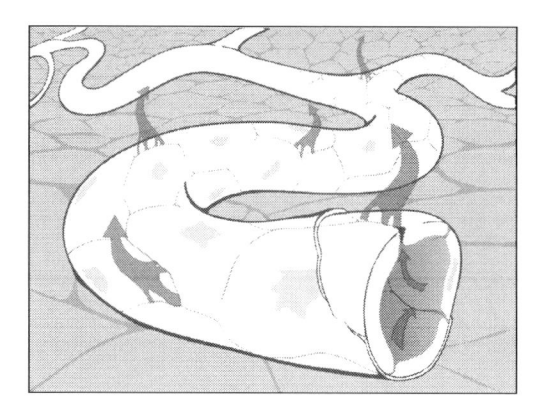

Peritoneal capillary vessels contain endothelial clefts and intercellular junctions that create fenestrations that allow for filtration of substances across the capillary wall

the capillary wall. Therefore, the capillary vascular surface area is the most important determinant of solute transport.

Several theoretical constructs have been described to help determine the transport of solutes across the peritoneal capillary bed. Two of the most discussed models are the:

1. The distributed model
2. Three pore model

The Distributed Model of Peritoneal Transport

The distributed model is used largely in the research setting and is much more complicated, mathematically, and not used clinically. In the distributed model, capillaries are described as being distributed throughout the peritoneal membrane and are at variable distances from the peritoneal cavity. Solute transport is therefore affected by the blood-dialysate distance (the amount of interstitium), the solute concentration gradient, and density of capillaries. Total solute transport requires the summation of partial distribution equations that take into consideration the spacing of capillaries within the interstitial matrix. The model factors different densities of capillaries within certain regions of the peritoneum and can take into consideration fibrotic changes in the interstitium that may occur during longer term PD. As mentioned, the technical nature of this model is for research purposes.

Three Pore Model of Peritoneal Transport

The most commonly discussed clinical model is the three pore model. In the three pore model, the main barrier to solute transport is the peritoneal capillary. The capillary endothelial cells are described as having 3 "pores" that allow for the movement of solute and water across the capillary.

These three pores are the trancellular aquaporins, small, and large pores. These pores have the following characteristics:

Pores	Size	Density
Aquaporins (AQP1)	R = 4-5 angstroms	Large
Small pores	R = 40-50 angstroms	Large
Large pores	R = >150 angstroms	Small

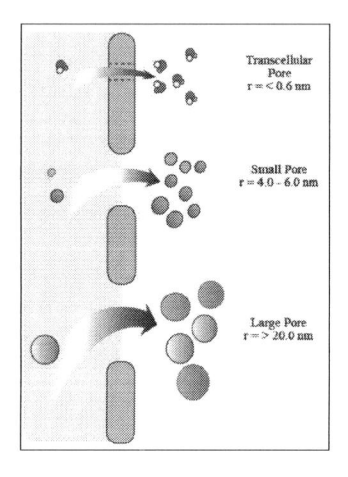

Capillary pores of three theoretical sizes explain solute and water transport across the capillary bed

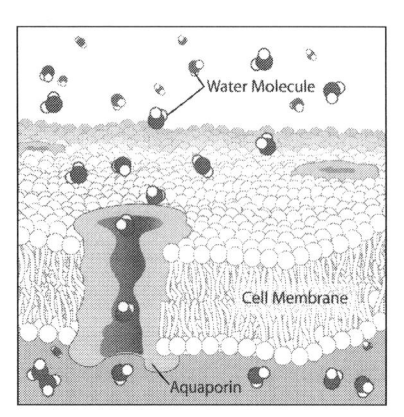

Aquaporin in peritoneal capillary

The aquaporins allow for only water transport across the cell and are a complete barrier to any solute transport across this pore. Aquaporins are stimulated by dialysate osmolality and are open when exposed to osmotically active dextrose solutions.

The small pores likely represent inter-endothelial clefts that allow for transport of small solutes such as urea, sodium, potassium, and creatinine dissolved in water. The large pores allow for transport of larger macromolecules such as proteins.

The three pore model allows for an understanding of the movement of water and solutes of varying sizes. This transport occurs due to two physiological processes that occur simultaneously:

1. Diffusion
2. Convection (Ultrafiltration)

Diffusion

Diffusion is the predominant mechanism of small solute transport in PD. Diffusive clearance is dependent on many variables:

1. The effective peritoneal membrane surface area
2. The solute concentration gradients from blood to dialysate
3. The dwell time of dialysate in the peritoneal cavity
4. The dialysate flow rates.

Diffusion occurs from the blood into the dialysate as well as from the dialysate into the blood. For example, uremic toxins diffuse down a concentration gradient into the dialysate while dialysate lactate and glucose diffuse into the capillary blood supply. Substances with smaller molecular weight diffuse more rapidly than those with larger molecular weight. Therefore, urea diffuses more rapidly than creatinine or middle molecules. Peritoneal diffusion of solutes can vary patient to patient and are determined by the vascularity of the peritoneal membrane and inflammatory state.

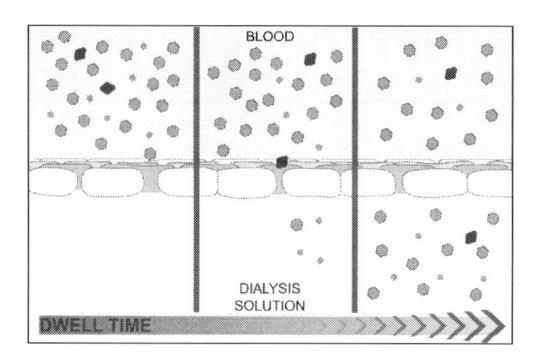

Convection

Convection occurs when dissolved solutes are small enough to move through the pores as water is moving across the capillary, in response to an osmotic force. More specifically, as dialysate glucose creates an osmotic force that attracts water from the capillary blood space, solutes that are dissolved in that water move into the dialysate, resulting in clearance of those solutes from the blood by this convection process- often called "solute drag". Middle molecules such as $B2$-microglobulin move into the peritoneal cavity predominantly by convection.

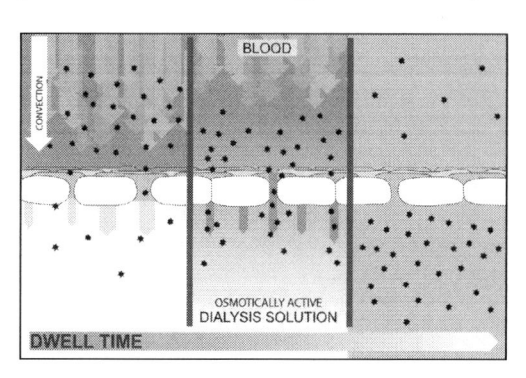

The combined diffusive and convective clearance of molecules can be modeled over varying time points.

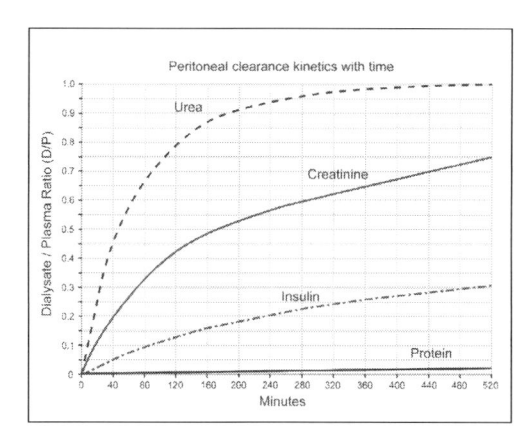

Ultrafiltration

Ultrafiltration refers to the process of fluid movement across the peritoneal membrane in response to an osmotic force. Ultrafiltration occurs across both the aquaporins and the small pores, with aquaporin mediated water movement accounting for

Substance size determines rate of clearance

40-50% of the total ultrafiltration and the small pores accounting for 50-60% of the total ultrafiltration.

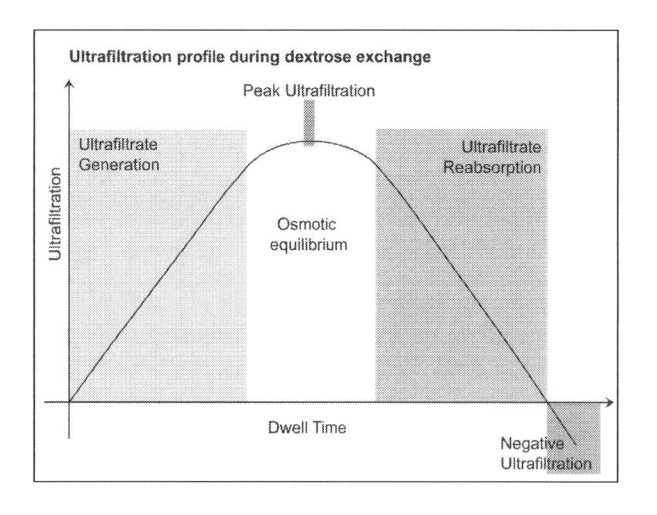

Three phases of dextrose-mediated UF:
   A. an early rapid UF
   B. osmotic equilibrium and cessation of UF
   C. reabsorption of UF over time

Ultrafiltration induced by crystalloid solutions shows a profile of three distinct phases. The initial phase is noted for rapid ultrafiltration as the osmotic gradient is large. The second phase is a noted for a plateau in ultrafiltration rate as the dextrose is absorbed across the peritoneal membrane and reaches osmotic equilibrium with the blood. The final stage is a period of reabsorption of the ultrafiltrate as continued dextrose absorption reduces the osmotic gradient further.

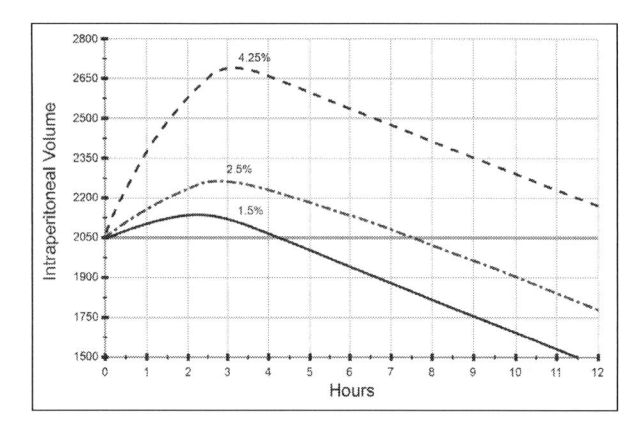

Ultrafiltration profile of different dialysate dextrose concentrations

Ultrafiltration volumes can be modified by use of different osmotically active PD solutions. Lower osmotic solutions (1.5% dextrose concentrations) can create a peak ultrafiltration of over one hundred mL. Higher osmotic forces (4.25% dextrose concentrations) result in larger movements of ultrafiltrate.

As dextrose is absorbed across the peritoneum and enters the capillary the osmotic gradient slowly dissipates, resulting in cessation of net ultrafiltration and an eventual re-absorption of dialysate. The efficacy of glucose as an osmotic agent is reflected in a term- "reflection coefficient". This term refers to the ability of a substance to pass thru a semi-permeable membrane and ranges from 1 (no passage) to 0 (free passage and no osmotic effect). The reflection coefficient for glucose is 0.03 demonstrating the poor ability of crystalloid solutions to generate a sustained osmotic effect.

Ultrafiltration Efficiency

Dextrose solutions result in carbohydrate absorption implying there is a metabolic consequence of the osmotically-driven ultrafiltration. This has been referred to as "ultrafiltration efficiency"- the volume of ultrafiltrate that results per gram of dialysate carbohydrate absorbed. Work by Finkelstein and colleagues demonstrated that use of hypertonic 4.25% dextrose solutions for the long exchange resulted in 77 grams of carbohydrate absorbed. Icodextrin exposure resulted in 56 grams of carbohydrate absorption despite increased ultrafiltration volumes. The ultrafiltration efficiency of icodextrin was determined to be 3-fold that of 4.25% dextrose solutions.

Lymphatic Fluid Absorption

Fluid in the peritoneal cavity can be absorbed via the lymphatic vessels. Lymphatic vessels are predominantly in the sub-diaphragmatic location and have transport rates of 1 to 2 mL/min or up to 2 liters per day that can vary by the degree of intraperitoneal hydrostatic pressure. Hydrostatic pressure is positional, with the greatest intra-abdominal pressure created in the sitting position compared to the lying position. The *net* fluid removal on PD is, therefore, the transcapillary ultrafiltration, in response to the dialysate osmotic force, minus the lymphatic re-absorption that has occurred.

Osmotic Conductance

Osmotic conductance refers to the movement of free water across the peritoneal membrane in response to an osmotic force. The osmotic properties induced by dextrose in the dialysate result in free water movement across the peritoneal capillary aquaporins, sodium sieving, and net free water movement into the dialysate. This free water movement, termed osmotic conductance, can be estimated by measuring the fall in the dialysate sodium concentration during the dwell. This determination can be made in the evaluation of ultrafiltration failure to assess the function of capillary aquaporins. Absence of osmotic conductance suggests peritoneal damage and loss of normal aquaporin function.

Sodium Sieving

As mentioned, aquaporins allow for up to 50% of total water movement across the capillary endothelium and, by definition, these pores allow for only water movement without solute. Therefore, any solute dissolved in the water is held back, or "sieved" at the aquaporin.

Rapid movement of water across the aquaporins, as can occur with rapid cycling of PD fluid with an automated cycler device, can result in significant sieving of sodium (a

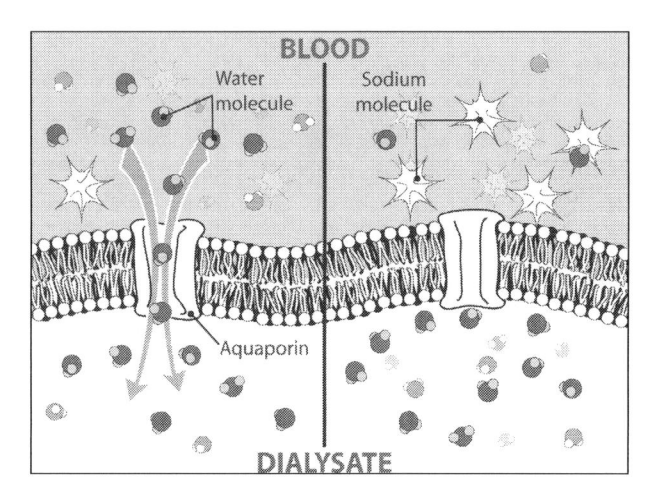

Aquaporins allow for transit of water molecules across the membrane and prevent sodium transit- termed "sodium sieving"

build-up of sodium in the capillary) resulting in relative hypernatremia with increased thirst. Attempting to rapidly remove fluid with frequent rapid cycling of PD fluid may be ultimately unsuccessful as the resultant hypernatremia, increased thirst, and increased fluid ingestion, may nullify the expected benefits of ultrafiltration.

As concerning as sodium sieving may be, the affects are somewhat mitigated as sieving widens the concentration gradient for sodium between capillary and dialysate and thus increases diffusive movement of sodium into the dialysate. The full clinical implications of sodium sieving have yet to be determined but suggest that rapid cycling in APD patients, in an attempt to improve urea kinetics or enhance ultrafiltration, may result in more sodium sieving and less sodium removal with the risk of expanded extracellular fluid.

The degree of sodium sieving (and aquaporin function) can be determined by measuring the sodium concentration in the dialysate. The initial dialysate sodium concentration 132 mEq/L is usually diluted by pure water movement across the aquaporins. Dialysate sodium concentrations can fall to the 120's mEq/L in the first few hours of the dwell. A failure of dialysate sodium to decrease during use of hypertonic exchanges is evidence of aquaporin deficiency and is useful in the investigation of ultrafiltration failure.

As mentioned earlier, aquaporins are stimulated by the hyperosmolality of the dextrose containing solutions. Aquaporins are not activated by icodextrin which is an iso-osmolar solution. Sodium sieving has not been described with icodextrin.

Peritoneal Membrane Changes in Longer Term PD Therapy

Patients on longer term PD therapy are noted to develop many alterations in the peritoneal membrane. Over time, mesothelial cell mass is reduced. Mesothelial cells are noted to undergo epithelial-to-mesenchymal transition (EMT) with mesothelial cells transforming to fibroblastic cell lines. The new fibroblasts migrate to a sub-mesothelial location and elaborate growth factors such as transforming growth factor-B, resulting in an expansion of sub-mesothelial connective tissue (the sub-mesothelial compact zone).

Concurrently, increased numbers of peritoneal capillaries were noted. These vascular changes appear to be the result of dialysate-induced increases in vascular endothelial growth factor (VEGF). In patients demonstrating these vascular changes, the movement of solutes can be increased, resulting in more rapid peritoneal membrane transport status and increased absorption of glucose with loss of ultrafiltration capacity. Monitoring long-term peritoneal membrane transport status is recommended and if significant changes are detected the PD prescription will require adjustment.

These are basic principles of peritoneal membrane physiology and will serve as the foundation for future descriptions of peritoneal solute clearance and ultrafiltration. An understanding of these principles of membrane physiology is required for proper determination of the PD prescription.

References:

Devuyst O, Goffin E. Water and solute transport in peritoneal dialysis: models and clinical applications. Nephrol Dial Transplant 2008;23:2120-2123.

Devuyst O, Margetts PJ, Topley N. The pathophysiology of the peritoneal membrane. J Am Soc Nephrol 2010;21:1077-1085.

Finkelstein F, Healy H, Abu-Alfa A, et al. Superiority of icodextrin compared with 4.25% dextrose for peritoneal ultrafiltration. J Am Soc Nephrol 2005;16:546-554.

Gillerot G, Goffin E, Michel C, et al. Genetic and clinical factors influence the baseline permeability of the peritoneal membrane. Kidney Int 2005;67:2477-2487.

Goffin E. Peritoneal membrane structural and functional changes during peritoneal dialysis. Semin Dial 2008;21:258-265.

Hills BA, Birch S, Burke JR, LaMont AC. Spatial distribution of dialysate in patients and its implications to intradialysate diffusion. Perit Dial Int 2002;22:698-704.

Krediet RT, Struijk DG. Peritoneal changes in patients on long-term peritoneal dialysis. Nat Rev Nephrol 2013;9:419-429.

Loureiro J, Aguilera A, Selgas R, et al. Blocking TGF-*B*1 protects the peritoneal membrane from dialysate-induced damage. J Am Soc Nephrol 2011;22:1682-1695.

Nessim SJ, Perl J, Bargman JM. The renin-angiotensin-aldosterone system in peritoneal dialysis: is what is good for the kidney also good for the peritoneum? Kidney Int 2010;78:23-28.

Ni J, Verbavatz JM, Rippe A, et al. Aquaporin-1 plays an essential role in water permeability and ultrafiltration during peritoneal dialysis. Kidney Int 2006;69:1518-1525.

Parikova A, Smit W, Struijk DG, Krediet RT. Analysis of fluid transport pathways and their determinants in peritoneal dialysis patients with ultrafiltration failure. Kidney Int 2006;70:1988-1994.

Rippe B. A three-pore model of peritoneal transport. Perit Dial Int 1993;13 [Suppl 2]:S35-S38.

Rippe B. Free water transport, small pore transport and the osmotic pressure gradient three-pore model of peritoneal transport. Nephrol Dial Transplant 2008;23:2147-2153.

Rubin J, Jones Q, Planch A, et al. The importance of the abdominal viscera to peritoneal transport during peritoneal dialysis in the dog. Am J Med Sci 1986;292:203-208.

Van Biesen W, Mortier S, Lameire N, De Vriese A. Effects of peritoneal dialysis on the vascular bed of peritoneal membrane. Contrib Nephrol 2006;150:84-89.

Wang T, Waniewski J, Heimburger O, et al. A quantitative analysis of sodium transport and removal during peritoneal dialysis. Kidney Int 1997;52:11609-1616.

Williams JD, Craig KJ, Topley N, et al. Morphologic changes in the peritoneal membrane of patients with renal disease. J Am Soc Nephrol 2002;13:470-479.

Yang AH, Chen JY, Lin JK. Myofibroblastic conversion of mesothelial cells. Kidney Int 2003;63:1530-1539.

Yu MA, Shin KS, Kim JH, et al. HGF and BMP-7 ameliorate high glucose-induced epithelial-to-mesenchymal transition of peritoneal mesothelium. J Am Soc Nephrol 2009;20:567-581.

Chapter 3:
Peritoneal Permeability Tests

THE PERITONEAL EQUILIBRATION TEST (PET), dialysis adequacy and transport test (DATT) and peritoneal dialysis capacity (PDC) test have become invaluable tools for the evaluation of peritoneal membrane function and provide information useful for tailoring the PD prescription to the individual patient.

Peritoneal Equilibration Test (PET)

The PET was first described by Twardowski and colleagues in 1987. The test determines the membrane solute transport characteristics of the individual patient, as transport status can vary from patient to patient. Some patients demonstrate rapid movement of solutes across the peritoneal membrane and others may show only slower transport of solutes. Twardowski described solute movement occurring rapidly in those he labeled "High" transporters and those with slow solute transport were termed "Low" transporters. He noted 2 intermediate groups that were labeled 'High-Average" and "Low-Average" transporters. So, by performing a PET, the clinician determines peritoneal membrane solute transport characteristics and uses this information to design a PD prescription.

The traditional PET is performed as below:

> The patient presents to the PD office and is asked to completely drain the prior night's long dwell (the night dwell should be at least 8 hours in duration).

> A 2 liter bag of 2.5% dextrose is then infused while the patient is in the recumbent position and the patient is asked to intermittently roll from side to side during the infusion.
>
> A sample of the dialysate is taken immediately after complete infusion of the fluid, then at 2 and 4 hours and sent for measurements of urea, creatinine, glucose and sodium. The creatinine is determined after correction for glucose interference.
>
> A blood sample is taken at 2 hours and sent for urea, creatinine, glucose and sodium determinations.
>
> The patient is drained upright after 4 hours and the drain volume is recorded.

With the information obtained in the PET, the dialysate to plasma (D/P) ratio for urea, creatinine and glucose are calculated.

The four hour dialysate and plasma creatinine level is used to express a D/P creatinine. This result is applied to the PET template to determine peritoneal membrane transport characteristics.

D/P creat 0.81 - 1.03	High (fast) transporter
D/P creat 0.65 - 0.81	High-average transporter
D/P creat 0.50 - 0.65	Low-average transporter
D/P creat 0.34 - 0.50	Low (slow) transporter

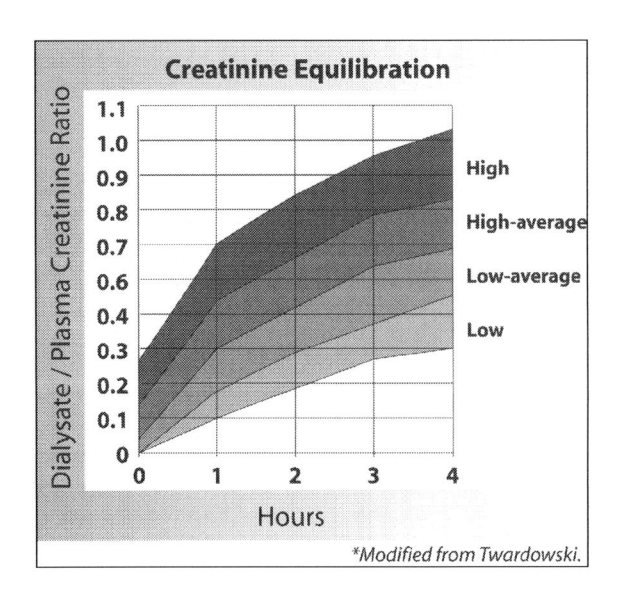

Creatinine Equilibration

Modified from Twardowski.

Similar determinations are made with the dialysate glucose concentration at time 0, 2, and 4 hours as an internal control to give independent validation of the membrane characteristics, using the parameter of glucose absorption, not creatinine removal.

Agreement in membrane transport classification using the D/P creatinine and D/D0 glucose should concur. The PET, by dialysate glucose concentrations, can be adversely

Glucose Equilibration

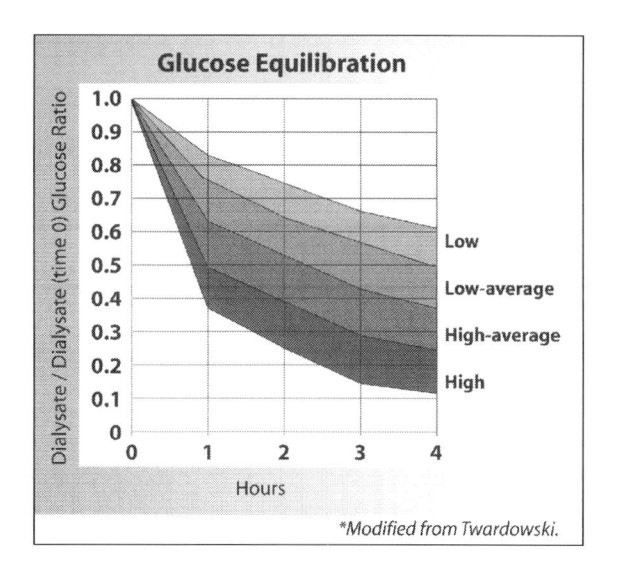

Modified from Twardowski.

affected by serum glucose greater than 235 mg/dL and ideally the test should be performed during reasonable control of the plasma glucose level.

With this information, the clinician can better understand that patients with high to high-average transport status have more rapid movement of solute and will have better daily clearance with multiple exchanges of shorter dwell times. High transporters will have more rapid absorption of glucose and dissipation of the osmotic gradient, making ultrafiltration compromised in longer exchanges- again suggesting that higher transporters should be treated with exchanges of shorter dwell times. Low transporters diffuse solute more slowly and will require longer dwells to reach significant equilibrium. Low transporters will have sustained ultrafiltration as the glucose osmotic gradient is maintained for a longer period of time. Again, low transporters are better suited to longer exchanges that allow more time for solute to move into the dialysate. Having this information allows the clinician to tailor the PD prescription for each unique patient. These principles are covered in Chapter 10.

The PET should be performed 4 to 6 weeks after the initiation of PD. Performing the PET earlier can introduce error, as peritoneal membrane transport characteristics change appreciably during the first weeks of PD therapy. Testing before 4 weeks was shown to poorly correlate with membrane characteristics later in time.

The PET was originally described in patients on CAPD with long night dwells. Patients on APD, however, have night exchanges that are more rapid or present to the PD office for testing while perhaps carrying no fluid during the day. Investigations in these APD patients determined that the PET did have variation based on the proceeding dwell status but the investigators believed that, for determining membrane status, APD patients did not have to convert to a long night dwell prior to the PET and results remained valid in APD patients.

Underlying Membrane Anatomy of PET Categories

The PET defines 4 types of peritoneal membrane transport characteristics- high, high-average, low-average, and low transport. The anatomic implications of these transport properties have been further characterized. Solute clearance (diffusion) occurs across the capillary wall and the total surface area of the peritoneal capillaries determines, in large part, the transport properties. Patients with relatively scant peritoneal capillary density have lower vascular surface area and are lower transporters. Patients with dense, rich peritoneal capillary beds and high vascular surface area are higher transporters.

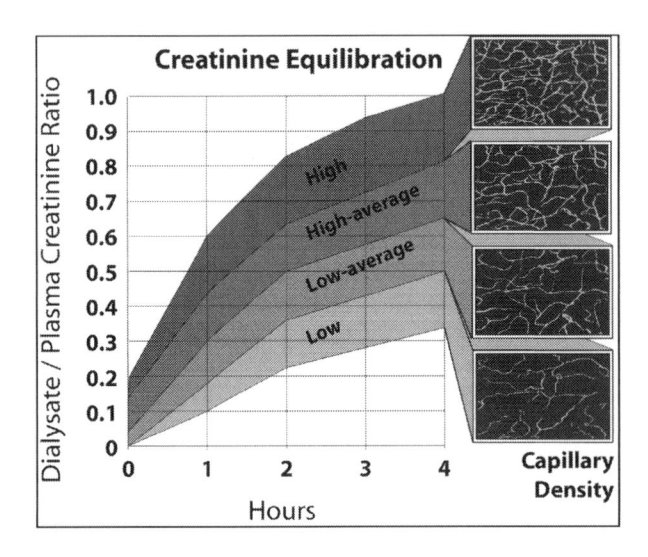

Capillary density (vascular surface area) of the peritoneal membrane is associated with the transport property

This suggests that the PET is a test that gives indirect anatomic information about the peritoneal capillary bed and vascular surface area. As the PET categories reflect varying vascular surface areas, it becomes more clear why high transport patients have increased creatinine clearance across the larger capillary bed but also absorb the dextrose more rapidly across these same vessels. Lower transport patients have fewer capillary vessels to diffuse creatinine and absorb dextrose.

Patients on longer term PD may migrate to higher transport properties, over time, due to neovascularization of the peritoneal membrane. This migration to higher transport property is induced by vascular endothelial growth factor (VEGF), analogous to the pathophysiology of diabetic retinopathy.

An understanding of this underlying peritoneal membrane vascularity can assist the clinician in devising the appropriate PD prescription as discussed in Chapter 10.

Discrepancies in the PET

Occasionally the transport properties determined by the D/Do glucose can differ from the transport determined by the D/P Creatinine. There are several factors that can explain these discrepancies. Prowant and colleagues determined that hyperglycemia can result in discrepancies between the creatinine and glucose PET categories. Serum glucoses levels above 235 mg/dL were associated with PET discrepancies. Due to this effect of the serum glucose on the D/Do glucose determination, clinicians who encounter transport characteristics that vary by one transport type should rely on the D/P creatinine as the more reliable result. A difference in one category is acceptable but creatinine results varying by 2 categories from the glucose result indicate an error has occurred in the test.

Transport properties that differ by two categories indicate a collection error or data entry error and the test should be repeated.

Fast PET

In this variation of the PET, only the 4-hour creatinine and glucose values are determined and not the baseline or 2-hour determinations. This test is less labor intensive for the nursing staff and was found to allow peritoneal membrane transport determinations similar to the traditional PET.

Modified PET

In the evaluation of suspected ultrafiltration failure, some authors have advocated use of the modified PET. These authors reasoned that a patient demonstrating possible membrane failure, with poor ultrafiltration, should be evaluated by exposing the membrane to the maximal osmotic stimulus during the study period. Therefore, in this circumstance, it was recommended to use a 4.25% dextrose solution during the 4 hour PET.

Besides use of a 4.25% dextrose solution during the test, the modified PET varies from the traditional PET as blood samples are taken at time 0, then at 60 minutes and 240 minutes. The baseline dialysate testing is done from fluid taken at the end of the infusion. Then, after the infusion of 2 liters of dialysate, dialysate is drained and sampled at 1, 60 and 240 minutes.

The test gives 2 metrics for evaluation of the membranes capacity to respond to an osmotic stimulus. If the net ultrafiltration is less than 400 mL during the 4 hour modified PET this is evidence that the peritoneal membrane has lost the capacity to remove ultrafiltrate to a degree that would support adequate volume control with dextrose solutions. Icodextrin should be added to test for improved ultrafiltration to allow for PD to continue or the patient should be evaluated for transfer to HD. If, however, the modified PET results in greater than 400 mL of ultrafiltration, the membrane itself remains responsive to an osmotic challenge.

The second metric is an evaluation of the aquaporin function of the peritoneal capillary bed. Normal capillary aquaporins would allow for pure water movement across the aquaporin into the dialysate. This water movement should dilute the dialysate sodium concentration significantly. Therefore, the D(0) sodium concentration is compared to the one-hour dialysate sodium concentration- to assess the dilution of the dialysate sodium. Failure to dilute the dialysate sodium concentration of approximately 132 mEq/L to 123-127 mEq/L would be indirect evidence that the aquaporin capacity to respond to an osmotic stimulus has been lost. Clinicians can use this information to try to determine if a patient who presents with chronic volume overload is demonstrating true membrane failure or is volume overloaded from other mechanisms such as excessive salt and fluid intake.

Mini-PET

The mini-PET was described by La Milia and colleagues as a one-hour test that could describe aquaporin and small pore-mediated free water transport as well as small solute transport. The authors found that there was reasonable agreement in the one-hour test as with the full 4-hour 4.25% dextrose modified PET.

DATT

In patients who are treated with CAPD, some centers use the dialysis adequacy and transport test (DATT) to determine peritoneal membrane transport status. Compared to the PET, the DATT is simpler to perform requiring only a single blood test and an aliquot of the pooled 24-hour CAPD dialysate. An additional advantage of the DATT is that daily ultrafiltration information is recorded. Studies have shown reasonable correlation between the PET and DATT in determining peritoneal transport status.

To perform the DATT, the CAPD patient collects all drained volume during a 24 hour period. A 10 ml aliquot is obtained from this pooled dialysate and a blood test is obtained in the morning of the following day to determine the plasma creatinine. The 24 hr D/P creatinine is used to determine transport status. Then, if needed, daily solute removal and ultrafiltration can be determined.

Peritoneal Dialysis Capacity (PDC) Test

The PDC test is used by some centers, largely outside of the USA. The test is used to determine peritoneal membrane characteristics using computer modeling based on parameters obtained from fluid collections. By using estimates of the MTAC, D/P creat, determinants of fluid reabsorption and large pore flow, peritoneal transport properties can be determined. The PDC has been evaluated by Van Biesen and colleagues and interested readers are referred to the publication noted below.

Standard Peritoneal Permeability Analysis (SPA)

The SPA is a permeability test used in certain research centers in Europe. The test is based on a 4-hr dwell using the instillation of 4.25% dextrose. After initial infusion, the dialysate is drained at multiple time points for sampling (time 10,20,30,60,120,180,240 min) then re-infused. Peritoneal transport properties are determined. Dextran 70 is added to the test solution to allow for determination of residual renal and peritoneal fluid kinetics.

Conclusions

Many tests are employed to determine the dialysate-to-plasma ratio of creatinine (D/P Cr). Knowledge of this parameter allows for classification of peritoneal membrane properties and individualization of the PD prescription. Knowledge of the D/P creat assures that the PD prescription matches the transport properties of the individual patient. A mismatch of PD prescription with transport properties can lead to underdialysis and problems maintaining adequate ultrafiltration. The basic concept is that patients with peritoneal membranes showing higher solute transport would benefit from dialysis exchanges that are more frequent. Patients with lower transport membranes should be managed with PD prescriptions with longer dwell-time exchanges.

References:

Bernardo AP, Bajo MA, Santos O, et al. Two-in-one protocol: simultaneous small-pore and ultrasmall-pore peritoneal transport quantification. Perit Dial Int 2012;32:537-544.

Cnossen TT, Smit W, Konings CJ, et al. Quantification of free water transport during the peritoneal equilibration test. Perit Dial Int 2009;29:523-527.

Heimburger O. How to assess peritoneal transport: which test should we use? Contrib Nephrol 2009;163:82-89.

Johnson DW, Mudge DW, Blizzard S, et al. A comparison of peritoneal equilibration tests performed 1 and 4 weeks after PD commencement. Perit Dial Int 2004;24:460-465.

Lilaj T, Vychytil A, Schneider B, et al. Influence of the preceding exchange on peritoneal equilibration test results: a prospective study. Am J Kidney Dis 1999;34:247-253.

La Milia V, Di Filippo S, Crepaldi M, et al. Mini-peritoneal equilibration test: a simple and fast method to assess free water and small solute transport across the peritoneal membrane. Kidney Int 2005:68:840-846.

La Milia V, Limardo M, Virga G, et al. Simultaneous measurement of peritoneal glucose and free water osmotic conductances. Kidney Int 2007;72:643-650.

La Milia V. Peritoneal transport testing. J Nephrol 2010;23:633-647.

Paniagua R, Amato D, Correa-Rotter R, et al. Correlation between peritoneal equilibration test and dialysis adequacy and transport test, for peritoneal transport type characterization. Perit Dial Int 2000;20:53-59.

Pannekeet MM, Imholz AL, Struijk DG, et al. The standard peritoneal permeability analysis: a tool for the assessment of peritoneal permeability characteristics in CAPD patients. Kidney Int 1995;48:866-875.

Perez-Fontan M, Rodriguez-Carmona A, Barreda D, et al. Peritoneal protein transport during the baseline peritoneal equilibration test is an accurate predictor of outcomes of peritoneal dialysis. Nephron Clin Pract 2010;116:c104-c113.

Prowant BF, Moore HL, Twardowski ZJ, Khanna R. Understanding discrepancies in peritoneal equilibration test results. Perit Dial Int 2010;30:366-370.

Rocco MV, Jordan JR, Burkart JM. Determination of peritoneal transport characteristics with 24-hour dialysate collections: dialysis adequacy and transport test. J Am Soc Nephrol 1994;5:1333-1338.

Rocco MV, Jordan JR, Burkart JM. 24-hour dialysate collection for determination of peritoneal membrane transport characteristics: longitudinal follow-up data for the dialysis adequacy and transport test (DATT). Perit Dial Int 1996;16:590-593.

Seo JJ, Kim YL, Park SH, et al. Usefulness of the dialysis adequacy and transport test in peritoneal dialysis. Adv Perit Dial 2005;21:25-30.

Szeto CC, Wong T, Chow K, et al. Dialysis adequacy and transport test for characterization of peritoneal transport type in Chinese peritoneal dialysis patients receiving three daily exchanges. Am J Kidney Dis 2002;39:1287-1291.

Twardowski ZJ, Nolph KD, Khanna R, et al. Peritoneal equilibration test. Perit Dial Bull 1987;7:138-147.

Twardowski ZJ. Clinical value of standardized equilibrium tests in CAPD patients. Blood Purif 1989;7:95-108.

Twardowski ZJ. The fast peritoneal equilibration test. Semin Dial 1990;3:141-142.

Van Biesen W, Heimburger O, Krediet R, et al. Evaluation of peritoneal membrane characteristics: a clinical advice for prescription management by the ERBP working group. Nephrol Dial Transplant 2010;25:2052-2062.

Van Biesen W, Van Der Tol A, Veys N, et al. The peritoneal dialysis capacity test is superior to the peritoneal equilibration test to discriminate inflammation as the cause of fast transport status in peritoneal dialysis patients. Clin J Am Soc Nephrol 2006;1:269-274.

Van Biesen W, Van Der Tol A, Veys N, et al. Evaluation of the peritoneal membrane function by three letter word acronyms: PET, PDC, SPA, PD-Adequest, POL: what to do? Contrib Nephrol 2006;150:37-41.

Chapter 4:
Kinetic Modeling / Adequacy of Dialysis

OVER THE LAST 30 years, the concept of "adequacy" of dialysis has been quite controversial. Many clinicians would believe that an adequate dialysis therapy is one in which the patient can feel well and maintain good nutrition, maintain a balance between the therapy itself and overall quality of life, and maintain the life-sustaining internal milieu of balanced electrolytes, hematologic and nutritional parameters. Yet, over the decades, adequate dialysis has been defined by mathematical extrapolations of urea and creatinine clearance - by a "number", not a clinical state of being. This "number" was to be associated with patient survival, without any consideration of the quality of the life survived. For this and other reasons, the concept of "adequacy" of dialysis stirs debate.

Early Studies in Urea Clearance Applied to PD

In 1981, a well-designed, multicenter prospective randomized study of 160 hemodialysis patients attempted to examine the relationship of dialysis dose and clinical outcomes such as hospitalization, uremic symptoms, and survival. This study, The National Cooperative Dialysis Study (NCDS), involved hemodialysis patients who were dialyzed for the same treatment time. By altering the dialyzer size and flux, the investigators were able to compare groups maintained with a BUN of 100 mg/dL to a group at 50 mg/dL. The study was terminated early due to excess morbidity in the higher BUN group. This study suggested there was a minimal dose of dialysis that must be delivered to improve outcomes and ushered in the era of defining "adequacy" of dialysis as a certain clearance target.

The primary data from the NCDS was examined by Gotch and Sargent and used to determine the urea clearance of peritoneal dialysis treatments. They established the concept of urea clearance expressed as the Kt/V where the K was the total dialysate and urinary urea clearance, t represented the time, and this time-averaged clearance was normalized to the patient's volume of distribution of urea - the V. Therefore Kt/V calculations could be used to give a mathematical number to a clearance target for peritoneal dialysis therapy.

Subsequently, several small studies examining the utility of the Kt/V formula to predict morbidity and mortality on PD gave inconsistent results. For example, Teehan and colleagues studied 51 PD patients for a 5 year period and determined that those patients who were prescribed a weekly Kt/V of 1.89 had a 90% five year survival compared to only 50% survival in those prescribed a lower dose of urea clearance. Yet Blake and colleagues could find no consistent predictive power to the Kt/V in 71 patients. Other studies were similarly conflicted and all were limited by small size, high rates of dropout, and retrospective design. It was clear that, as these smaller studies gave inconsistent results, a larger prospective study was needed.

The CANUSA Peritoneal Dialysis Study Group, a conglomeration of 10 Canadian and 4 USA PD centers, organized the CANUSA trial - a multicenter prospective observational study involving 680 PD patients in Canada and the USA. The trial noted a 78% 2-year survival at Kt/V of 2.1 and a 5% increase in the relative risk of death for every 0.1 decrease in the total Kt/V. The overall conclusion of the CANUSA study was that the dose of peritoneal dialysis should achieve a total weekly Kt/V of 2.1.

After the original CANUSA study published in 1996, the Ad Hoc Advisory Committee of the National Kidney Foundation's Dialysis Outcomes Quality Initiative (NKF-DOQI) met to make recommendations on adequacy targets based on this validated Kt/V measurement. The committee determined that patients on CAPD therapy should maintain a weekly total Kt/V of 2.0. Due to concerns of the peak urea concentration hypothesis, patients who did not have continuous prolonged exposure of the peritoneum to dialysate, such as those using only nightly cycler intermittent therapy (NIPD), were recommended to achieve a higher weekly total Kt/V of 2.2, and cyler patients with a day dwell were felt to be a hybrid therapy that could have a target Kt/V of 2.1. In 1997, the NKF-DOQI committee published clinical practice guidelines for peritoneal dialysis adequacy and established the following targets for total weekly Kt/V and weekly creatinine clearance:

CAPD Kt/V 2.00   CrCl 60 L/wk/m^2
CCPD Kt/V 2.10   CrCl 63 L/wk/m^2
NIPD Kt/V 2.20   CrCl 66 L/wk/m^2

In 2001, after several editorials questioned the original CANUSA findings, a follow-up publication reanalyzing the CANUSA data showed that the contribution of residual kidney function to the total Kt/V was more predictive of survival than the peritoneal component. This suggested that the peritoneal and renal components of the total Kt/V were not equivalent and simply additive. Rather, the authors concluded that the renal component was much more physiologically important and they noted that for every 5 liters per week of residual GFR the relative risk of death was reduced by 12% and for every 250 mL of urine output the death rate was reduced by 36%. This somewhat surprising observation led to recommendations that clinicians take special measures to attempt to preserve the residual kidney function in peritoneal dialysis patients.

Subsequent Studies Challenged Urea Clearance Targets

Additional studies began to raise questions about the 1997 DOQI Kt/V recommendations. The ADEMEX trial published in 2002 randomized CAPD patients in Mexico to 2 levels of solute clearance. The control group received their usual 8 L CAPD regimen and the intervention group was administered additional fluid to target higher peritoneal clearance targets. No survival benefit could be seen to increasing the total Kt/V above approximately 1.6. An additional study published in Hong Kong randomized CAPD patients to one of three clearance targets: a Kt/V of 1.5 -1.7 vs. 1.7 - 2.0 vs. > 2.0. No statistically significant survival advantage was noted between the three groups. The KDOQI committee also noted results of the HEMO study, as the study did not demonstrate a survival difference in the group assigned to higher hemodialysis urea clearances.

After reviewing the ADEMEX study, the Hong Kong study, the HEMO study and others, the K/DOQI committee felt that a revision was needed in clearance targets. In retrospect, several members of the committee felt that prior adequacy targets were unduly complicated and burdensome, the creatinine clearance targets added very little to the urea targets, and that an overall simplification in their recommendations was needed. In 2006, the committee issued their revised targets de-emphasizing weekly creatinine clearances and simply stated:

> "The minimal "delivered" dose of total small-solute clearance should be a total (peritoneal and renal) Kt/V urea of at least 1.7 per week."

They further recommended that the Kt/V should be measured within the first month of starting PD and monitored every 4 months thereafter.

A Quantified Dose of Peritoneal Dialysis

Today, the current established expression for the dose of peritoneal dialysis is the Kt/V. As mentioned, this expression represents a mathematical model of the total urea nitrogen clearance from the volume of distribution of urea.

Therefore:

Kt = peritoneal and residual kidney clearance in liters
V = urea volume of distribution, which is total body water (TBW).

Determining the Peritoneal Contribution to the Total Kt/V

To determine the peritoneal Kt the clinician measures the urea concentration in the total drained dialysate (D) and measures the urea concentration in the blood (P) and expresses the clearance of urea as a fraction (D/P) multiplied by the total dialysate volume in liters:

Peritoneal urea clearance = (D/P urea) x liters of dialysate.

For example:

A male CAPD patient performs 4 exchanges a day with 2 L solutions. This results in a net ultrafiltration of 1.5 liters for a total volume of the drained dialysate of 8 L + 1.5 L = 9.5L.

The Kt calculation would, therefore, be determined by measuring the urea concentration in each of the 4 drained bags. In this hypothetical example the values will be:

Exchange #1 - Dialysate urea 72 mg/dL
Exchange #2 - Dialysate urea 68 mg/dL
Exchange #3 - Dialysate urea 74 mg/dL
Exchange #4 - Dialysate urea 72 mg/dL

The mean dialysate urea is therefore (72 + 68 + 74 + 72) / 4 = 72 mg/dL.

The urea concentration is measured in the blood and found to be 80 mg/dL which is the (P).

Therefore, daily peritoneal urea clearance is the D/P x dialysate volume
(72/80) x 9.5 L = 8.6 L

The total body V is typically determined from a nomogram, the Watson formula, or simply estimated as 0.58 x ideal body weight in kilograms. The Watson nomogram is recommended in the obese patient.

In the above hypothetical example, assume that the male CAPD patient is 70 kilograms and is at an ideal body weight. The total body water, therefore, would be simply estimated at 0.58 x 70 = 40.6 L.

The daily peritoneal Kt/V calculation becomes:

8.6L/ 40.6L = 0.21 - a unitless expression of the daily urea clearance. It was suggested that this value be expressed as a weekly value, therefore the 0.21 is multiplied by 7 to express the weekly peritoneal urea clearance of 7 x 0.21 = 1.47.

Determining the Renal Contribution to the Total Kt/V

A similar calculation is done to determine the residual kidney Kt/V. In our example, assume the patient has a residual urine output of 1 liter a day. The urea concentration in this volume is measured and found to be 180 mg/dL. The residual kidney Kt would be (U/P urea) x U volume = 180/80 x 1 L = 2.25 L and the daily renal Kt/V would be 2.25L/40.6L = 0.055. Multiplying this by 7 would give the weekly renal Kt/V of 0.38

Adding the weekly peritoneal Kt/V to this residual renal weekly Kt/V would give the total weekly Kt/V of 1.47 + 0.38 = 1.85.

Determining the Weekly Kt/V in the Patient on Automated PD

Determination of the total weekly Kt/V is done differently in the patient using a cycler machine for automated PD (APD). These patients have multiple shorter dwells at night followed by a long dwell during the day. The multiple cycles at night are drained into a single drain bag and an aliquot can be taken to determine the urea concentration.

For example, if the same patient described above is a cycler patient who performs 4 exchanges at night that results in 1 liter of ultrafiltration- the drained dialysate overnight would contain 8 L + 1 L = 9 L. If the aliquot taken from this bag reveals a urea concentration of 58 mg/dL the Kt for the cycler component is:

(D/P urea) x 9 L or (58/80) x 9 L = 6.5 L

The long day dwell values are then determined by measuring the urea in the long dwell. Assuming the long day dwell is 2 liters and results in 1 liter of ultrafiltration, for a total volume of 3 liters, and the measured urea in this exchange is 75 mg/dl. The Kt for this exchange would be:

(D/P urea) x 3 L or (75/80) x 3 L = 2.8 L

The cycler Kt is added to the long dwell Kt to give the peritoneal Kt of 6.5L + 2.8L = 9.3L. This value is divided by the total body water (V) and multiplied by 7 to give the total weekly peritoneal Kt/V: 9.3L/40.6L = 0.23 x 7 = 1.61. Adding this to the total weekly residual kidney Kt/V of 0.38 results in a total weekly Kt/V of 1.99.

Calculating volume (V) using the Watson formula

The Watson formula for estimating total body water (TBW) and therefore the V was published in 1980 but still remains the most common formula for this calculation. These researchers collected data from 458 men and 265 women who underwent formal determinations of TBW by dilution methods using diluents with no permeability barrier such as deuterium, tritium oxide, or antipyrine. From these dilution studies they developed a simple prediction equation that could accurately estimate TBW knowing the patients height in centimeters, weight in kilograms, age, and gender. The original publication also includes 2 nomograms that can be used to visually determine the TBW. Limitations of the Watson formula are that it was not validated in the Asian population, in the grossly obese and was determined in healthy volunteers or hospitalized patients with only minor illnesses - not the target population of often overhydrated PD patients. Nevertheless, this formula is commonly used to estimate V.

The Watson formulae are:

For males:
V (liters) = 2.447 - (0.09516 x age) + (0.1074 x height in cm) + (0.3362 x weight in kg)

For females:
V (liters) = -2.097 + (0.1069 x height in cm) + (0.2466 x weight in kg)

An additional example of an adequacy calculation in a cycler patient is below. In this example, clinicians calculated V by the Watson formula:

Another Example of the Kt/V Calculation in a Cycler (APD) Patient

The patient is a 70 year old male with a weight of 188 pounds and is 5 feet 9 inches tall. He is moderately obese and has residual kidney function. He has been placed on a cycler machine with 3 exchanges of 2.5 liters and a 2 liter day dwell.

The PD unit requests a 24-hour urine, a sample from the overnight large drain bag and a careful measurement of the volume of the drained overnight bag. The clinic appointment is later in the afternoon and his day exchange has been dwelling for 8 hours. The staff drain out the day exchange, weigh the bag, and send a sample to the laboratory. The patient is then asked to go to the laboratory for a blood draw.

Serum blood urea nitrogen concentration 78 mg/dL
24 hour urine volume 900 mL
Urine urea concentration 160 mg/dL

Cycler bag urea concentration 40 mg/dL
Cycler bag volume 8.5L (7.5 dialysate and 1 L ultrafiltrate)

Day dwell urea concentration 60 mg/dL
Day dwell volume 1.8 L (patient absorbed some of the fluid)

The total daily residual kidney Kt is calculated to be (160/78) x 0.9 L = 1.85. The patient's total body V is determined from the Watson formula or by using a nomogram. With the Watson formula:

V (liters) in males = [2.447 - (0.09516 x age)] + (0.1074 x height in cm) + (0.3362 x weight in kg) therefore:

V in this patient = 2.447 - (0.09516 x 70) + (0.1074 x [69 inches x 2.54 cms/inch]) + (0.3362 x [188 pounds /0.45 kg/pound]) = 43 L

Therefore the weekly renal Kt/V is 1.85/43 = 0.043 x 7 = 0.30
The peritoneal Kt = 40/78 x 8.5L added to 60/78 x 1.8L = 5.74
The weekly Kt/V = 5.74/43 x 7 = 0.93

Total Kt/v is peritoneal Kt/V added to renal Kt/V therefore 0.93 + 0.30 = 1.23.

This result is below current Kt/V targets so the prescription should be examined and could be adjusted by increasing the night exchanges from 3 to 4 and increasing the day dwell to be similar to the night dwells of 2.5 L.

Dietary Indicators of Adequate Peritoneal Dialysis

A well dialyzed patient would be expected to have an adequate appetite and be free of nausea and vomiting that limit the ingestion of adequate nutrition. Assuming steady state, since urea nitrogen is a breakdown product of protein it is possible to use the daily urea clearance to determine the daily protein intake. Urea generation is proportional to protein breakdown, termed the normalized protein equivalent of nitrogen appearance (nPNA). In stable patients, the nPNA is reflective of dietary protein intake.

Earlier balance studies determined that negative nitrogen balance would occur in a PD patient ingesting less than 1.1 grams of protein/kg/day. Patients ingesting >1.4

grams/kg/day were in definite positive nitrogen balance. A PNA calculation is completed using dialysate urea nitrogen and, if there is significant residual kidney function, 24-hour urine collections. The two results are added to give an estimation of daily protein intake in gms/kg/day. This PNA is normalized to ideal body weight using anthropometric tables to give the nPNA (Frisancho AR. Am J Clin Nutr).

Therefore, using the dialysate urea nitrogen values, employed in the Kt/V calculation, the clinician can calculate the estimated protein intake as follows:

nPNA (g/24 hrs) = 15.1 + 6.95(urea nitrogen apprearance in g/24 hrs) added to any protein losses, then normalized to ideal body weight

Example:

A 70 kg patient on CAPD with 10 liters of daily dialysate containing 65 mg/dL urea nitrogen would have total urea nitrogen content of 10L x 65mg/dL x 10 dL/L = 6500 mgs or 6.5 grams of urea nitrogen. The 24-hour urine obtained showed 400 mL of urine containing 640 mg/dL urea nitrogen for 2.56 grams of urea nitrogen. Added together the urea nitrogen appearance in g/24 hrs is 6.5 + 2.5 = 9 grams/24 hr. The dialysate contains 6 grams of protein per day.

The nPNA is 15.1 + 6.95(9) + 6 = 83.65 grams day/70 kg (assuming patient is at ideal body weight) = 1.19 g/kg/day

The patient has a borderline estimated dietary protein intake and requires ongoing monitoring and recommendations to increase protein intake.

Conclusions

In PD patients, to achieve target urea clearances, urea kinetic modeling can help ensure adequate delivery of dialysis and allow estimates of dietary protein intake. There should be no overt uremic symptoms with sufficient intake of protein and other nutrients, suggesting the dialysis prescription is "adequate". While control of small molecules is important, it is emphasized that the PD prescription, designed to meet these targets, should not be unduly complex lest the patient may burn out, or become non-compliant. Creative use of time and dialysate volume will be required. The marked importance of residual kidney function, in achieving adequacy targets and as an independent predictor of survival, suggests that all prudent measures should be taken to preserve remaining kidney function.

References:

Blake PG, Bargman JM, Brimble KS, et al. Canadian Society of Nephrology Guidelines/Recommendations.Clinical practice guidelines and recommendations on peritoneal dialysis adequacy 2011. Perit Dial Int 2011;31:218-239.

Bargman JM, Thorpe KE, Churchill DN. Relative contribution of residual renal function and peritoneal clearance to adequacy of dialysis: a reanalysis of the CANUSA study. J Am Soc Nephrol 2001;12:2158-2162.

Bergstrom J, Heimburger O, Lindholm B. Calculation of the protein equivalent of total nitrogen appearance from urea appearance. Which formulas should be used/ Perit Dial Int 1998;18:467-473.

Burkart JM. The ADEMEX study and its implications for peritoneal dialysis adequacy. Semin Dial 2003;16:1-4.

Churchill DN, Taylor DW, Keshaviah PR for the CANUSA Peritoneal Dialysis Study Group. Adequacy of dialysis and nutrition in continuous peritoneal dialysis: association with clinical outcomes. J Am Soc Nephrol 1996;7:198-207.

Frisancho AR. New standards of weight and body composition by frame size and height for assessment of nutritional status of adults and elderly. Am J Clin Nutr 1984;40:808-819.

Gotch FA, Sargent JA. A mechanistic analysis of the National Cooperative Dialysis Study (NCDS). Kidney Int 1985;28:526-534.

Guest S, Akonur A, Ghaffari A, et al. Intermittent peritoneal dialysis: urea kinetic modeling and implications of residual kidney function. Perit Dial Int 2012;32:142-148.

NKF-KDOQI Guideline 2. Peritoneal dialysis solute clearance targets and measurements. Am J Kidney Dis 2006;48 [Suppl 1];S103-S116.

Lo WK, Bargman JM, Burkart J, et al. Guideline on targets for solute and fluid removal in adult patients on chronic peritoneal dialysis. Perit Dial Int 2006;26:520-522.

NKF-KDOQI clinical practice guidelines for peritoneal dialysis adequacy. Am J Kidney Dis 2006;48 [supple 1]: S91-S158.

Nolph KD, Keshaviah P, Popovich R. Problems in comparisons of clearances prescriptions in hemodialysis and continuous ambulatory peritoneal dialysis. Perit Dial Int 1991:11:298-300.

Teehan BP, Schleifer CR, Brown J. Assessment of dialysis adequacy and nutrition by urea kinetic modeling. Perit Dial Int 1994;14[Suppl 3]:S99-104.

Teehan B, Schleifer CR, Brown J. Urea kinetic modeling is an appropriate assessment of adequacy. Semin Dial 1992;5:189-192.

Van Olden RW, Krediet RT, Struijk DG, Arisz L. Measurement of residual renal function in patients treated with continuous peritoneal dialysis. J Am Soc Nephrol 1996;7:745-748.

Watson PE, Watson ID, Batt RD. Total body water volumes for adult males and females estimated from simple anthropometric measurements. Am J Clin Nutr 1980;33:27-39.

Chapter 5:
Residual Kidney Function in PD

THE OVERALL PROGNOSIS AND well-being of the PD patient is closely linked to the degree of residual kidney function (RKF) present at the start and maintained during PD therapy. Compared with patients without significant RKF, patients who maintain significant RKF have better overall survival, better hematologic and nutritional parameters, better blood pressure control, better control of extracellular volume, and reduced left ventricular hypertrophy. These benefits of RKF mandate that attempts be made to preserve RKF in the patient initiating dialysis.

Survival Implications

The importance of RKF in prolonging survival was noted in a reanalysis of the landmark Canada-USA (CANUSA) study, originally published in 1996. As mentioned, the CANUSA study was a prospective observational study to determine the total urea clearance targets that correlated with improved survival. The study reported that the best survival could be maintained in PD patients who were prescribed therapy that delivered a total weekly Kt/V urea of 2.0 to 2.25. Subsequent editorials suggested that as all CANUSA study patients were on a similar CAPD regimen and, therefore, had minimal differences in their peritoneal contribution to urea clearance, survival differences were based solely on the RKF component of clearance. In 2001, a reanalysis of the CANUSA database was published and showed that for every 5 mL/min of residual kidney glomerular filtration rate (GFR) there was a 12% decrease in the relative risk of death and for every 250 mL of urine the relative risk was reduced by 36 percent.

This led to the wider recognition that the residual kidney component of the total Kt/V has a greater impact on survival than does the peritoneal component and that these 2 components, peritoneal and residual kidney, should not be considered equal and additive when determining the total weekly Kt/V.

Impact of Residual Kidney Function on the Internal Milieu

Residual kidney function contributes to daily loss of salt and water and therefore improved indices of volume status such as blood pressure control and the extent of edema. Residual kidney function contributes significantly to the clearance of middle molecules and RKF is associated with lower beta-2-microglobulin and *p*-cresol levels. Dialysis patients that reach anuria have worsened anemia with erythropoietin resistance, inflammation and aggravated mineral imbalances. A recent report noted loss of normal endothelial function in patients losing residual kidney function, suggesting preservation of RKF could prevent endothelial dysfunction and impact cardiac risk.

Clinical Consequences of Loss of Residual Kidney Function

Reduced survival
Worsened blood pressure control
Increased risk of volume expansion with edema formation
Worsened cardiac hypertrophy
Reduced middle molecule clearance
Erythropoietin resistance
Lower serum albumin levels
Elevated calcium-phosphorus product
Endothelial dysfunctioin

Preservation of Residual Kidney Function

This suggests that active measures should be taken to avoid nephrotoxic insults and that strategies should be considered to intervene and attempt to preserve the residual kidney's clearance capabilities and ability to excrete salt and water.

Many clinical recommendations can be made to attempt to preserve RKF in patients on PD. These recommendations are summarized below:

> **Strategies to Preserve Residual Kidney Function**
>
> Avoid prolonged use of aminoglycosides
> Cautious and limited use of non-steroidal anti-inflammatory agents
> Avoidance or cautious use of iodinated contrast agents
> Precautions taken before contrast studies
> Antagonism of the renin-angiotensin system
> Use of diuretics
> Hypertension control
> Avoidance of intravascular volume depletion
> Avoid urinary tract obstruction

Aminoglycoside Use

Concern over the nephrotoxicity of aminoglycosides led to a revision of the 2000 ISPD guidelines for the treatment of peritonitis. In the 1997 guidelines, empiric use of ceftazadime or aminoglycosides to cover gram negative organisms was recommended. The subsequent revision precautioned against prolonged use aminoglycosides in patients with significant RKF. Of note, 2 subsequent retrospective analyses could not demonstrate loss of RKF with limited use of gentamicin or netilmicin yet it seems prudent to caution against prolonged use of aminoglycosides. Aminoglycoside use is limited to regimens involving once-daily dosing with careful monitoring of drug levels to minimize the chance of tubular toxicity.

Iodinated Contrast Agents

Both iodinated contrast media and gadolinium have been associated with loss of RKF in dialysis patients. In dialysis patients, the added risk of nephrogenic systemic fibrosis (NSF) makes the use of gadolinium particularly contraindicated. Recommendations for use of iodinated contrast material in PD patients would be the same as for those with advanced CKD- limited dye exposure, consideration of iso-osmotic agents, and avoidance of dye in the setting of intravascular volume depletion. In patients who must receive iodinated contrast agents, careful pre-hydration and administration of n-acetyl cysteine may be prudent.

Antagonism of the Renin-Angiotensin-Aldosterone System

Medications that antagonize the actions of the renin-angiotensin-aldosterone system (RAAS) have been a mainstay in the treatment of patients with CKD, by lowering the degree of proteinuria and slowing progression of disease. Several studies have demonstrated that patients on PD can benefit from these agents, despite markedly reduced renal function. Li and colleagues randomized PD patients to ramipril vs control and noted the treated group had greater preservation of function at 12 months. The beneficial effects appeared after 6 months, but the interpretation of the study has been complicated by an inadequate randomization of some patient variables. This study was followed by an additional trial comparing use of the angiotensin receptor blocker valsartan to an untreated control group. At 2 years, the valsartan group maintained creatinine clearance and urine volumes to a greater extent. The authors concluded that antagonism of the RAAS system could be of benefit despite advanced renal disease. The Kidney Disease Outcomes Quality Initiative (KDOQI) has issued treatment guidelines for preservation of residual kidney function in PD patients and recommends use of RAAS inhibitors in patients initiated on PD to attempt to slow progression toward anuria.

Diuretics

In general, the use of diuretics in PD patients is much more common outside of the USA and at doses that would seem surprisingly high. Daily doses of oral furosemide from 250 mg to thousands of milligrams are employed to attempt to maintain urine output in the remnant kidney. These doses have been formally studied and determined to better stimulate urine output compared to untreated controls. Higher doses may be required due to development of many "mechanisms of resistance" in patients with advanced chronic kidney disease. At least 6 mechanisms of resistance may play a role in making the kidney refractory to lower doses of loop diuretics.

Mechanism 1: Delayed and reduced gastric absorption of medication
Mechanism 2: Reduced delivery of medication to the kidney
Mechanism 3: Hypoalbuminemia
Mechanism 4: Proteinuria
Mechanism 5: Competition from organic anions
Mechanism 6: Distal tubule hypertrophy

An understanding of these physiologic mechanisms of diuretic resistance mandate that higher doses of loop diuretics may be required for the remnant kidney to respond, if at all.

Mechanism #1: Patients on PD often have delayed gastric emptying and diabetics may have concurrent gastroparesis. Glucose absorption from the dialysate has been shown to delay gastric motility and the physical presence of dialysate in the abdomen causes the gas filled stomach to be elevated, changing the normal gastro-esophageal junction that can result in reflux and delay in normal gastric transit times. These changes can reduce the absorption of oral diuretics leading to reduced plasma levels.

Mechanism #2: Once absorbed, there may be decreased delivery of the drug to the renal parenchyma. In patients with cardiomyopathy, reduced effective delivery of loop diuretics has been demonstrated.

Mechanism #3: Loop diuretics are highly protein-bound in the plasma and patients with hypoalbuminemia may have more free, unbound drug in the circulation that is not retained in the blood compartment and distributes through total body water, effectively reducing plasma concentrations.

Mechanism #4: The loop diuretic that remains bound to albumin is absorbed by specialized cells in the proximal tubule that un-couple the diuretic from the albumin, return the albumin to the circulation, and directly secrete the drug into the tubular lumen. In patients with significant proteinuria, urinary albumin re-binds the diuretic, within the tubule lumen, effectively preventing free drug from binding the target site in the ascending loop on Henle. Hypoalbuminemia and proteinuria can significantly reduce the likelihood of the expected diuretic response to loop diuretics.

Mechanism # 5: Patients with advanced kidney disease have accumulation of organic anions. Diuretics are themselves anions and the accumulating organic anions compete with diuretic receptor sites for tubular transport in the nephron and diminish the response of the nephron to the diuretic.

Mechanism #6: In patients that have been on loop diuretics chronically, the initial desired natriuresis stimulates the distal tubule cells to hypertrophy and assemble luminal sodium transporters in an attempt to counter the natriuresis. This "distal hypertophy" increases sodium reabsorption at that site and further counters a net diuresis.

Due to these mechanisms, higher doses of loop diuretics are advised. In patients who demonstrate a gradual loss of urine volume, the diuretic dosing should be re-evaluated with an increase in dose considered. The estimated ototoxic plasma level of furosemide is 85 mg/L and in a study involving dialysis patients chronically administered furosemide 250-1000 mg daily the plasma furosemide level was below 35 mg/L, suggesting larger oral doses of furosemide in this refractory population do not risk ototoxicity. Appropriate use of diuretics to maintain residual urine output can augment urine production allowing for use of less hypertonic glucose solutions.

Withdrawal of Transplant Immunosuppression

According to USRDS data, 16% of patients with a failed kidney transplant elect PD as their post-transplant dialysis modality. These patients are noted to have a more rapid decline in RKF compared to transplant naïve patients. Due to the survival benefit of RKF, certain strategies have been discussed to attempt to preserve RKF in the post-transplant population.

After initiation of PD, should transplant immunosuppression be rapidly weaned? Perhaps not. Jassel and colleagues examined whether maintenance of immunosuppression, to preserve residual kidney transplant function, affected the survival of the post-transplant PD patient. The authors developed a probability model based on multiple inputs from the published literature and administrative data bases. Their model predicted that life expectancy, in the post-transplant PD patient, would be longer if allograft function was maintained by continued immunosuppression. More work is needed in this area and clear clinical recommendations are lacking.

Conclusions

Preservation of residual kidney function is a clinical priority in patients on PD. Maintenance of residual kidney function has been linked to survival and ease of maintenance of volume, hematologic, and nutritional targets. At the initiation of dialysis, clinicians should review the medication list and evaluate for the need to resume medications that may have been discontinued prior to dialysis, such as those that inhibit the renin-angiotensin system. Diuretic dosing should be re-evaluated frequently and possibly increased to maintain urine volume. In those with remaining RKF, avoidance of nephrotoxins remains important.

References:

Bammens B, Evenepoel P, Verbeke K, Vanrenterghem Y. Removal of middle molecules and protein-bound solutes by peritoneal dialysis and relation with uremic symptoms. Kidney Int 2003;64:2238-2243.

Bargman JM, Thorpe KE, Churchill DN. Relative contribution of residual renal function and peritoneal clearance to adequacy of dialysis: a reanalysis of the CANUSA study. J Am Soc Nephrol 2001;12:2158-2162.

Fan SL, Pile T, Punzalan S, et al. Randomized controlled study of biocompatible peritoneal dialysis solutions: effect on residual renal function. Kidney Int 2008;73:200-206.

Han SH, Lee SC, Ahn SV, et al. Reduced residual renal function is a risk of peritonitis in continuous ambulatory peritoneal dialysis patients. Nephrol Dial Transplant 2007;22:2653-2658.

Han SH, Lee SC, Kang EW, et al. Reduced residual function is associated with endothelial dysfunction in patients receiving peritoneal dialysis. Perit Dial Int, 2012;32:149-158.

Jansen MA, Hart AA, Korevaar JC, et al. on behalf of the NECOSAD Study Group. Predictors of the rate of decline of residual renal function in incident patients. Kidney Int 2002;62:1046-1053.

Jassal SV, Lok CE, Walele A, Bargman JM. Continued transplant immunosuppression may prolong survival after return to peritoneal dialysis: results of a decision analysis. Am J Kidney Dis 2002;40:178-183.

Johnson DW, Mudge DW, Sturtevant JM, et al. Predictors of decline of residual renal function in new peritoneal dialysis patients. Perit Dial Int 2003;23:276-283.

Kooman JP, Cnossen N, Konings CJ, et al. Is there a competition between urine volume and peritoneal ultrafiltration in peritoneal dialysis patients? Contrib Nephrol 2006;150:111-118.

Lang SM, Bergner A, Topfer M, Schiffl H. Preservation of residual renal function in dialysis patients: effects of dialysis-technique-related factors. Perit Dial Int 2001;21:52-57.

Liao CT, Chen YM, Shiao CC, et al. Rate of decline of residual renal function is associated with all-cause mortality and technique failure in patients on long-term peritoneal dialysis. Nephrol Dial Transplant 2009;24:2909-2914.

Li PK, Chow KM, Wong TY, et al. Effects of an angiotensin-converting enzyme inhibitor on residual renal function in patients receiving peritoneal dialysis. A randomized, controlled study. Ann Intern Med 2003;139:105-112.

Lysaght MJ, Vonesh EF, Gotch F, et al. The influence of dialysis treatment modality on the decline of remaining renal function. ASAIO Trans 1991;37:598-604.

Marron B, Remon C, Perez-Fontan, et al. Benefits of preserving residual renal function in peritoneal dialysis. Kidney Int 2008;73:S42-51.

Medcalf JF, Harris KPG, Walls J. Role of diuretics in the preservation of residual renal function in patients on continuous ambulatory peritoneal dialysis. Kidney Int 2001;59:1128-1133.

Moist LM, Port FK, Orzol SM, et al. Predictors of loss of residual renal function among new dialysis patients. J Am Soc Nephrol 2000;11:556-564.

Moranne O, Willoteaux S, Pagniez D, et al. Effect of iodinated contrast agents on residual renal function in PD patients. Nephrol Dial Transplant 2006;21:1040-1045.

Noordzij M, Voormolen N, Boeschoten E, et al. Disordered mineral metabolism is not a risk factor for loss of residual renal function in dialysis patients. Nephrol Dial Transplant 2009;24:1580-1587.

Perl J, Bargman JM. The importance of residual kidney function for patients on dialysis: a critical review. Am J Kidney Dis 2009;53:1068-1081.

Rocco MV, Frankenfield DL, Prowant B, et al. Risk factors for early mortality in U.S. peritoneal dialysis patients: impact of residual renal function. Perit Dial Int 2002;22:371-379.

Rosenthal DI, Becerra CR, Toto RD, et al. Reversable renal toxicity resulting from high single doses of the new radiosensitizer gadolinium texaphyrin. Am J Clin Oncol 2000;23:593-598.

Shemin D, Bostom AG, Laliberty P, Dworkin LD. Residual renal function and mortality risk in hemodialysis patients. Am J Kidney Dis 2001;38:85-90.

Suda T, Hiroshige K, Ohta T, et al. The contribution of residual renal function to overall nutritional status in chronic haemodialysis patients. Nephrol Dial Transplant 2000;15:396-401.

Suzuki H, Kanno Y, Sugahara S, et al. Effects of angiotensin II receptor blocker, valsartan, on residual renal function in patients on CAPD. Am J Kidney Dis 2004;43:1056-1064.

Tam P. Peritoneal dialysis and preservation of residual renal function. Perit Dial Int 2009;29(S2):S108-S110.

Van Biesen W, Lameire N, Verbeke F, Vanholder R. Residual renal function and volume status in peritoneal dialysis patients: a conflict of interest? J Nephrol 2008;21:299-304.

Van den Wall Bake AWL, Kooman JP, Lange JM, Smit W. Adequacy of peritoneal dialysis and the importance of preserving residual renal function. Nephrol Dial Int 2006;21 [suppl 2]: ii34-ii37.

Van Olden RW, Krediet RT, Struijk DG, Arisz L. Measurement of residual renal function in patients treated with continuous ambulatory peritoneal dialysis. J Am Soc Nephrol 1996;7:745-750.

Van Olden RW, Guchelaar HJ, Struijk DG, et al. Acute effects of high-dose furosemide on residual renal function in CAPD patients. Perit Dial Int 2003;23:339-347.

Wang AY, Lai KN. The importance of residual renal function in dialysis patients. Kidney Int 2006;69:1726-1732.

Wang AY, Wang M, Woo J, et al. A novel association between residual renal function and left ventricular hypertrophy in peritoneal dialysis patients. Kidney Int 2002;62:639-647.

Wang AY, Wang M, Woo J, et al. Inflammation, residual kidney function, cardiac hypertrophy are interrelated and combine adversely to enhance mortality and cardiovascular death risk of peritoneal dialysis patients. J Am Soc Nephrol 2004;15:2186-2194.

Wang AY, Woo J, Sea MM, et al. Hyperphosphatemia in Chinese peritoneal dialysis patients with and without residual kidney function: what are the implications? Am J Kidney Dis 2004;43:712-720.

Wang AY, Sea MM, Ip R, et al. Independent effects of residual renal function and dialysis adequacy on actual dietary protein, calorie, and other nutrient intake in patients on continuous ambulatory peritoneal dialysis. J Am Soc Nephrol 2001;12:2450-2457.

Wang AYM, Lam CWK, Wang M, et al. Is valvular calcification a part of the missing link between residual kidney function and cardiac hypertrophy in peritoneal dialysis patients? Clin J Am Soc Nephrol 2009;4:1629-1636.

Chapter 6:
Peritoneal Dialysis Solutions

A VARIETY OF PD solutions are in clinical use. The solutions include the traditional dextrose-based solutions, non-dextrose solutions and dextrose solutions felt to be more biocompatible due to a neutral pH or lower content of glucose degradation products (GDPs). This chapter will review each of these solutions and briefly explain the rationale for their development, constituents, clinical indications and experience.

Traditional Dextrose-Based Solutions

Worldwide, dextrose-based solutions (such as *Dianeal*, Baxter Healthcare; *Delflex*, Fresenius Medical Care) are the most common solutions for PD therapy. The solutions contain dextrose in varying concentrations to create osmotic gradients to drive ultrafiltration and convective solute removal.

The constituents of these solutions are below:

Dextrose (g/dL)	1.5, 2.5, 4.25
Sodium (mEq/L)	132
Chloride (mEq/L)	96-102
Calcium (mEq/L)	3.5, 2.5
Magnesium (mEq/L)	0.5-1.5
L-Lactate (mEq/L)	35, 40

Osmolality (mOsm/kg)	346-485
pH	5.2

As shown, currently available dextrose concentrations of 1.5% (1.5 g/dL dextrose), 2.5% (2.5 g/dL), and 4.25% (4.25 g/dL) allow for varying osmotic stimuli to the peritoneum. By varying the dextrose concentration, clinicians can obtain a desired daily ultrafiltration.

Dialysate bags should be stored in cool areas, as heat exposure can degrade glucose and increase the concentration of glucose degradation products. The pH is lowered to prevent carmelization during heat sterilization.

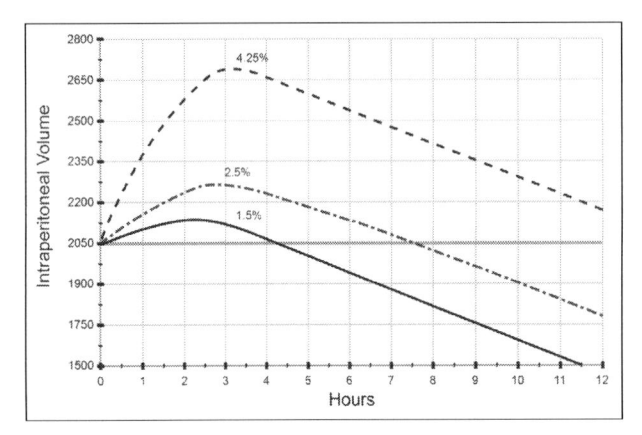

By altering the dextrose concentration and dwell time clinicians can prescribe a desired ultrafiltration volume

Dianeal-N (Baxter Healthcare) is a solution available in Japan that contains L-histidine as a pH adjuster, to achieve a neutral pH. The solution contains the typical lactate buffer but the addition of low amounts of L-histidine allows for the normalization of the pH.

Solutions with Lower Glucose Degradation Products and/or Neutral pH

Glucose degradation products (GDPs) are produced during the heat sterilization process. Changes to the solution bags have allowed for a reduction in GDPs produced and several lower GDP solutions are available outside of the USA (*Physioneal*, Baxter Healthcare; *Balance*, Fresenius Medical Care; *Gambrisol Trio*, Gambro; *BicaVera*, Fresenius Medical Care). Low GDP solutions are expected in the USA soon.

Electrolytes	Physioneal	Balance	BicaVera	Gambrisol Trio
Sodium	132	134	134	132
Calcium	2.5	3.5	2.5	2.6
Magnesium	0.5	1.0	1.0	0.5
Lactate	15	35	0	40

Bicarbonate	25	2.5	34	0
pH	7.4	7.0	7.4	6.3
% Glucose	1.5 – 4.25	1.5 – 4.25	1.5 – 4.25	1.5 – 4.25

There may be slight variations in preparations from different regions.

The technical advances that led to the development of these solutions were the use of dual chambers within the bags, allowing for separation of the dextrose. A dextrose/electrolyte compartment is maintained at a much lower pH during the heat sterilization process, to reduce the formation of GDPs. Before use, the patient manually separates a septum within the bag that allows admixture of the lower pH /dextrose component with the other higher pH bicarbonate or lactate /electrolyte compartment to create the low GDP final solution. The dual chambers also allow for bicarbonate to be used as a buffer, allowing separation of bicarbonate from electrolytes to prevent calcium and magnesium carbonate precipitation.

Studies using animal models have shown that low-GDP solutions appear to preserve peritoneal membrane integrity to a greater extent than traditional dextrose solutions. A large clinical trial, the Euro-Balance trial, showed that these newer solutions resulted in higher levels of peritoneal CA-125 levels, suggesting improved mesothelial cell homeostasis. However, besides these more local effects, there is no convincing information that use of lower GDP solutions confers a survival advantage. Some, but not all, studies suggest possible preservation of residual kidney function during treatment with lower GDP solutions. Also noted, however, in some of these studies was a reduction in ultrafiltration, raising concern that volume expansion may have contributed to the augmented urine output. Further research is needed to clarify the role of lower GPD solutions in improving long-term PD outcomes.

Icodextrin

Icodextrin (Extraneal, Baxter Healthcare) is the product of enzymatic dissolution of corn starch that is then subjected to fractionalization to create polymers of varying size (typically 13 to 19 kdaltons).

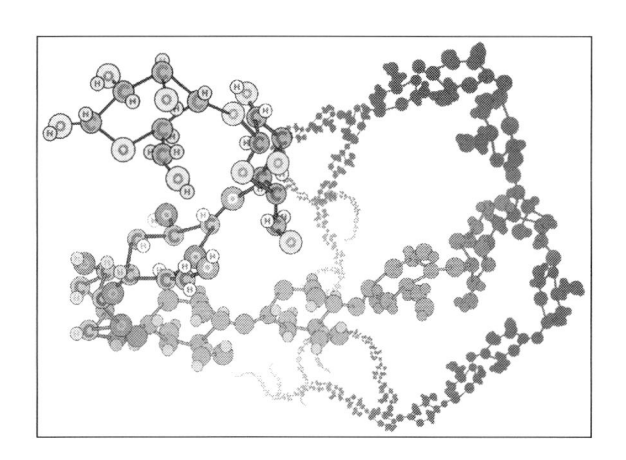

Chemical structure of glucose that allows polymerization into chains of dextrin molecules to form icodextrin

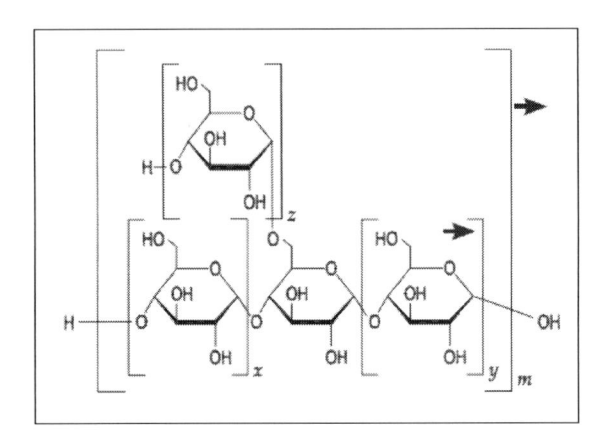

Glucose molecule can be repeated in polymerized chains

The large polymers consist of repeating chains of glucose molecules in a 1,4 linkage.

These macromolecules have high reflection coefficients and induce water movement across the small pores in endothelial cells. It is important to recognize that icodextrin solutions are iso-osmotic and therefore do not activate capillary aquaporins. No water movement occurs across the capillary aquaporin and therefore no sodium ions are sieved. Increased net sodium removal occurs by convection through the small pores.

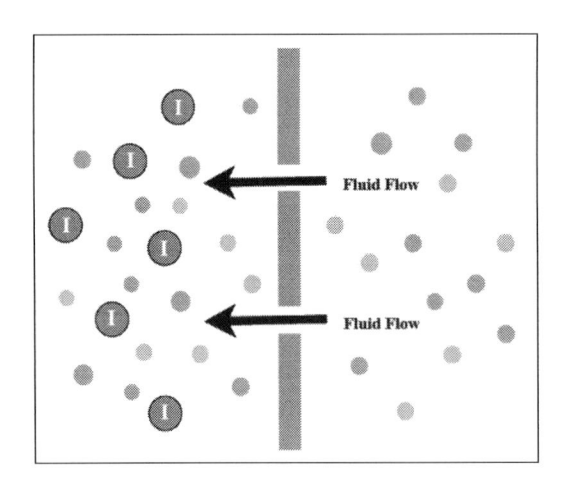

Icodextrin creates a colloidal osmotic pressure resulting in fluid movement across the small and large capillary pores. Capillary aquaporins are not activated as icodextrin is iso-osmotic

The glucose chains confer an oncotic property so that ultrafiltration across the peritoneal membrane is due to a colloidal osmotic pressure similar to albumin.

The solution has been considered more biocompatible as there is no glucose exposure to the peritoneum and the solution is iso-osmolar.

The formulation of icodextrin is below:

Icodextrin (g/dL)	7.5
Sodium (mEq/L)	132
Chloride (mEq/L)	96
Calcium (mEq/)	3.5
Magnesium (mEq/L)	0.5

Lactate (mEq/L)	40
Dextrose (g/dL)	0
Osmolality (mOsm/kg)	282-286
pH	5.2

The icodextrin molecules remain in the peritoneum for long periods of time allowing for sustained ultrafiltration. The metabolic fate of icodextin involves the slow absorption of a fraction of the infused concentraton. Icodextrin is not absorbed across the peritoneal membrane (due to the large size) but, rather, is absorbed via the lymphatics, then appears in the circulation and is subjected to degradation by serum amylase to maltose. Maltose transports into the cells of the body and is converted by maltase to glucose where it is used for cellular energy. Therefore, icodextrin is a non-glucose solution in the sense that the peritoneal membrane and plasma are not exposed to glucose during the dwell time.

Icodextrin has a unique ultrafiltration curve that illustrates the sustained convection that can occur:

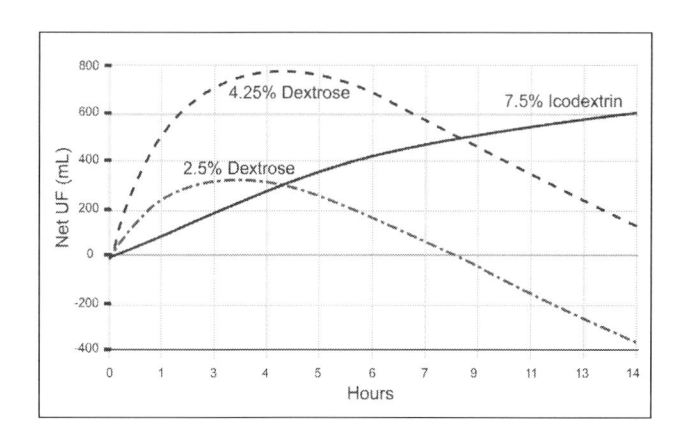

There are several important precautions that should be taken in patients using icodextrin. The most significant clinical issue is the interference of icodextrin metabolites (maltose) with certain devices used in diabetic testing. Some glucose testing devices are not specific for glucose and will read maltose as glucose and give an artificially elevated reading that could lead to the inadvertent administration of insulin. Excess insulin administration has led to serious hypoglycemia that can be life threatening. Not all glucose monitors read maltose as glucose and this depends on the chemical reagent used in the monitors. Those monitors that use glucose dehydrogenase with pyrroloquinolinequinone (GDH-PQQ) or the glucose-dye-oxidoreductase-based reagents will be contraindicated in patients using icodextrin as these reagents will give false glucose readings. The reagents that should be used for these patients are glucose oxidase, glucose dehydrogenase with nicotinamide adenine dinucleotide or flavin-adenine dinucleotide as the active ingredients. Precautions should be made to ensure that the patient, hospital ward, and emergency room personnel are aware of this device interaction.

Fortunately, glucose oxidase based monitors are commonly employed monitors in the USA. Nevertheless, this important interaction requires that clinicians check on their local testing devices. This is a potentially serious drug-device interaction and patients themselves should be educated by the PD nurses and given wallet cards and other identifiers to notify hospital staff of this potential interaction. The FDA has added a black box warning of this drug-device interaction on icodextrin product labeling. More information is available at **glucosesafety.com** as well as a list of glucose monitors that are not glucose specific.

Icodextrin is derived from corn starch and some patients present with hypersensitivity skin rashes. The incidence of skin rash may be as high as 10%. The rash is macular papular and most commonly appears on the trunk and extremities. No Stevens-Johnson reactions have been described. In patients developing rash, icodextrin should be discontinued.

An additional nuance associated with the use of icodextrin is an interference with the serum amylase determination. As mentioned, icodextrin, absorbed via the lymphatics, enters the circulation and is degraded to maltose by serum amylase. As the amylase enzyme is partially consumed by degrading icodextrin to maltose, less of the free enzyme is available to react with a reagent used in laboratory testing. This competitive inhibition results in a falsely lowered serum amylase determination. In patients using icodextrin, if pancreatitis is suspected, a serum lipase should be used to confirm the diagnosis. There is no icodextrin interference with lipase.

Amino Acid-Based Solutions

An amino acid (AA) based solution (Nutrineal, Baxter Healthcare) is available outside of the USA. This solution contains an electrolyte solution and mixture of 9 essential and 6 non-essential amino acids at a total concentration of 1.1%.

Sodium (mEq/L)	132
Chloride (mEq/L)	105
Calcium (mEq/L)	2.5
Magnesium (mEq/L)	0.5
Lactate	40
Dextrose (g/dL)	0
Amino acids	1.1%
Osmolality	Similar to 1.5%
pH	6.5

The amino acid components of Nutrineal:

Essential Amino Acids	Non-essential Amino Acids
Valine	Serine
Leucine	Alanine
Isoleucine	Arginine glycine
Methionine	Proline
Lysine	Glycine
Histidine	Tyrosine
Threonine	
Phenylalanine	
Tryptophan	

The amino acids are osmotically active and confer the same osmotic properties as a dextrose 1.5% solution. Nutrineal contains no glucose and has no GDP concentrations or potential for advanced glycation end-product (AGE) formation. Nutrineal increases protein absorption and reduces carbohydrate absorption so may be more metabolically favorable compared to dextrose-based solutions. Use of AA solutions has resulted in lower serum phosphorus values as these solutions are a phosphorus sparing source of protein. Use is limited to one exchange per day as more frequent use worsens uremia and metabolic acidosis.

Nutrineal was developed as a nutritional supplement for PD patients. While short term studies showed improvement in nitrogen and protein balance, no longer term nutritional benefit was consistently observed. These studies often failed to control for the state of inflammation or degree of metabolic acidosis - both potent stimuli of protein breakdown. In addition, adequate delivery of calories was not controlled which may have led to breakdown of amino acids as an energy source and prevented incorporation into protein stores.

The most vigorous study by Li and colleagues involved a 3-year prospective, randomized study using one exchange of AA-based solutions compared to traditional all dextrose solutions in 60 CAPD patients with signs of malnutrition. This study could show no impact of AA solutions on survival, hospitalization rate, or peritonitis rate. Over the three years of the study there appeared to be only modest, if any, improvement in nutritional parameters. Current use of AA solutions may be driven by strategies designed to avoid dextrose exposure, rather than for any proven nutritional impact.

Recent Solution Trials

Several recent solution trials have attempted to clarify the role of the newer solutions, often used in combination. The BALANZ trial was published in 2012. This trial enrolled incident PD patients with residual renal function who were randomized to receive conventional solutions or a biocompatible solution with neutral pH (Balance). Total enrollment was 185 patients and patients were followed for 2 years. The study intended to evaluate whether these newer solutions had favorable impact on residual renal function. At the 2-year endpoint there was no difference in the decline of GFR between the two groups but the neutral cohort had a delay in onset of complete anuria. A secondary endpoint of peritonitis rate suggested that the neutral solution cohort had a lower peritonitis rate during the study.

The most recent trials were the IMPENDIA and EDEN trials. The results of these 2 studies were combined and reported in 2013. The studies examined whether a low-glucose PD regimen could improve metabolic control in diabetic patients on PD. Patients were randomly assigned to conventional solutions or a low-glucose cohort that employed a traditional dextrose, icodextrin, and amino-acid combination (IMPENDIA) or a biocompatible dextrose, icodextrin, and amino-acid combination (EDEN). The combined study population consisted of 251 patients with the primary endpoint being change in glycated hemoglobin from baseline. The results of these combined studies were surprising. While there was an improvement in glycated hemoglobin in the intervention group and improvement in serum triglyceride levels, there were more deaths and serious adverse events in the intervention group. Many of the adverse events were related to hypertension and extracellular volume expansion. The implications of these studies are now being debated in the global PD community.

Conclusions

A variety of peritoneal dialysis solutions are available worldwide. The traditional dextrose-based solutions are used most commonly but alternatives to these include icodextrin, amino acid based solutions, and dextrose solutions produced to reduce GDP formation. Many randomized controlled trials have demonstrated the benefit of icodextrin in enhancing ultrafiltration in patients with higher membrane transport properties.

Clinical studies have not fully clarified the benefit of the newer solutions on long term membrane function, technique success, and preservation of residual kidney function. Animal models have demonstrated protection of the peritoneal membrane with lower GDP solutions but the full translation of this benefit to humans is yet to be convincing.

References:

Traditional dextrose based solutions

Erixon M, Wieslander A, Linden T, et al. Take care in how you store your PD fluids: actual temperature determines the balance between reactive and non-reactive GDPs. Perit Dial Int 2005;25:583-590.

Biocompatible, low GDP dextrose solutions

Fan SLS, Pile T, Punzalan S, et al. Randomized controlled study of biocompatible peritoneal dialysis solutions: effect on residual renal function. Kidney Int 2008;73:200-206.

Haag-Weber M, Kramer R, Haake R, et al. Low-GDP fluid (Gambrosol trio) attenuates decline of residual renal function in PD patients: a prospective randomized study. Nephrol Dial Transplant 2010;25:2288-2296.

Han SH, Ahn SV, Yun JY, et al. Mortality and technique failure in peritoneal dialysis patients using advanced peritoneal dialysis solutions. Am J Kidney Dis 2009;54:711-720.

Ho-dac-Pannekeet MM, Schouten N, Langendijk MJ, et al. Peritoneal transport characteristics with glucose polymer based dialysate. Kidney Int 1996:50:979-986.

Hoff CM. In vitro biocompatibility performance of Physioneal. Kidney Int 2003;64[Suppl 88]:S57-S74.

Li PKT, Culleton BF, Ariza A, et al. Randomized, controlled trial of glucose-sparing peritoneal dialysis in diabetic patients. J Am Soc Nephrol 2013;24:1889-1900.

Montenegro J, Saracho R, Gallardo I, et al. Use of pure bicarbonate-buffered peritoneal dialysis fluid reduces the incidence of CAPD peritonitis. Nephrol Dial Transplant 2007;22:1703-1708.

Mortier S, Faict D, Schalkwijk CG, et al. Long-term exposure to new peritoneal dialysis solutions: effects on the peritoneal membrane. Kidney Int 2004;66:1257-1265.

Mortier S, Faict D, Lameire NH, De Vriese AS. Benefits of switching from a conventional to a low-GDP bicarbonate/lactate-buffered dialysis solution in a rat model. Kidney Int 2005;67:1559-1565.

Szeto CC, Chow KM, Lam CW, et al. Clinical biocompatibility of a neutral peritoneal dialysis solution with minimal glucose-degradation products - a 1- year randomized control trial. Nephrol Dial Transplant 2007;22:552-559.

Tranaeus A. A long-term study of bicarbonate/lactate-based peritoneal dialysis solution-clinical benefits. Perit Dial Int 2000;20:516-523.

Williams JD, Topley N, Craig KJ, et al. The Euro-Balance Trial: the effect of a new biocompatible peritoneal dialysis fluid (balance) on the peritoneal membrane. Kidney Int 2004;66:408-418.

Icodextrin

Babazono T, Nakamoto H, Kasai K, et al. Effects of icodextrin on glycemic and lipid profiles in diabetic patients undergoing peritoneal dialysis. Am J Nephrol 2007;27:409-415.

Cho KH, Do JY, Park JW, Yoon KW. Effect of icodextrin dialysis solutions on body weight and fat accumulation over time in CAPD patients. Nephrol Dial Transplant 2010;25:593-599.

Davies SJ, Woodrow G, Donovan K, et al. Icodextrin improves the fluid status of peritoneal dialysis patients: results of a double-blind randomized controlled trial. J Am Soc Nephrol 2003;14:2338-2344.

Davies SJ, Brown EA, Frandsen NE, et al. Longitudinal membrane function in functionally anuric patients treated with APD: data from EAPOS on the effects of glucose and icodextrin prescription. Kidney Int 2005;67:1609-1615.

Finkelstein F, Healy H, Abu-Alfa A, et al. Superiority of icodextrin compared with 4.25% dextrose for peritoneal ultrafiltration. J Am Soc Nephrol 2005;16:546-554.

Gokal R, Moberly J, Lindholm B, Mujais S. Metabolic and laboratory effects of icodextrin. Kidney Int 2002;62[Suppl 81]:S62-S71.

Konings CJ, Kooman JP, Schonck M, et al. Effect of icodextrin on volume status, blood pressure and echocardiographic parameters: a randomized study. Kidney Int 2003;63:1556-1563.

Lee JH, Reddy DK, Saran R, et al. Peritoneal accumulation of advanced glycosylation end-products in diabetic rats on dialysis with icodextrin. Perit Dial Int 2000;20[Suppl 5]:S39-47.

Lin A, Qian J, Li X, et al. Randomized controlled trial of icodextrin versus glucose containing peritoneal dialysis fluid. Clin J Am Soc Nephrol 2009;4:1799-1804.

Mistry CD, Gokal R, Peers E. A randomized multicenter clinical trial comparing isosmolar icodextrin with hyperosmolar glucose solutions in CAPD. Kidney Int 1994;46:496-503.

Paniagua R, Ventura M, Avila-Diaz M, et al. Icodextrin improves metabolic and fluid management in high and high-average transport diabetic patients. Perit Dial Int 2009;29:422-432.

Rodriguez-Carmona A, Perez Fontan M, Garcia Lopez E, et al. Use of icodextrin during nocturnal automated peritoneal dialysis allows sustained ultrafiltration while reducing the peritoneal glucose load: a randomized crossover study. Perit Dial Int 2007;27:260-266.

Takatori Y, Akagi S, Sugiyama H, et al. Icodextrin increases technique survival rate in peritoneal dialysis patients with diabetic nephropathy by improving body fluid management: a randomized controlled trial. Clin J Am Soc Nephrol 2011;6:1337-1344.

Wolfson M, Piraino B, Hamburger RJ, Morton AR. A randomized controlled trial to evaluate the efficacy and safety of icodextrin in peritoneal dialysis. Am J Kidney Dis 2002;40:1055-1065.

Wolfson M, Ogrinc F, Mujais S. Review of clinical trial experience with icodextrin. Kidney Int 2002;62[Suppl 81]:S46-S52.

Amino acid-based solutions

Jones M, Hagen T, Boyle CA, et al. Treatment of malnutrition with 1.1% amino acid peritoneal dialysis solution: results of a multicenter outpatient study. Am J Kidney Dis 1998;32:761-769.

Le Poole CY, Welten AG, Weijmer MC, et al. Initiating CAPD with a regimen low in glucose and glucose degradation products, with icodextrin and amino acids (NEPP) is safe and efficacious. Perit Dial Int 2005;25[Suppl 3]:S64-S68.

Li FK, Chan LY, Woo JC, et al. A 3-year, prospective, randomized, controlled study on amino acid dialysate in patients on CAPD. Am J Kidney Dis 2003;42:173-183.

Tjiong HL, Swart R, van den Berg JW, Fieren MW. Amino acid-based peritoneal dialysis solutions for malnutrition: new perspectives. Perit Dial Int 2009;29:384-393.

Tjiong HL, Swart R, van den Berg J, Fieren MW. Amino acid-based peritoneal dialysis solutions for malnutrition: new perspectives. Perit Dial Int 2009;29:384-393.

Recent solution trials

Johnson DW, Brown FG, Clark M, et al. Biocompatible versus standard peritoneal dialysis fluid- the balANZ trial. J Am Soc Nephrol 2012;23:1097-1107.

Li PKT, Culleton BF, Ariza A, et al. Randomized, controlled trial of glucose-sparing peritoneal dialysis in diabetic patients. J Am Soc Nephrol 2013;24:1889-1900.

Chapter 7:
Catheters and Placement Techniques

CRITICAL TO THE SUCCESS of PD therapy is reliable long-term access to the peritoneal cavity. Current PD catheters exist in a variety of materials, configurations, lengths and are placed by a variety of procedures. This chapter will review PD catheters and best demonstrated placement techniques.

Catheter Materials

The earliest access devices were metal followed by crude plastic materials. In the 1960s, work with silicone rubber helped to determine that this material was superior to other plastics and less irritating to the peritoneal membrane. In 1968, Tenckhoff and colleagues added a Dacron cuff to the catheter material to allow for tissue in-growth and reduced leaks. Catheters presently in use are made of silicone (siliconized rubber). Polyurethane catheters were discontinued in 2009.

Catheter Configurations and Lengths

Peritoneal dialysis catheters are made in a variety of shapes and sizes. The intraperitoneal segment is in a straight configuration or in a coiled design, often termed "pigtailed". The catheter material often has a barium impregnation to provide a radiopaque marker for x-ray identification.

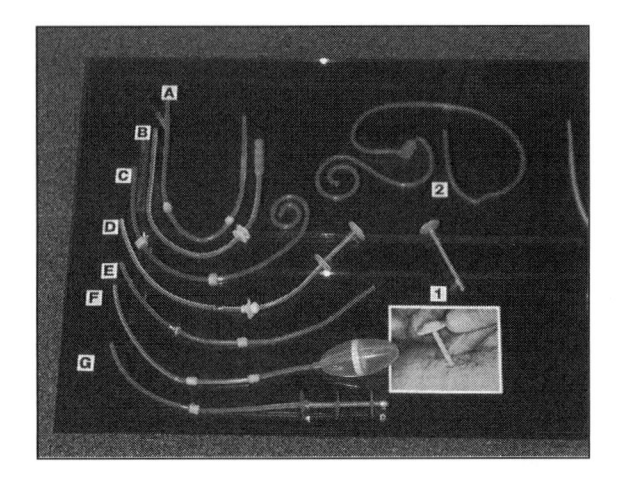

Historically there have been a variety of PD catheter configurations and materials

A polyurethane catheter (Cruz Catheter) had a larger internal diameter to allow for more rapid fluid transit but had limitations due to the polyurethane material itself, which was noted to degrade and fracture when exposed to a topical mupirocin antibiotic ointment. As mentioned, these catheters were discontinued in 2009.

The available siliconized rubber catheters vary in length and configuration of the intraperitoneal and tunneled segments. As mentioned, the intraperitoneal segment can be either straight or coiled. The straight intraperitoneal segment is widely used but has been described to create a direct fluid stream during infusion that can result in mild infusion pain. The straight segment has been rarely described to erode into and eventually perforate bowel viscera and to migrate into adhesion pockets, limiting flow of fluid.

For these reasons, the coiled intraperitoneal segment was designed to better disperse the infused dialysate to limit infusion discomfort and lessen chances that the most distal catheter tip could erode into viscera or migrate into collections of adhesion tissue. The coiled design could theoretically protect the catheter holes from tissue obstruction due to bowel or omentum. This design also gives added weight to the coiled tip to encourage the dependent pelvic location of the catheter. Some studies suggest that longer catheter survival occurs with the coiled catheters, compared to the straight configuration.

The coiled adult catheter lengths can vary from 57 cm to 62 cm. The internal diameter can vary from 2.5 mm to 3.5 mm. The more obese patient with a larger true peritoneal capacity may require the 62 cm length to reach the deep pelvic location and care should be taken to select the appropriate longer length of catheter if the abdominal cavity is large. The subcutaneous portion of the catheters can be a straight or angled configuration, termed a "swan neck" design.

Besides the straight and coiled configurations, other variations include deep cuff replacement by a disc or bead, by the internal catheter segment having discs attached to extrude bowel or omentum, or a tungsten weight to allow self locating into the pelvis.

Catheter	Configuration	Label
Silicone	Coiled	Tenckhoff
Silicone	Added discs	Toronto-Western-Hosp
Silicone	Internal weight added	Di Paolo
Silicone	Short internal segment	Vincenza
Silicone	Internal balloon added	Valli
Silicone	T-fluted	Ash
Silicone	Bead and disc	Missouri
Silicone	Swan neck embedded	Moncrief-Popovich
Polyurethane	Coiled	Cruz

Images of commonly employed catheters:

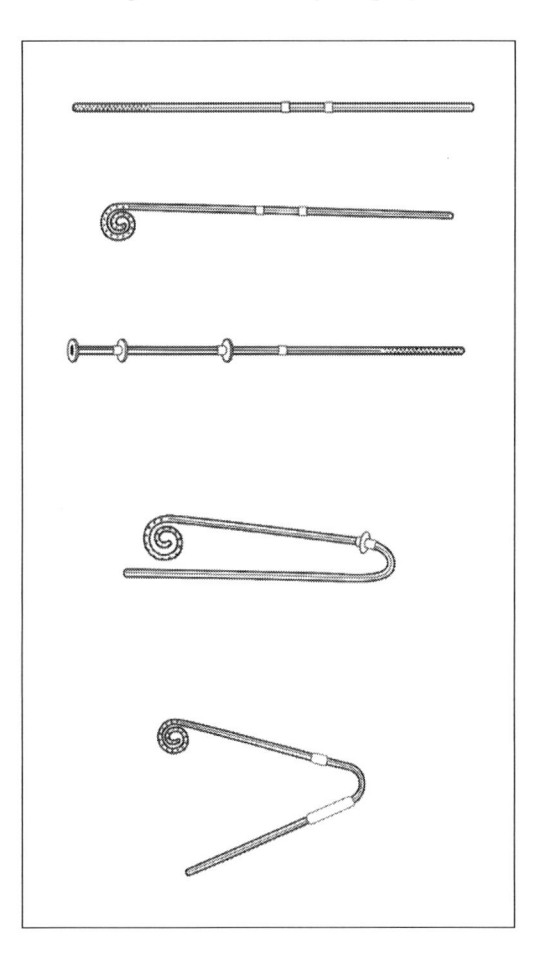

Double cuffed straight catheter

Coiled "pig-tail" double cuff catheter

Column-disc Toronto-Western catheter

Swan neck catheter

Moncrief-Popovich swan neck catheter with elongated cuff

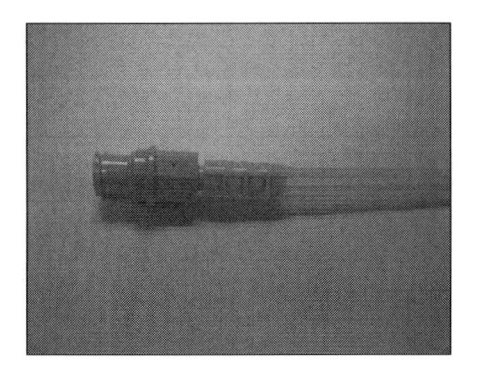

Adapters made from plastic or titanium are inserted into the distal catheter to allow screw on attachment of the patient's transfer set and sterile cap

At the external catheter tip, an adapter is attached - made of either titanium or plastic. Adapters are made to fit into the internal diameter of the catheter. The adapters allow for a screw-on attachment of the transfer sets made by various dialysis solution vendors. Therefore the entire apparatus, placed in the operative setting, is the catheter with the inserted adapter and attached transfer set.

The catheters described can be used for acute PD, but a variation of an acute catheter is the straight uncuffed catheter with an internal rigid stylet. The rigidity of the stylet allows for puncture of the abdominal wall to enter the peritoneum where the stylet is then removed and the catheter secured to begin exchanges.

Initial Planning for Catheter Placement

Proper positioning of the catheter requires pre-operative assessment and skin marking. The abdomen should be examined for locations of skin creases, pannus locations, the presence of any abdominal wall hernias, surgical scars, as well as the belt line. The exam should note these landmarks in both the lying and standing position as the anatomy may shift in these different positions.

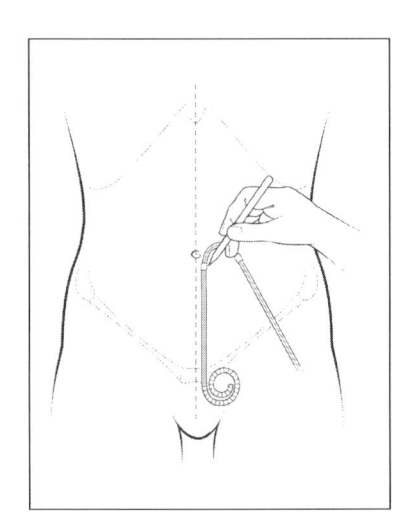

The catheter's coiled end should align with the upper border of the symphysis pubis and the deep cuff position marked at the rectus muscle for placement of the deep cuff in the rectus sheath.

A curved tunnel position can be marked toward the superficial cuff. The exit site can be planned by marking a skin exit approximately 3 to 4 centimeters away from the cuff. The exit site should be planned to have a lateral and downward position to allow natural cleansing of the site during showering.

Positioning of the Deep Cuff

The catheter deep Dacron cuff is ideally placed within the rectus sheath to allow more tissue in-growth into the cuff. This lessens the chance of leak and subsequent hernia

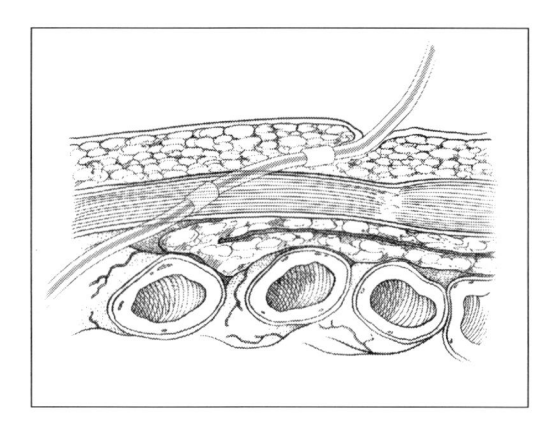

The deep cuff should be placed within the rectus muscle to allow muscle tissue in-growth into the Dacron cuff to minimize changes of subsequent leaks and hernia formation

formation. Placement of the deep cuff in the mid-line linea alba has been associated with more complications.

Proper Positioning of the Exit Site

Patients should be examined while sitting and standing to determine the ideal exit site. Exit sites should be oriented laterally and/or inferiorly. An upward directed exit site can lead to the accumulation of cellular debris, sweat, and water within the catheter-skin

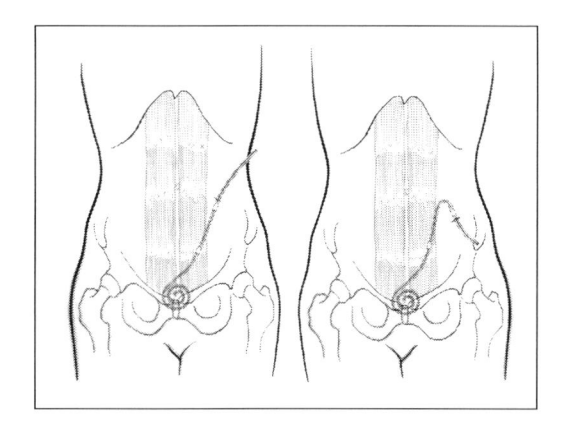

Upward facing exit sites are not preferable, as the site can collect debris and moisture. A downward facing exit site allows for better cleansing of the site during showering

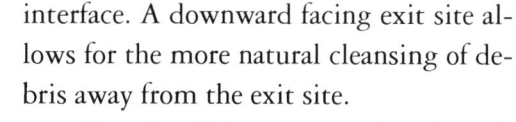

interface. A downward facing exit site allows for the more natural cleansing of debris away from the exit site.

Care should be taken to place the exit site in a position that will avoid the belt line. Females tend to have the belt line above the umbilicus so a sub-umbilical exit site is preferred. The design of the swan-neck catheter easily allows for this exit site orientation.

The catheter exit site should avoid the belt line and many females keep the belt line above the umbilicus.

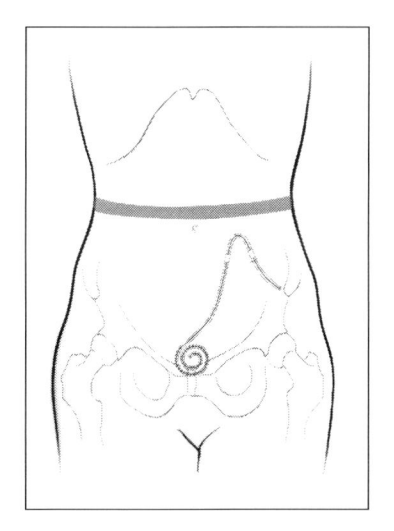

Swan neck catheter design allows for downward oriented exit site location that avoids the belt line

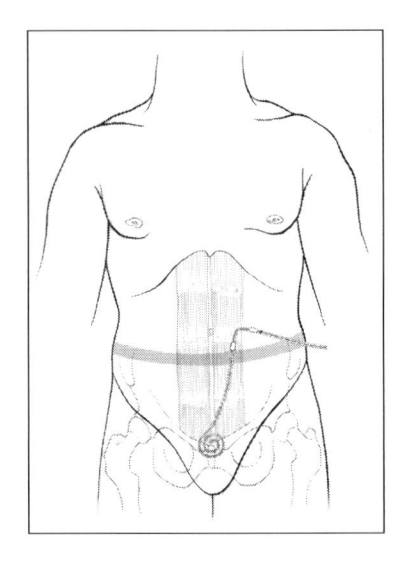

Exit site location in males should avoid the belt line and have a lateral/inferior orientation

Males tend to wear the belt line below the umbilicus and the exit site can be placed laterally and superior to the belt line.

The catheter can be elongated by a titanium adapter that allows for the connection of a second catheter. The second catheter can be trimmed to any desired length to allow for an exit site in the upper abdomen, chest, or back.

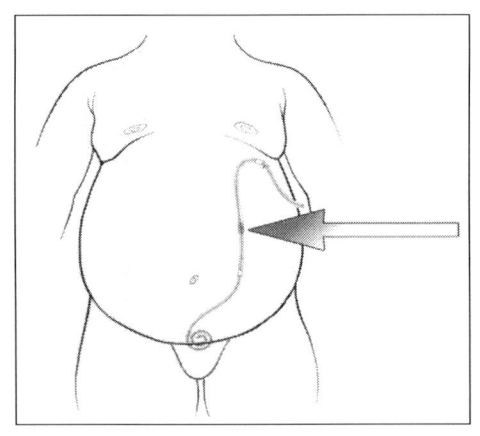

Titanium adapter allows connection to a second catheter for an exit site away from the lower abdomen

Catheter exit sites can be in the pre-sternal or posterior sub-scapular location (used for patients with dementia or other mental impairment and a history of picking or pulling of the catheter).

These non-traditional exit site locations have been demonstrated to have wide patient acceptance, lower exit site infection rates, and allow for the enjoyment of sitting in hot tubs.

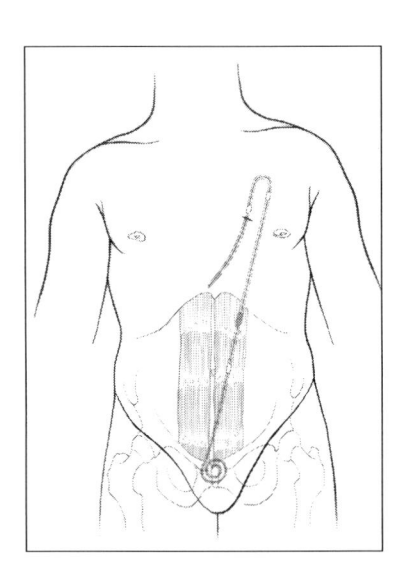

The pre-sternal exit site location is ideal for the obese patient, patients with gastrostomies, colostomies, or patients with body image concerns in the lower abdomen

Pre-Operative Management

A distended colon can complicate catheter placement and initial function so it is recommended to administer a stimulant suppository or non-phosphorus or magnesium containing enema prior to surgery. Laxatives may need to be administered for several days pre-operatively in patients with a history of chronic constipation.

Patients are kept fasted for 8 hours prior to surgery but in catheters placed percutaneously, under local anesthesia, fasting may be omitted. Usual medications can be taken with a small amount of water prior to the procedure. Patients can be advised to shower on the day of the procedure and wash with a chlorhexidine soap scrubbing of the abdomen. Patients are asked to completely empty the bladder just prior to the procedure and in patients with a history of neurogenic bladder a bladder catheter may be inserted. Prophylactic antibiotics are given intravenously within hours of the procedure - typically a first generation cephalosporin or, in those allergic or at risk of MRSA colonization, vancomycin may be administered. The role of antibiotic prophylaxis has been controversial but in surgeries involving the placement of a foreign body the role of prophylaxis may be greater. A prospective randomized study by Gadallah and colleagues showed that a single pre-operative dose of vancomycin 1000 mg reduced post-operative peritonitis compared to cefazolin and a control group.

Post-Operative Management

After catheter placement the exit site and new catheter, with transfer set, are covered with a sterile, semi-occlusive dressing, which is left in place for one week. (If acute PD is required the exit site can be dressed sterilely, with the catheter tubing exempted to allow access to the transfer set.) The post-operative dressing is changed at one week and the catheter is flushed with sterile saline. Flushing the catheter with dialysate has been reported to lead to fibrin occlusion, possibly due to irritation from the inherently less biocompatible dialysate. Weekly dressing changes and flushes can continue for 2 to 3 weeks. These initial bandage

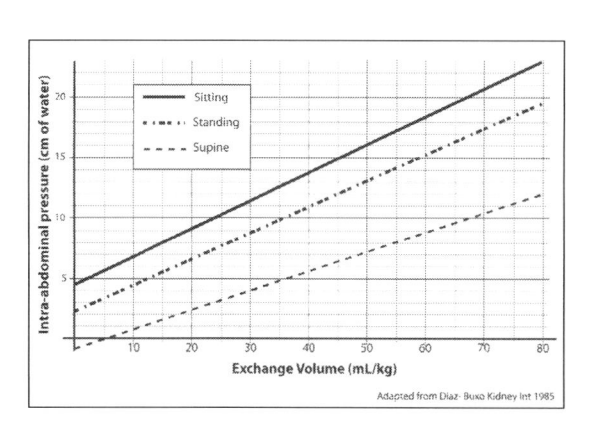

Intraabdominal pressure is highest in the sitting position and lowest in the supine position. If a new catheter is used more urgently dialysis should take place in the supine position to lessen the chance of early dialysate leak

changes should be done under sterile conditions with mask and gloves. After 3 weeks, routine daily exit site care can begin, with local cleansing with soap and water and administration of a topical antibiotic. The exit site should be covered with gauze or a transparent semi-permeable dressing and the catheter secured to the skin with tape, to avoid trauma. Showering should be avoided for 4 weeks after implantation to promote wound healing and allow the exit site to remain dry.

If possible, PD should be deferred for 10 to 14 days to allow for tissue in-growth to reduce the chance of early leak. If urgent initiation of PD is required the patient should be kept in the recumbent position with low volume dwells, then dry when upright and ambulating. Use of a cycler machine for supine, low volume dwells has been used for urgent start PD regimens.

Percutaneous Placement Techniques

The earliest catheter placement techniques involved percutaneous placement of a metal trochar into the peritoneal cavity. These straight trocar insertions were used predominantly for acute PD. With the development of more flexible siliconized rubber catheters, placement can be commonly performed with the Seldinger technique. Insertion kits come complete with catheters, introducer needles, wire and dilators that allow for easy insertion under local anesthesia. These percutaneous techniques can be used for both acute and chronic PD catheter initiation. Typical materials in insertion kits, such as the Quinton catheter kit made by Covidian (Kendall) appear below:

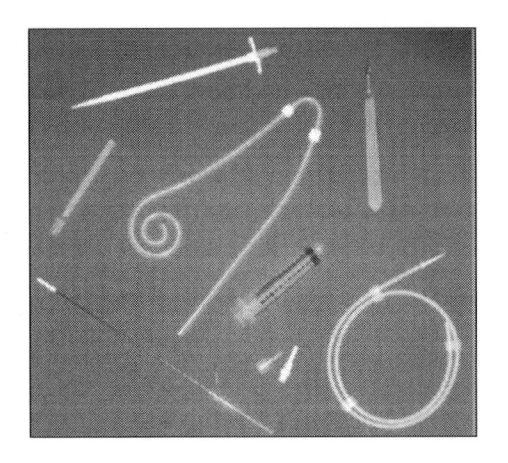

Catheter related components used for percutaneous or surgical catheter placement including introducer needles and syringe, introducer guidewires and dilators, scalpel, catheter, and tunneling tool

A variation of the blind Seldinger technique is to place catheters percutaneously using ultrasound guidance to assist in peritoneal cavity entry and then fluoroscopy to guide in proper catheter placement into the pelvis. Fluoroscopically guided PD catheter placement is done by interventional radiologists or interventional nephrologists and these techniques are notable for the low complication rates, ease in scheduling without the need for anesthesia clearance, operating or recovery room time. Percutaneous placement is cost-effective and requires only local anesthesia. PD programs that have developed the capability to place PD catheters by an interventional nephrologist or radiologist have described rapid growth in patient numbers due to ease of scheduling and patient acceptance. Placing a purse string suture at the deep cuff entry site in the rectus sheath has allowed acute dialysis with minimal leaking after these percutaneous procedures.

Recent reports of initiating PD urgently after percutaneous catheter placement have demonstrated that patients presenting late in the course of disease can avoid temporary vascular access catheters and successfully initiate PD by clinical pathways that allow for percutaneous catheter placement followed by lower volume, recumbent prescriptions.

Peritoneoscopy

Another technique for placing PD catheters is by peritoneoscopy. In this technique, a small rigid scope (Y-Tec; Merit Medical Systems, Inc, South Jordan, Utah, USA) is inserted into the abdomen that allows for visual inspection of the abdominal space to guide catheter placement.

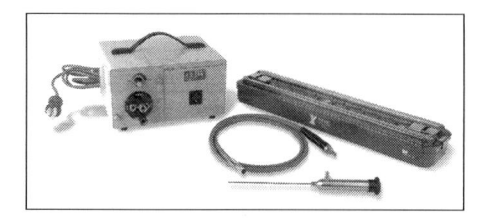

Peritoneoscope with sterilizing tray and light source (Y-Tec, Merit Medical Systems)

After surgical scrub, creation of a sterile field, a prophylactic antibiotic, and mild intravenous sedation, if required, a local anesthetic is administered. The surgeon or nephrologist makes a 2 cm paramedian incision to allow for blunt dissection down to the

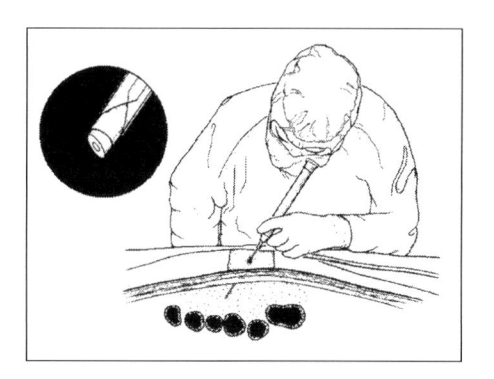

The peritoneoscope allows for direct visualization of the abdomen and placement of the catheter tip in a location that avoids adhesions or omentum

rectus sheath. The peritoneal cavity is entered first by a small trocar with sheath. The trocar is removed and the Y-Tec scope is inserted via the sheath. The scope confirms the peritoneal position. The scope and sheath, under direct visualization, are directed into an intra-abdominal site that avoids adhesions or omentum.

Use of a peel away sheath (Quill catheter guide; Merit Medical Systems) allows for placement of the catheter after the rigid scope has identified the ideal location for the distal catheter.

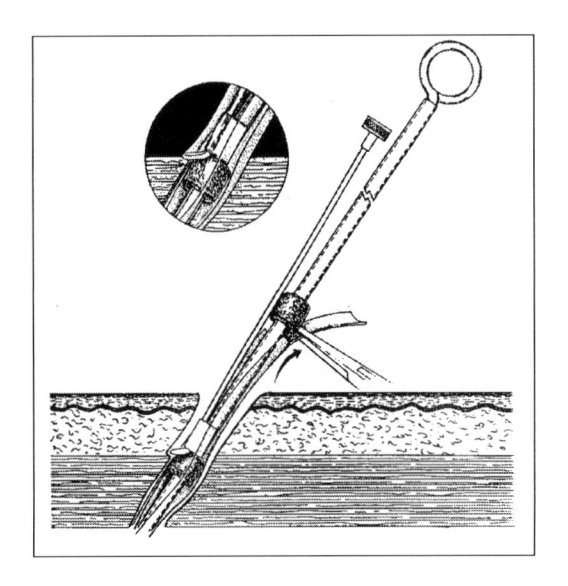

Catheter being advanced through a peel away sheath with deep cuff placement within the rectus sheath

The deep cuff is placed within the rectus sheath and a tunneling tool is used to create the subcutaneous tract and exit site. The 2 cm entrance site is sutured but no suture is placed at the exit site. The catheter and exit site is covered with a semi-occlusive dressing. The patient is observed for several hours prior to decisions regarding discharge home. Many publications document the use of peritoneoscopy for successful catheter placement and many centers employ this strategy as a means of expeditiously placing catheters without incurring the obstacles and delays often involved with scheduling surgical and operating room time.

Open Laparotomy

In the USA, the most common method for PD catheter placement is open laparotomy by surgeons. A preoperative bowel preparation is given to reduce the chances of colonic distention risking injury to the colon or catheter interference. The patient is taken to the operating room after an 8 hour fast and chlorhexidine abdominal wash. The patient is asked to void urine or an in-dwelling catheter is placed. A sterile field is created and under regional or general anesthesia, a paramedian incision is made to expose the rectus sheath. The catheter, over a rigid introducer, is placed into the peritoneum and directed toward the pelvis. The introducer is then removed and the catheter is flushed to assure patency. The deep cuff is placed within the rectus sheath and many surgeons place a reinforcing suture around the rectus sheath entry site to lessen the chance of leak should the catheter to be used acutely. This is followed by creation of a subcutaneous tract and exit site. The catheter is secured with tape and exit site covered with an semi-occlusive dressing. One limitation of open laparotomy placement is the lack of direct visualization of the intra-abdominal catheter location. In the operation room, it is important that surgeons ensure normal catheter function prior to ending the procedure.

Basic and Advanced Laparoscopic Techniques

The introduction of laparoscopic techniques to PD catheter placement allowed for direct visualization of the peritoneal cavity. After similar bowel preparation, surgical scrub and anesthesia, a laparoscope is introduced into the peritoneum which allows for identification and avoidance of adhesions or omental tissue that may interfere with catheter flow. The catheter tip can be visually directed into the deep pelvis. The deep cuff is placed within the rectus muscle as with open laparotomy.

Several advanced laparoscopic procedures have been recommended as complementary procedures to enhance long term catheter function and viability. One such procedure is termed "rectus sheath tunneling".

In rectus sheath tunneling the surgeon uses the rectus muscle sheath itself to direct the catheter downward into the pelvis. A tunneling device enters the rectus muscle sheath and instead of immediately entering the peritoneal cavity the surgeon tunnels inferiorly within the rectus sheath to place a segment of catheter within the sheath before entering the peritoneal cavity. This orients the catheter toward the pelvis and prevents catheter migration out of the pelvis. The rectus sheath tunneling procedure also lowers the risk of pericatheter leaks and eliminates pericatheter hernias.

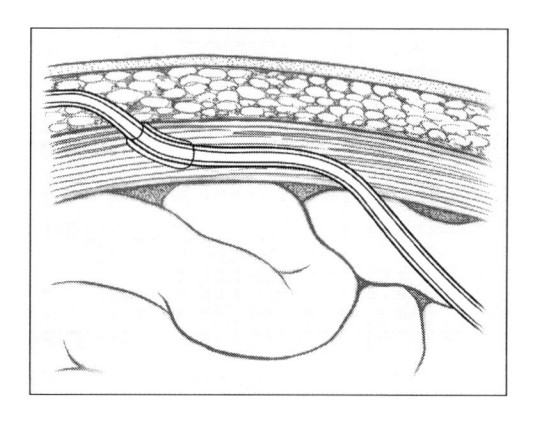

The deep cuff is placed in the rectus muscle with a portion of the catheter tunneled inferiorly within the rectus sheath to direct the catheter toward the pelvis

In addition to rectus sheath tunneling, laparoscopic surgeons can visualize and lyse pre-existing adhesions. Adhesions result in compartmentalization of the peritoneal cavity. These compartments prevent free contact and dispersion of dialysate and can lead to catheter kinking or occlusion. If detected during PD catheter placement, adhesions should be lysed by heat cautery to create a more open peritoneal cavity for free flow of PD fluid.

In omentopexy procedures the surgeon laparoscopically inspects the abdomen for evidence of redundant omental tissue and if detected the tissue is folded upon itself and tacked with a restraining suture to keep the omentum restricted to the upper portions of the abdomen. This procedure lessens the chance that free omentum enters the pelvic region where entrapment of the catheter tip could occur.

By using these advanced laparoscopic techniques long-term catheter function has been documented. PD centers that are experiencing difficulties with catheter placement and function may want to introduce advanced laparoscopic techniques to ensure greater overall success.

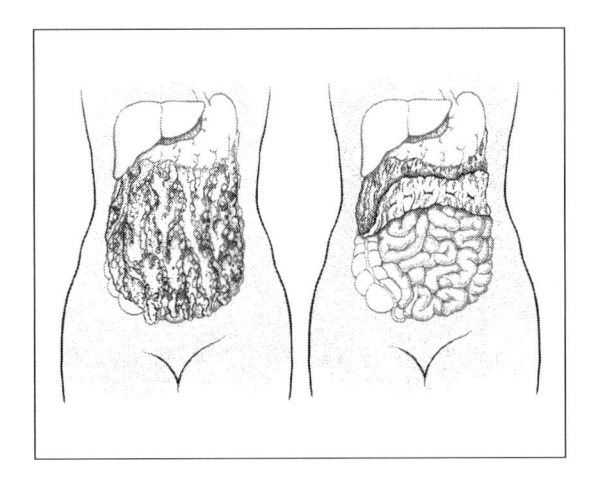

Redundant omental tissue that reaches the pelvis can be folded or tacked up superiorly in an omentopexy procedure to reduce the incidence of omental occlusion

If catheters are placed using a laparoscope, surgeons should take advantage of the operative setting and inspect the abdomen to detect any small hernias that have escaped clinical detection. If at all possible, surgeons are advised to repair these pre-existing hernias at the time of catheter implantation to prevent the need for a subsequent hernioplasty.

Laparoscopic placement of PD catheters is typically performed via multiple abdominal ports to allow for insufflation of the abdomen and surgical instrumentation. As an alternative, a recently published single port laparoscopic technique has been described.

Embedded Catheter Techniques

An alternate technique for PD catheter placement has been termed the embedded or buried catheter, initially described by Moncrief and Popovich. Embedding is done at the time of the original catheter placement. In this procedure the surgeon or interventionalist places the PD catheter in the usual fashion and verifies the patency with flushes. Then the operator tunnels the external catheter under the skin completely. The catheter's deep rectus cuff and subcutaneous cuff heal while the catheter remains completely under the skin. When the decision is made to initiate PD, a small incision is made approximately 3 cm distal to the subcutaneous cuff and the catheter is externalized at this incision to initiate PD. At the time of externalization the operator must be careful to avoid cutting or puncturing the catheter. This buried PD catheter is analogous to a HD fistula in which an access is created, in advance of starting dialysis, and allowed to mature until needed.

With embedded catheter placement, the advanced planning of PD access can commit the patient to PD and lessen the chance of subsequent drop out to HD. Should the patient's medical condition deteriorate unexpectedly the catheter can be externalized and used for immediate full-dose PD therapy. This reduces the chance that HD would be needed as a "bridge therapy" until a PD catheter can be placed.

Embedded catheters allow for certain operational efficiencies. The buried catheter can be placed electively, weeks to months before the initiation of PD. This allows for more elective scheduling of the surgical consultation and operating room. The embedded catheter, being completely buried, does not require flushing by the nursing staff, lessening the demands on nursing time in the pre-training period. Finally, as mentioned, the buried catheter lessens the chance that hemodialysis would need to be arranged in the patient with unexpected deterioration in renal function.

Clinical benefits of the embedded catheter are unclear. No consistent trends in the literature suggest that embedded catheters lead to less peritonitis. Mechanical complications of leak and primary non-function are still described. A recent review of 349 embedded catheters by Brown and McCormick noted a primary failure rate of 9.4% in catheters

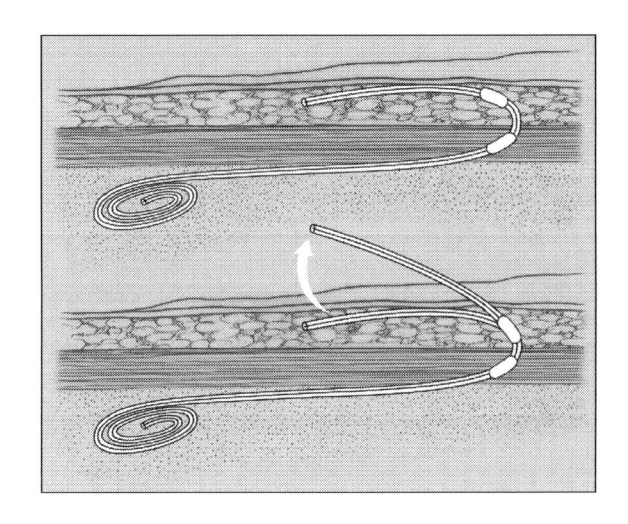

Catheter that has been embedded at the time of placement and then externalized weeks or months later to initiate PD - analogous to the fistula in HD

buried for more than 134 days, leading the authors to conclude that mechanical complications and catheter loss with embedded catheters can be minimized if the catheters can be externalized and used between 6 weeks to 5 months of insertion. Crabtree and Burchette published a recent series of 84 embedded catheters. Mean duration of embedment was 13.9 months and immediate function was noted in 85.7% of catheters after externalization. Interestingly, catheter dysfunction occurred exclusively in embedded catheters that were of the 2-piece extended variety. The authors were unclear as to why extended catheters systems would show reduced function rates after embedment but speculated that the longer catheters may be affected by position, catheter lock solution leakage, or systemic inflammation as these catheters were predominantly placed in obese or diabetic patients.

Conclusions

Successful peritoneal dialysis relies on dependable, long-term access to the peritoneal cavity. A variety of catheter materials and configurations are available and the siliconized rubber, dual cuff, coiled catheter is commonly used. Catheter placement by percutaneous Seldinger technique, peritoneoscopy, laparotomy, and laparoscopic techniques are common. Successful results have been achieved by all approaches depending, predominantly, on the skill of the operator. However, laparoscopy allows for important adjuvant procedures such as adhesiolysis, omentopexy, and hernia repair that have been documented to improve long-term success.

The catheter exit site should be carefully considered to avoid the belt line and be directed in a lateral to inferior direction. Patients, especially the obese, can consider an upper abdominal or pre-sternal exit site location. Catheters can be buried for elective use weeks to months after implantation.

References:

General Catheter Placement and Catheter Care

Dell'Aquila R, Chiaramonte S, Rodighiero MP, et al. Rational choice of peritoneal dialysis catheter. Perit Dial Int 2007;27[Suppl 2]:S119-125.

Dombros N, Dratwa M, Feriani M, et al. European best practice guidelines for peritoneal dialysis. Peritoneal access. Nephrol Dial Transplant 2005;20[Suppl 9]:ix8-ix12.

Gadallah MF, Ramdeen G, Mignone J, et al. Role of preoperative antibiotic prophylaxis in preventing postoperative peritonitis in newly placed peritoneal dialysis catheters. Am J Kidney Dis 2000;36:1014-1019.

Eklund B, Honkanen E, Kyllonen L, et al. Peritoneal dialysis access: prospective randomized comparison of single-cuff and double-cuff straight Tenckhoff catheters. Nephrol Dial Transplant 1997;12:2664-2666.

Figueiredo A, Goh BL, Jenkins S, et al. Clinical practice guidelines for peritoneal access. Perit Dial Int 2010;30:424-429.

Flanigan M, Gokal R. Peritoneal catheters and exit-site practices toward optimum peritoneal access: a review of current developments. Perit Dial Int 2005;25:132-139.

Keshvari A, Fazeli MS, Meysamie A, et al. The effects of previous abdominal operations and intraperitoneal adhesions on the outcome of peritoneal dialysis catheters. Perit Dial Int 2010;30:41-45.

Nielsen PK, Hemmingsen C, Friis SU, et al. Comparison of straight and curled Tenckhoff peritoneal dialysis catheters implanted by percutaneous technique: a prospective randomized study. Perit Dial Int 1995;15:18-21.

Twardowski ZJ, Prowant BF, Nichols K, et al. Six-year experience with swan neck presternal peritoneal dialysis catheter. Perit Dial Int 1998;18:598-602.

Twardowski ZJ. History of peritoneal access development. Int J Artif Organs 2006;29:2-40.

Percutaneous Techniques

Abdel-Aal AK, Joshi AK, Saddekni S, Maya ID. Fluoroscopic and sonographic guidance to place peritoneal catheters: how we do it. Am J Roentgenol 2009;192:1085-1089.

Alvarez AC, Salman L. Peritoneal dialysis catheter insertion by interventional nephrologists. Adv Chronic Kidney Dis 2009;16:378-385.

Asif A. Peritoneal dialysis access-related procedures by nephrologists. Semin Dial 2004;17:398-406.

Banli O, Altun H, Oztemel A. Early start of CAPD with the Seldinger technique. Perit Dial Int 2005;25:556-559.

Brunier G, Hiller JA, Drayton S, et al. A change to radiological peritoneal dialysis catheter insertion: three-month outcomes. Perit Dial Int 2010;30:528-533.

Henderson S, Brown E, Levy J. Safety and efficacy of percutaneous insertion of peritoneal dialysis catheters under sedation and local anaesthetic. Nephrol Dial Transplant 2009;24:3499-3504.

Jo YI, Shin SK, Lee JH, et al. Immediate initiation of CAPD following percutaneous catheter placement without break-in procedure. Perit Dial Int 2007;27:179-183.

Maya ID. Ambulatory setting for peritoneal dialysis catheter placement. Semin Dial 2008;21:457-458.

Maya ID. Ultrasound/fluoroscopy-assisted placement of peritoneal dialysis catheters. Semin Dial 2007;20:611-615.

Medani S, Shantier M, Hussein W, et al. A comparative analysis of percutaneous and open surgical techniques for peritoneal catheter placement. Perit Dial Int 2012;32:628-635.

Niyyar V, Work J. Interventional nephrology: core curriculum 2009. Am J Kidney Dis 2009;54:169-182.

Perakis KE, Stylianou KG, Kyriazis JP, et al. Long-term complication rates and survival of peritoneal dialysis catheters: the role of percutaneous versus surgical placement. Semin Dial 2009;22:569-575.

Reddy C, Dybbro PE, Guest S. Fluoroscopically guided percutaneous peritoneal dialysis catheter placement: single center experience and review of the literature. Ren Fail 2010;32:294-299.

Sreenarasimhaiah VP, Margassery SK, Martin KJ, Bander SJ. Percutaneous technique of presternal peritoneal dialysis catheter placement. Semin Dial 2004;17:407-410.

Vaux EC, Torrie PH, Barker LC, et al. Percutaneous fluoroscopically guided placement of peritoneal dialysis catheters- a 10-year experience. Semin Dial 2008;21:459-465.

Voss D, Hawkins S, Poole G, Marshall M. Radiological versus surgical implantation of first catheter for peritoneal dialysis: a randomized non-inferiority trial. Nephrol Dial Transplant 2012;27:4196-4204.

Zaman F, Pervez A, Atray NK, et al. Fluoroscopy-assisted placement of peritoneal dialysis catheters by nephrologists. Semin Dial 2005;18:247-251.

Zaman F. Peritoneal dialysis catheter placement by nephrologist. Perit Dial Int 2008:28:138-141.

Peritoneoscopy

Ash S. Laparoscopy for PD catheter placement: advantages and disadvantages versus peritoneoscopy. Perit Dial Int 2005;25:541-543.

Asif A, Byers P, Vieira C, et al. Peritoneoscopic placement of peritoneal dialysis catheter and bowel perforation: experience of an interventional nephrology program. Am J Kidney Dis 2003;42:1270-1274.

Gadallah MF, Pervez A, el-Shahawy MA, et al. Peritoneoscopic versus surgical placement of peritoneal dialysis catheters: a prospective randomized study on outcomes. Am J Kidney Dis 1999;33:118-122.

Kelly J, McNamara K, May S. Peritoneoscopic peritoneal dialysis catheter insertion. Nephrology 2003;8:315-317.

Laparotomy

Stegmayr B. Advantages and disadvantages of surgical placement of PD catheters with regard to other methods. Int J Artif Organs 2006;29:95-100.

Laparoscopic Techniques

Ashegh H, Rezaii J, Esfandiari K, et al. One-port laparoscopic technique for placement of Tenckhoff peritoneal dialysis catheters: report of seventy-nine procedures. Perit Dial Int 2008;28:622-625.

Comert M, Borazan A, Kulah E, Ucan BH. A new laparoscopic technique for the placement of a permanent peritoneal dialysis catheter: the preperitoneal tunneling method. Surg Endosc 2005;19:245-248.

Crabtree JH, Fishman A. A laparoscopic method for optimal peritoneal dialysis access. Am Surg 2005;71:135-143.

Crabtree JH. Selected best demonstrated practices in peritoneal dialysis access. Kidney Int 2006;70[Suppl 103]:S27-37.

Crabtree JH, Burchette RJ. Effective use of laparoscopy for long-term peritoneal dialysis access. Am J Surg 2009;198:135-141.

Crabtree JH, Burchette RJ. Effect of prior abdominal surgery, peritonitis, and adhesions on catheter function and long-term outcome on peritoneal dialysis. Am Surg 2009;75:140-147.

Crabtree JH, Burchette RJ. Comparative analysis of two-piece extended peritoneal dialysis catheters with remote exit-site locations and conventional abdominal catheters. Perit Dial Int 2010;30:46-55.

Goh YH. Omental folding: a novel laparoscopic technique for salvaging peritoneal dialysis catheters. Perit Dial Int 2008;28:626-631.

Keshvari A, Najafi I, Jafari-Javid M, et al. Laparoscopic peritoneal dialysis catheter implantation using a Tenckhoff trocar under local anesthesia with nitrous oxide gas insufflations. Am J Surg 2009;197:8-13.

Ogunc G. Minilaparoscopic extraperitoneal tunneling with omentopexy: a new technique for CAPD catheter placement. Perit Dial Int 2005;25:551-555.

Penner T, Crabtree JH. Peritoneal dialysis catheters with back exit sites. Perit Dial Int 2013;33:93-96.

Embedded catheters

Brown PA, McCormick BB, Knoll G, et al. Complications and catheter survival with prolonged embedding of peritoneal dialysis catheters. Nephrol Dial Transplant 2008;23:2299-2303.

Crabtree JH, Burchette RJ. Peritoneal dialysis catheter embedment: surgical considerations, expectations, and complications. Am J Surg 2013;206:464-471.

Elhassan E, McNair B, Quinn M, Teitelbaum I. Prolonged duration of peritoneal dialysis catheter embedment does not lower the catheter success rate. Perit Dial Int 2011;31:558-564.

McCormick BB, Brown PA, Knoll G, et al. Use of the embedded peritoneal dialysis catheter: experience and results from a North American center. Kidney Int 2006;70:S38-S43.

Moncrief JW, Popovich RP, Broadrick LJ, et al. The Moncrief-Popovich catheter. A new peritoneal access technique for patients on peritoneal dialysis. ASAIO J 1993;39:62-65.

Chapter 8:
Catheter Dysfunction

TO ALLOW FOR LONG-TERM success of the therapy, proper catheter placement is a critical component of the care plan. Prior chapters have emphasized the importance of proper positioning of the intra-abdominal catheter as well as the deep and superficial cuffs. Despite initial successful function of the catheter, dysfunction can develop later in the course of patient care. Different clinical presentations of catheter dysfunction, such as slow fill or drain, obstruction, or catheter tip migration can interfere with proper dialysate flows needed for dialysis. This chapter will address the causes and treatment approaches to catheter dysfunction.

Delayed Fill or Drain Times

Occasionally the dialysate flows are initially adequate and then subsequently the patient describes delays in filling or draining of the dialysate. Slow fill or drain times can be due to a variety of scenarios. Experienced PD practitioners suggest there is one predominant reason why a previously functioning PD catheter begins to demonstrate poor flows - constipation. These practitioners often explain that there is limited "real estate" within the peritoneal cavity and proper flows of dialysate will be dependent on the colon not being distended with stool, directly occupy excessive "real estate" and impinging on the catheter itself, preventing adequate fluid movement to and from the catheter.

Patients receiving narcotics for reasons such as dental work, or due to other medical problems, may develop constipation and present with delayed flows. PD nurses should inquire as to the bowel habits of patients to ensure that proper control of constipation is emphasized. If the patient experiences a single day without movement of the bowels there should be the consideration of a laxative, to ensure that insidious constipation does not interfere with the peritoneal dialysis process. Laxative use should be considered with the understanding that patients with ESRD (or advanced kidney disease) should not take laxatives that contain phospho-soda or other phosphate compounds, and should have limited exposure to magnesium containing laxatives. Mineral oil based laxatives or lactulose are alternatives for the patient on peritoneal dialysis. Even if the patient reports a reasonable response to the laxative, abdominal x-rays often reveal significant residual stool, so repeated bowel cleansing treatments may be necessary to restore proper catheter flows.

If initial trials of laxative therapy do not restore normal catheter function the clinician should obtain an abdominal x-ray. Most PD catheters have an impregnated radiopaque stripe that allows for visualization of the intra-abdominal catheter on x-ray. The x-ray can better delineate whether poor catheter flows are due to residual stool, catheter migration out of the pelvic location, or an unusual kink in the catheter material. Catheters have been noted to migrate to different abdominal locations and still remain functional, so migration of the catheter in itself does not mean that the catheter will not function. But in a poorly functioning catheter, that is also noted to have migrated to an upper abdominal location, the clinician could suspect that there is a relationship between the poor function and the migration.

Catheter Migration

The desired location for the distal catheter segment is within the pelvic portion of the peritoneal cavity. As mentioned, catheter migration can be the result of distention of the colon by excess stool but also due to peristalsis of the intestine or omental tissue. Migration can occur in all patients as the distal catheter is typically not sutured into the pelvis and therefore able to move to different locations within the abdomen. This migration out of the pelvis can result in inflow or outflow dysfunction or pain.

Straight catheters that are bent, to create a downward facing tunnel and exit site, retain their "memory" and

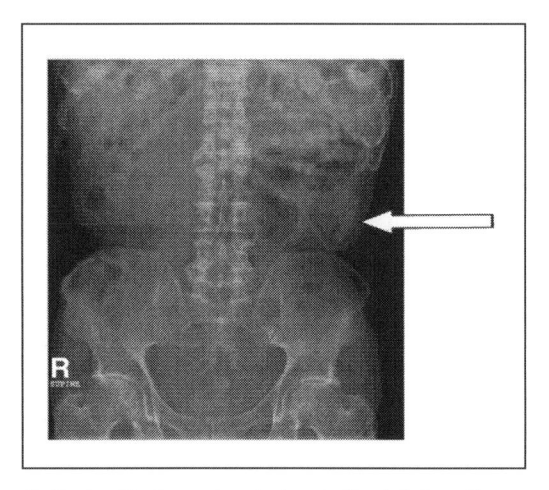

Catheter tip has migrated out of pelvic location

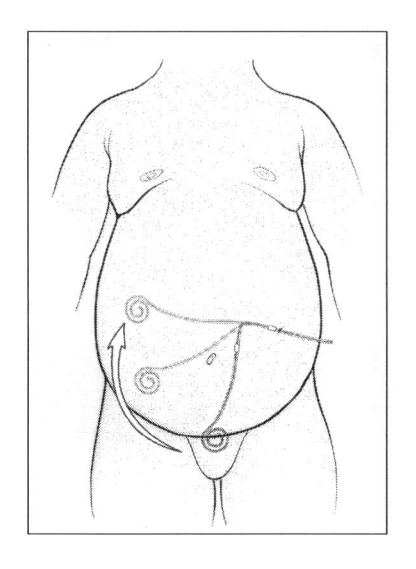

Straight catheters bent to create the tunnel and downward exit site can retain the straight "memory" resulting in migration of catheter pigtail out of the pelvis

can slowly resort to the straight position, leading to catheter migration. Swan neck catheters with a preformed bend may be less likely to straighten and migrate.

If the catheter has migrated out of the pelvis resulting in flow disturbances or discomfort and laxative therapy has not resolved the problem, other approaches may need to be considered. There are 3 general approaches to restoring catheter flow and/or repositioning a migrated PD catheter:

1. Interventionalist repositioning of the catheter with a Fogarty balloon catheter or stiff - wire manipulation
2. Laparoscopic surgical repositioning
3. Removal of original catheter and replacement with new catheter in different location

A variety of devices have been described to reposition catheters in a minimally invasive approach. An interventional radiologist or nephrologist, under fluoroscopic guidance can reposition the catheter by inserting semi-rigid rods or stiff wires. Another approach involves a 5 French urethral catheter threaded inside the catheter to attempt to expel obstructing material and then, if needed, to allow for the operator to attempt to reposition the catheter by inflating the balloon and applying traction. The success rate for catheter repositioning by this non-surgical approach is operator dependent.

Recently Miller and colleagues described a single-center experience with 70 consecutive fluoroscopic manipulations of malfunctioning PD catheters. Sixty three percent of the migrated catheters were successfully repositioned with restoration of flow. Predictors of failure were the catheters that had migrated into the upper abdomen (as opposed to mid-abdomen) and catheters that had failed on initial attempts at use (as opposed to previously functioning catheters).

Laparoscopic surgery to reposition a PD catheter is associated with a higher success rate and is helpful to rule out other anatomic abnormalities that may have contributed to the catheter migration such as fibrotic adhesions or omentum. In cases where laparoscopic intervention is required to restore catheter position, serious consideration should be made to intervening on any anatomic factors that may lead to catheter dysfunction in the future. If adhesions or omentum are noted, the surgeon can perform adhesiolysis and/or omentopexy to reduce the chance of catheter dysfunction at a later point. During laparoscopic repositioning, the deep and superficial cuffs are left in place allowing the more rapid resumption of PD.

Fibrin Occlusion

Temporary drain problems or catheter obstruction can occur due to obstruction from fibrin. Mucinous fibrin lubricates the external bowel wall to aid in peristalsis. Fibrin can be suspended in the dialysate to create concretions that become lodged within the catheter obstructing the distal catheter or the side holes of the intra-peritoneal catheter. Fibrin production can often be significant and patients should be instructed to inspect their drainage bags. If fibrin is noted, consideration should be given to the temporary addition of heparin to the infusing dialysate as a method to reduce the viscosity of the

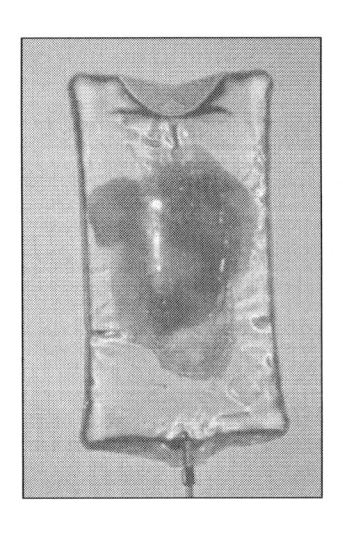

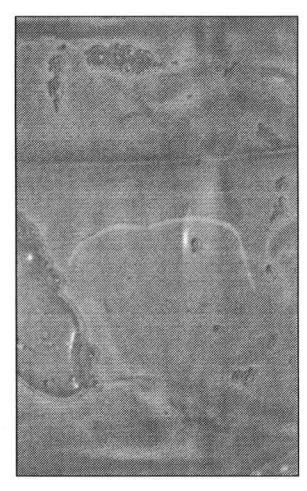

Fibrin appearing in drained dialysate

fibrin.

Typical heparin concentrations recommended are 1000 to 2000 units of heparin sulfate injected into the 2 liter dialysate bag's medication port. This heparin remains within the peritoneal cavity, is not systemically absorbed, and has not been described to affect systemic coagulation parameters. Heparin can be very effective in reducing the chances of fibrin-related catheter dysfunction. Typically, several days of heparin administration is sufficient to reduce this fibrin-related complication. If catheter flows are reduced due to fibrin deposits, flow can be restored by forceful flushing of the catheter or by inserting a sterile 5 French urologic catheter to attempt to expel the fibrin into the peritoneal cavity.

Thrombolytics have been used to disrupt fibrin lodged within the catheter lumen. Typically, low dose tissue plasminogen activator (TPA) suspended in normal saline is slowly infused by syringe into the catheter lumen, allowed to sit as a "locking" solution for one hour, followed by aspiration and further attempts to restore normal catheter flow. The locking solution can be repeated if residual fibrin is deemed present. TPA doses of 1 to 5 mg have been used as catheter locking solutions.

Omental Wrap

Redundant omental tissue can obstruct catheter flow. The omentum can occlude both the distal catheter and side holes completely obstructing dialysate flow. Attempts to free the catheter by saline flushes, thrombolytics, and stiff wire manipulations are largely unsuccessful. Oftentimes surgical intervention with omentopexy or omentectomy is required. Initial catheter placement with omentopexy can prevent this complication.

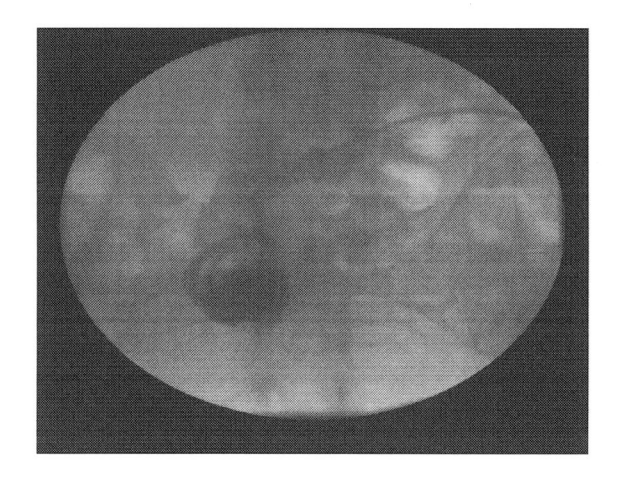

Catheter injection with iodinated contrast material showing omental encasement of the distal coiled catheter- "omental wrap"

To diagnose an omental encasement, often termed "omental wrap", non-ionic contrast material can be sterilely injected into the catheter under fluoroscopy. If the contrast material does not freely disperse within the peritoneal cavity and is noted to be contained within a loculated compartment an omental wrap can be suspected.

Superficial Cuff Erosion

The subcutaneous cuff can erode through the skin and create a chronically irritated exit site that is painful, has drainage, and is prone to exit site infection. A partially extruding cuff is a constant source of irritation of the exit site and only when the cuff is fully extruded does the exit site have the ability to heal properly. Once extruded, some clinicians have advocated removing the cuff carefully with scissors or sand paper obtained at the local hardware store. The cuff that has extruded is no longer sterile so using non-sterile sand paper to carefully scrape off the Dacron cuff has been successful. The subcutaneous cuff erodes through the skin due to significant weight loss or improper initial cuff placement.

Infusion pain

Rarely, patients can complain of a painful sensation during infusion of dialysate. This discomfort has been attributed to a variety of potential causes including a forceful stream of dialysate creating a painful "jetty" against peritoneal structures or the acidic pH of standard solutions. Slowing the infusion rate can oftentimes reduce discomfort. Infusion pain may also result from constipation and may be reduced by laxative treatments. Bicarbonate addition to the dialysate, just prior to infusion, can treat infusion pain due to the acidic pH but risks contamination of the dialysate and subsequent peritonitis. Use of tidal PD regimens can oftentimes eliminate infusion pain.

Drain Pain

Patients on PD occasionally experience abdominal pain during the phase of the dialysis exchange when fluid is draining from the peritoneal cavity. Commonly referred to as "drain pain", this discomfort is attributed to contact between the lining of the peritoneal membrane or intestines and the siliconized rubber dialysis catheter. Drainage of the peritoneal fluid can contract the peritoneal membrane and allow contact with the catheter, stimulating peritoneal nerves resulting in abdominal discomfort.

A variety of recommendations have been made to reduce or eliminate drain pain. These include positional changes during the drain phase of the exchange, changing the drain logic of the cycler machine so that the machine does not excessively "search" for fluid to drain, changing the drain pressure created by the cycler by raising the cycler relative to the patient up to 12 inches (but not more), decompression of the colon with laxatives, dietary changes to prevent constipation, and therapy prescription changes that allow some of the fluid to remain in the abdomen to act as a "cushion" and prevent complete drainage of the abdomen. These prescription changes often use a Tidal regimen in patients on APD and can be achieved in the CAPD patient by manual cessation of the drain at the point of abdominal discomfort. Success reducing drain pain has been described with these maneuvers.

Summary Recommendations for Catheter Flow Dysfunction

A series of recommendations can be made to address the catheter that is demonstrating inflow or outflow obstruction, often associated with migration.

Approach to Catheter Dysfunction

1. Aggressive laxative administration to treat constipation that may be contributing to catheter dysfunction

2. If no improvement, a trial of tissue plasminogen activator (TPA) to attempt to lyse obstructing biofilm or fibrin

3. Obtain a flat plate abdomen x-ray to identify the intra-abdominal catheter segment, document any possible catheter migration, examine for any obvious catheter kink, and better view for residual stool impaction

4. If persistent dysfunction and catheter noted to be migrated, consider catheter manipulation with Fogarty catheter or stiff wire by interventional nephrology or radiology

5. If persistent dysfunction, consider surgical repositioning. Laparoscopic repositioning with possible omentopexy and adhesiolysis would be ideal with care given to leaving both catheter cuffs intact so that low volume PD could be resumed in 48 hours to 72 hours

References:

Bunchman TE, Ballal SH. Treatment of inflow pain by pH adjustment of dialysate in peritoneal dialysis. Perit Dial Int 1991;11:179-180.

Crabtree JH, Burchette RJ. Effect of prior abdominal surgery, peritonitis, and adhesions on catheter function and long-term outcome on peritoneal dialysis. Am Surg 2009;75:140-147.

Diaz-Buxo JA. Management of peritoneal catheter malfunction. Perit Dial Int 1998;18:256-259.

Gadallah MF, Arora N, Arumugam R, Moles K. Role of Fogarty catheter manipulation in management of migrated, nonfunctional peritoneal dialysis catheters. Am J Kidney Dis 2000;35:301-305.

Goedde M, Sitter T, Schiffl H, et al. Coagulation- and fibrinolysis-related antigens in plasma and dialysate of CAPD patients. Perit Dial Int 1997;17:162-166.

Juergensen PH, Lola Murphy A, Pherson KA, et al. Tidal peritoneal dialysis to achieve comfort in chronic peritoneal dialysis patients. Adv Perit Dial 1999;15:125-126.

Jwo SC, Chen KS, Lee CM, Huang CY. Correction of migrated peritoneal dialysis catheters using Lunderquist guidewire: a preliminary report. Perit Dial Int 2001;21:619-621.

Kappel JE, Ferguson GM, Kudel RM, et al. Stiff wire manipulation of peritoneal dialysis catheters. Adv Perit Dial 1995;11:202-207.

Keshvari A, Fazeli MS, Meysamie A, et al. The effects of previous abdominal operations and intraperitoneal adhesions on the outcome of peritoneal dialysis catheters. Perit Dial Int 2010;30:41-45.

Kim HJ, Lee TW, Ihm CG, Kim MJ. Use of fluoroscopy-guided wire manipulation and/or laparoscopic surgery in the repair of malfunctioning peritoneal dialysis catheters. Am J Nephrol 2002;22:532-538.

Kim SH, Lee DH, Choi HJ, et al. Minilaparotomy with manual correction for malfunctioning peritoneal dialysis catheters. Perit Dial Int 2008;28:550-554.

McLaughlin K, Jardine AG. Closed stiff-wire manipulation of malpositioned Tenckhoff catheters offers a safe and effective way of prolonging peritoneal dialysis. Int J Artif Organs 2000;23:219-220.

Miller M, McCormick B, Lavoie S, et al. Fluoroscopic manipulation of peritoneal dialysis catheters: outcomes and factors associated with successful manipulation. Clin J Am Soc Nephrol 2012;7:795-800.

Moreiras-Plaza M, Caceres-Alvarado N. Peritoneal dialysis catheter obstruction caused by Fallopian tube wrapping. Am J Kidney Dis 2004;44:e28-E30.

Ogunc G. Malfunctioning peritoneal dialysis catheter and accompanying surgical pathology repaired by laparoscopic surgery. Perit Dial Int 2002;22:454-462.

Ozyer U, Harman A, Aytekin C, et al. Correction of displaced peritoneal dialysis catheters with an angular stiff rod. Acta Radiologica 2009;50:139-143.

Santarelli S, Zeiler M, Marinelli R, et al. Videolaparoscopy as rescue therapy and placement of peritoneal dialysis catheters: a thirty-two case single centre experience. Nephrol Dial Transplant 2006;21:1348-1354.

Santos CR, Branco PQ, Martinho A, et al. Salvage of malpositioned and malfunctioning peritoneal dialysis catheters by manipulation with a modified Malecot introducer. Semin Dial 2010;23:95-99.

Savader SJ, Lund G, Scheel PJ, et al. Guide wire directed manipulation of malfunctioning peritoneal dialysis catheters: a critical analysis. JVIR 1997;8:957-963.

Savader SJ. Radiologic manipulation of failed peritoneal dialysis catheters. Semin Dial 1998;11:382-386.

Stegmayr BG, Hedberg B, Norrgard O. Stylet with a curved tip to facilitate introduction of new Tenckhoff catheters and reposition of displaced ones. Surgical technique. Eur J Surg 1993;159:495-497.

Stegmayr BG, Wikdahl AM, Bergstrom M, et al. A randomized clinical trial comparing the function of straight and coiled Tenckhoff catheters for peritoneal dialysis. Perit Dial Int 2005;25:85-88.

Tu W, Su Z, Shan Y. An original non-traumatic maneuver for repositioning migrated peritoneal dialysis catheters. Perit Dial Int 2009;29:325-329.

Vanderperren B, Hammer F, Malaise J, et al. Poor ultrafiltration shortly after peritoneal dialysis initiation. Nephrol Dial Transplant 2002;17:2265-2267.

Yilmazlar T, Kirdak T, Bilgin S, et al. Laparoscopic findings of peritoneal dialysis catheter malfunction and management outcomes. Perit Dial Int 2006;26:374-379.

Zorzanello MM, Fleming WJ, Prowant BF. Use of tissue plasminogen activator in peritoneal dialysis catheters: a literature review and one center's experience. Nephrol Nurs J 2004;31:534-537.

Chapter 9:
PD in Acute Kidney Injury or the Late-Referred ESRD Patient

PD THERAPY CAN BE initiated acutely for the patient with acute kidney injury (AKI) or for the late-referred CKD patient requiring an urgent start to dialysis. PD can be initiated rapidly due to bedside or interventional suite catheter insertion followed by low volume, recumbent exchanges. Recent publications have demonstrated the adequate clearances that can be achieved by various acute PD regimens.

Acute PD was more commonly employed in the USA in the 1990's, but has declined in parallel to the overall decline in PD utilization for ESRD. Many other countries rely solely on acute PD as the treatment for AKI. Acute PD offers many potential benefits in acute renal failure such as avoidance of temporary vascular access and systemic heparinization, greater hemodynamic stability, can be performed despite relative hypotension, and is cost-effective. In the ESRD patient requiring urgent start dialysis, placement of a dual cuff PD catheter creates the acute dialysis access that becomes the chronic access - all in a single procedure. This would be an alternative to the patient urgently initiating HD and requiring placement of a temporary vascular access followed by additional surgeries for creation of longer term access.

Contraindications for acute PD include ileus or other intra-abdominal conditions such as appendicitis, ischemic bowel, intestinal obstruction or perforation. Patients with relative contraindications to acute PD include those with known bacterial or fungal peritonitis, new aortic grafts, known abdominal or diaphragmatic fistulae, or abdominal burns or cellulitis. Marked hypercatabolic states, profound metabolic acidosis, and most drug intoxications are better suited for acute hemodialysis sessions.

Catheter Placement in Acute PD

Various acute PD catheter placement techniques have been described. A stiff acute catheter placed over a rigid rod has been used in some centers (Trocath catheters). The catheter is placed blindly in the infra-umbilical midline linea alba to avoid vascular structures. It seems reasonable to have a bladder catheter placed to reduce the chance of a distended bladder compromising dialysate flows or risking bladder entry. After sterile preparation and local anesthesia, a small incision of less than 2 cm is made in the planned entry site, followed by blunt dissection to identify the underlying muscle fascia. While asking the patient to tense the abdominal muscles, the rigid catheter is used to puncture into the peritoneal cavity. During the puncture procedure, the trochar can be held at the distal end by one hand and several centimeters from the expected peritoneal cavity entrance by the other hand to avoid deeper puncture of the abdomen. Some practitioners use a modification of this puncture technique by puncturing into the peritoneum first with a 14 to 16 g angiocath, then removing the needle and infusing 2 liters of dialysate into the abdomen prior to placement of the larger rigid acute catheter. The rigid catheter is then attached to a transfer set to allow exchanges to occur. The straight midline catheter may develop dialysate leaks during use so bulky compression bandages are placed around the entry site and then taped securely in place.

An alternative to the rigid temporary acute catheter is the paramedian placement of a double cuff Tenckhoff catheter that can be used for both acute and chronic PD. These catheters are placed by blind surgical laparotomy, laparoscopy, or by various percutaneous techniques. As AKI patients are typically not stable for operative procedures, a percutaneous placement, either at the bedside or in an interventional suite, is preferable. In this technique, after sterile preparation and local anesthesia, a small incision is made to allow blunt dissection to the fascia, a 16 gauge needle is inserted into the peritoneum, oriented toward the coccyx, followed by a flexible wire advanced into the pelvis. The needle is then removed over the wire and a dilator is passed to widen the entry tract. The dilator is removed over the wire and a peel-away sheath is passed. The wire is then removed leaving the peel-away sheath oriented into the deeper pelvis. The double cuff catheter is submerged into a bowl of saline to extrude air bubbles from the Dacron cuffs, then lubricated on the outside, then passed within the peel-away sheath. During insertion, care must be taken to align the radiopaque stripe as a positioning guide to avoid kinking or twisting of the catheter internally or along the subcutaneous tunnel. Once the catheter has been advanced to allow the deep cuff to rest at the rectus sheath, the peel away sheath is removed, and hemostat forceps or other device is used to push the deep cuff into the rectus sheath. Once the deep cuff has entered the rectus sheath some practitioners describe use of a purse-string suture at the fascia entry point. With this modification, pericatheter leaks occurred in only 1.9% of catheters placed percutaneously. The tunnel and proper exit site is then created followed by

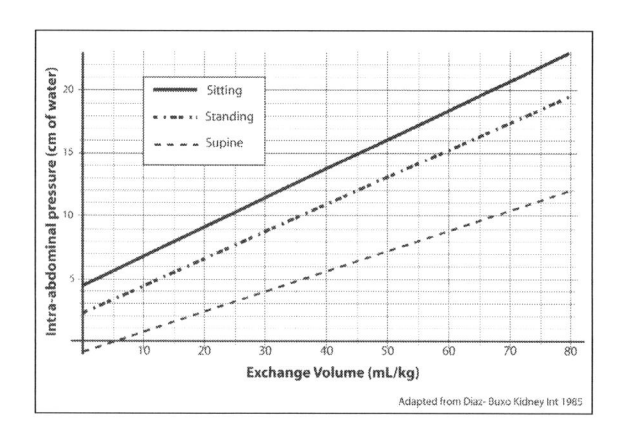

Intra-abdominal pressure is lowest in the supine position which lessens chance of dialysate leak after acute catheter placement

suture closing of the initial abdominal incision.

Leaks are minimized by smaller initial dialysate volumes of 500 mL to 1 liter, with exchanges being done only in the supine position. Should the patient need to sit up or stand the dialysate is drained, to minimize the risk of subcutaneous leak. Intra-abdominal pressure is the lowest in the supine position and acute PD with a new catheter will have less chance of leaking if the patient is maintained in this recumbent position.

PD Prescription in Acute Kidney Injury

Solute clearances in PD are determined by the dwell volume, peritoneal membrane permeability and the peritoneal surface area. Urea, being a small molecule, is more rapidly cleared into the dialysate.

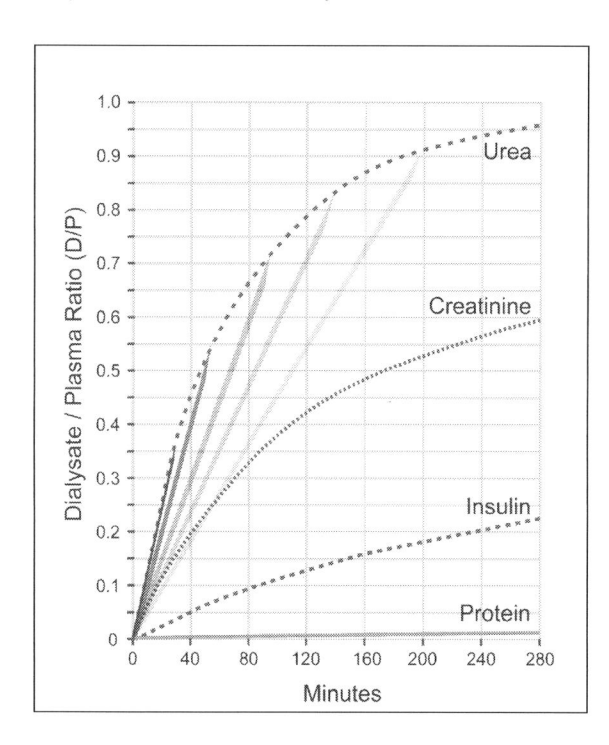

The acute PD prescription should be based on this rapid urea clearance. Dialysate should be infused to allow for the rapid initial diffusion, then drained to allow for new dialysate to be re-infused to again allow for rapid urea diffusion. These short, repeated cycles can maximize clearance of smaller molecules and allow for the most efficient treatment of uremic symptoms.

In most patients, a dwell can reach 50% urea saturation in 30

Urea, being a smaller molecule, more rapidly diffuses into the dialysate

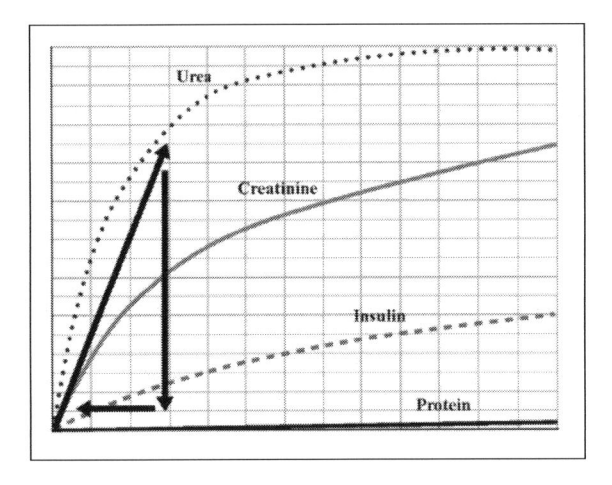

To achieve the greatest clearances in AKI, cycles should be shortened to maximize urea clearances, typically 30 to 50 minute dwell times

minutes. Dwell times ranging from 30 to 50 minutes have been suggested as ideal for the AKI patient requiring higher clearance targets. Estimated urea clearances can be calculated from this estimated D/P urea of 0.5 per 2L infused if the dwell time is between 30 to 50 minutes. For example, if eighteen exchanges of 2L were performed daily, the approximate urea clearance would be 18 L and would represent a weekly Kt/V of at least 2.1 in a 60 kg patient. The exchanges typically require a 10 minute infusion time and 20 minute drain time.

Ultrafiltration requirements are individualized using the available dialysate osmolalities of 1.5%, 2.5%, and 4.25% dextrose. If hypertonic solutions are required, careful monitoring of the blood glucose is advised, as many patients may not give a history of glucose intolerance. If rapid fluid removal is required, several 4.25% exchanges can be given with minimal dwell times of 10 to 15 minutes, as peak ultrafiltration occurs in the initial 15 to 30 minutes of an exchange. The solutions should be warmed as with the chronic PD population. The addition of potassium to the dialysate is individualized as is the calcium concentration.

Careful monitoring of acute dialysis is required. Pre-printed order templates and the use of a standardized flow sheet can assist in the documentation of initial prescription orders, actual dwell times, dialysate concentrations, net ultrafiltration, and medications administered.

Patient Name: _____   Date: _____

Medical Record Number: _____

Lab Values: Potassium _____   BUN: _____

Prescription: <u>1 liter dwells, 1.5% dextrose, dwell time 50 minutes, total volume 12 L/d</u>

Exchange Number	% Dextrose	Infusion Start Time	Infused Volume	Drained Volume	Net UF	Cumulative UF
1	1.5	8 A.M.	1 L	1.2 L	200 ml	200 ml
2	1.5	9:20 A.M.	1 L	0.9	-100 ml	100 ml
3	1.5	10:40 A.M.	1 L	1.3	300 ml	400 ml
4	1.5	12:00 P.M.	1 L	1.2	200 ml	600 ml

If acceptable volume and metabolic parameters have been reached with the shorter dwell times, the prescription can be altered to a longer dwell time of 3 to 4 hours. Patients should be monitored daily for signs and symptoms of peritonitis.

Clinical Experiences in AKI

Gabriel and colleagues recently published 2 descriptions of continuous PD therapy for the treatment of AKI. In a prospective randomized trial, 120 patients were treated with either PD or daily HD for acute tubular necrosis. The primary end point was hospital survival and kidney function recovery and secondary end points were metabolic control. The group also determined the delivered clearances of both modalities. PD catheters were placed by blind placement of a flexible Tenckhoff catheter using a rigid trochar, inserted in the infra-umbilical, midline location. PD was delivered continuously for 24 hours, seven days a week. Two liter exchanges were performed using a cycler, with 35 to 50 minute dwell times. A total of 36 to 44 liters were administered in 18 to 22 exchanges. This was considered high volume acute PD and the delivered weekly Kt/V was 3.6, with similar clearance and ultrafiltration volumes per session compared to the HD cohort. Metabolic control was similar in the two treatment groups. Infectious complications were not significantly different, with peritonitis occurring in 18% of the patients compared to similar rates of temporary vascular access infections. If dialysis leaks were encountered the dwell volume was reduced to 1500 mL. Mortality and recovery of kidney function was similar in both groups, duration of treatment was shorter in the PD group as recovery of renal function occurred at 7 versus 10 days. This larger description of acute PD therapy for AKI documents the adequate clearances and outcomes that can be achieved in higher dose acute PD therapy. Gabriel and colleagues have now published multiple descriptions of use of acute PD for the treatment of AKI.

Phu and collegues had less success with acute PD in the treatment of AKI associated with severe falciparum malaria or sepsis. The authors used 30 minute dwell times possibly compromising the achievable clearances. This emphasizes the need to allow for dwell volumes and exchange intervals that allow for reasonable solute saturation of the dialysate.

Chitalia et al. evaluated 2 methods of PD for the treatment of AKI in 87 patients with mild to moderate catabolism. Manual exchanges with 2 L and 3.5 hour dwell times were compared to APD with a tidal regimen of 2 L initial fill followed by 750 mL infusion/drains after 10 minute dwells. Both groups received 12.5 L per day. The tidal regimen was shown to enhance solute clearance to a greater extent and the authors recommended APD for the treatment of AKI.

These studies, and others, support the conclusion that acute PD is an acceptable treatment modality for AKI.

Urgent-Start PD for the Late-Referred ESRD patient

Patients reaching ESRD without prior dialysis access are often given temporary vascular access and initiated on HD. The benefits of PD, however, such as better preservation of residual kidney function, quality of life, early survival advantage in many patient groups, lower risk of sepsis and Hepatitis B and C transmission, and preservation of vascular access for future options, all suggest that initiation of dialysis with PD should be considered. In the late-referred ESRD patient, PD can be initiated urgently and temporary HD access can be avoided. With dual cuff catheter placement, the PD access can be used for both the acute/urgent start to PD and then matured to become the chronic access - avoiding the multiple procedures involved with converting temporary HD access to permanent access.

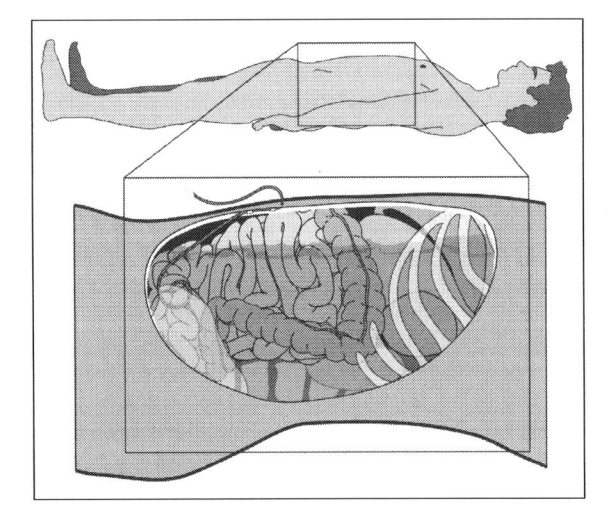

The patient requiring an urgent start to PD, soon after catheter placement, can be initiated on PD using the recumbent position and lower dwell volumes. This reduces the risk of early leak and allows for the initiation of PD without the usual break-in

Initiating PD in the recumbent position with lower dwell volumes reduces the risk of leak in patients with newly placed catheters

period to allow for tissue in-growth into the catheter's Dacron cuffs. To reduce the likelihood of early leak further the surgeon or interventionalist can place a purse string suture around the rectus entry site of the deep cuff.

Ghaffari described an urgent-start PD program and reported on 18 patients who presented at ESRD without prior renal care. Typically these patients were treated with temporary vascular access followed by urgent HD. An alternative urgent-start PD algorithm was developed requiring initial evaluation of the patient's social support and home setting, followed by modality education. In patients deemed suitable candidates for home therapy, the recommendation was made to initiate dialysis with PD. If this recommendation was accepted by the patient a PD catheter was placed in the interventional radiology suite followed by the initiation of recumbent, low volume, staff-assisted PD, performed on an intermittent schedule. This intermittent PD (IPD) was initiated in the hospital or outpatient setting depending on clinical judgment. Once control of the uremia had been addressed by IPD the patients were trained to perform self-care. The urgent-start PD group was compared to a cohort of PD patients started electively. The urgent-start patients experienced higher rates of leak, but most were minor and resolved with temporary interruption of PD. Outcomes at 90 days were felt to be comparable to patients initiating PD electively.

A subsequent publication in the USA by Casaretto and colleagues described the urgent initiation of PD, within hours or days after laparoscopic catheter placement. No patients experienced subcutaneous leaks. The PD prescriptions, similar to that described above, were based on lower volume, recumbent dialysis sessions on an alternate day (IPD) schedule. Urea-kinetic modeling of IPD sessions has demonstrated that adequacy targets of Kt/V of 1.7 are achievable in patients with residual kidney function of 6.0 to 7.6 mL/min.

Outside of the USA, several earlier publications on urgent-start PD are notable. Povlsen and Ivarsen described their experience with offering PD to patients referred late to a nephrologist or were known CKD patients who experienced an unexpected loss of kidney function. Patients and their relatives were given detailed explanations of dialysis modalities and required access procedures. Acceptable patients, agreeable to start PD, were initiated on urgent start PD. Coiled double cuff catheters were placed by open laparotomy and within 24 hours of catheter placement APD was initiated with a standard prescription of 12 hour, overnight APD in the recumbent position. Patients remained in bed during the treatments but then were able to ambulate with dry abdomens during the day. The maximum dwell volume was 1.2 to 1.5 liters, depending on body weight, and a total volume of 10 liters a night was administered. A tidal regimen was used with 50 to 75% of the initial infused volume drained and infused on subsequent exchanges. At 10 to 14 days the patients converted to traditional 8 hr APD regimens. In 52 urgent starts, PD technique success was over 85%.

In a similar publication, Lobbedez and colleagues described urgent start PD in 34 of 60 late-referred dialysis patients. PD was initiated a median of 4 days after catheter insertion with APD regimens as described above. Only two patients had dialysate leaks and the physicians elected to hold PD for a week. All 34 patients were discharged and maintained on stable, chronic APD therapy. Lastly, Koch and colleagues recently described 66 incident unplanned dialysis patients who initiated PD urgently. These patients were either late-referrals to a nephrologist or experienced unexpected deterioration in renal function with uremia or volume concerns. Catheters were placed surgically and were used within 12 hours of surgery. PD was delivered in an in-center nocturnal unit on an intermittent basis, using a cycler device for 12-hour treatments with lower volumes. Outcomes of these 66 urgent PD patients were compared to 57 urgent HD patients treated with the tradition temporary vascular catheter and in-center HD. There was no significant difference in 6-month mortality between groups, the PD patients had less bacteremia episodes, and peritonitis episodes did not differ between the groups.

Patients with advanced CKD presenting emergently were offered PD by Ilabaca-Avendano and colleagues. They reported 4 patients with undiagnosed ESRD who presented to the emergency room in critical condition with uremia and varying degrees of hyperkalemia and metabolic acidosis. If required, emergent treatment of hyperkalemia was initiated with insulin, glucose, calcium gluconate and diuretics. Bedside Tenckhoff catheter placement was then performed followed immediately by automated PD therapy. The patients recovered and were discharge home on APD. The authors concluded that APD therapy could be a frontline treatment option even for the emergency room presentation of critical, advanced uremia. They emphasized the importance of a coordinated approach between emergency room and nephrology staff to expedite the delivery of care. An alternate approach in these emergent cases, has been a very short exposure to a temporary vascular catheter followed by several HD sessions, to gain control of metabolic and volume parameters. The catheter is then discontinued (reducing infectious risk) and the patient receives a permanent PD catheter then enters an urgent-start clinical pathway. This latter approach, in the emergent case, has been termed a "bimodal" pathway.

Conclusions

PD can be initiated acutely for the treatment of AKI or the late-presenting patient with advanced CKD. Initiating PD within hours to days after catheter insertion is possible by employing supine, lower dwell volume exchanges. Percutaneous PD catheter placement can oftentimes be expeditious and avoid delays in catheter placement often associated with surgical referrals and operating room scheduling. Urgent catheters have been placed by nephrologists or interventionalists and can facilitate the urgent initiation of PD. However, even surgically placed catheters have been used soon after surgery to initiate PD.

With an urgent catheter placement capability, many late-referred patients with advanced CKD may avoid temporary vascular access catheters and be offered PD therapy more urgently. Initiating PD in the late-referred patient may allow these patients to benefit from the lifestyle implications of PD, preserve residual kidney function, and spare their arms for future vascular access options.

References:

PD in Acute Kidney Injury

Ash SR. Peritoneal dialysis in acute renal failure of adults: the under-utilized modality. Contrib Nephrol 2004;144:239-254.

Burdmann EA, Chakravarthi R. Peritoneal dialysis in acute kidney injury: lessons learned and applied. Semin Dial 2011;24:149-156.

Chitalia VC, Almeida AF, Rai H, et al. Is peritoneal dialysis adequate for hypercatabolic acute renal failure in developing countries? Kidney Int 2002;61:747-757.

Gabriel DP, Nascimento GV, Caramori JT, et al. High volume peritoneal dialysis for acute renal failure. Perit Dial Int 2007;27:277-282.

Gabriel DP, Caramori JT, Martim LC, et al. High volume peritoneal dialysis vs daily hemodialysis: a randomized, controlled trial in patients with acute kidney injury. Kidney Int 2008;73[Suppl 108]:S87-S93.

Gabriel DP, Caramori JT, Martin LC, et al. Continuous peritoneal dialysis compared with daily hemodialysis in patients with acute kidney injury. Perit Dial Int 2009;29[Suppl 2]:S62-S71.

Himmelfarb J, Evanson J, Hakim RM, eta l. Urea volume of distribution exceeds total body water in patients with acute renal failure. Kidney Int 2002;61:317-323.

Passadakis PS, Oreopoulos DG. Peritoneal dialysis in patients with acute renal failure. Adv Perit Dial 2007;23:7-16.

Ponce D, Berbel MN, De Goes R, et al. High-volume peritoneal dialysis in acute kidney injury: indications and limitations. Clin J Am Soc Nephrol 2012;7:887-894.

Phu NH, Hien TT, Mai NT, et al. Hemofiltration and peritoneal dialysis in infection-associated acute renal failure in Vietnam. N Engl J Med 2002;347:895-902.

Sharma AP, Mandhani A, Daniel SP, Filler G. Shorter break-in period is a viable option with tighter PD catheter securing during the insertion. Nephrology 2008;13:672-676.

Stegmayr BG. Three purse-string sutures allow immediate start of peritoneal dialysis with a low incidence of leakage. Semin Dial 2003;16:346-348.

Steiner RW. Continuous equilibration peritoneal dialysis in acute renal failure. Perit Dial Int 1989;9:5-7.

Urgent-Start PD for ESRD

Ilabaca-Avendano MB, Yarza-Solorzano G, Rodriguez-Valenzuela J, et al. Automated peritoneal dialysis as a lifesaving therapy in an emergency room: report of four cases. Kidney Int 2008;73[Suppl 108]:S173-S176.

Banli O, Altun H, Oztemel A. Early start of CAPD with the Seldinger technique. Perit Dial Int 2005;25:556-559.

Casaretto A, Rosario R, Kotzker WR, et al. Urgent-start peritoneal dialysis: report from a U.S. private nephrology practice. Adv Perit Dial 2012;28:102-105.

Ghaffari A. Urgent-start peritoneal dialysis: a quality improvement report. Am J Kidney Dis 2012;59:400-408.

Guest S, Akonur A, Ghaffari A, et al. Intermittent peritoneal dialysis: urea kinetic modeling and implications of residual kidney function. Perit Dial Int 2012;32:142-148.

Jo YI, Shin SK, Lee JH, et al. Immediate initiation of CAPD following percutaneous catheter placement without break-in procedure. Perit Dial Int 2007;27:179-183.

Koch M, Kohnle M, Trapp R, et al. Comparable outcome of acute unplanned peritoneal dialysis and haemodialysis. Nephrol Dial Transplant 2012;27:375-380.

Lobbedez T, Lecouf A, Ficheux M, et al. Is rapid initiation of peritoneal dialysis feasible in unplanned dialysis patients? A single-center experience. Nephrol Dial Transplant 2008;23:3290-3294.

Povlsen JV, Ivarsen P. How to start the late referred ESRD patient urgently on chronic APD. Nephrol Dial Transplant 2006;21[Suppl 2]:ii56-ii59.

Chapter 10:
Prescribing Chronic PD Therapy

THE PRESCRIPTION FOR A chronic PD regimen is part science, part art. The science of the prescription is in the understanding of the patient's membrane transport status, daily required small solute removal, and residual kidney function (RKF). The art of a PD prescription is in designing a regimen that is sensitive to and compliments the patient's lifestyle, sleep patterns, work, travel, and family obligations.

Modality Selection

The first step in designing the PD prescription is determining the therapy modality - manual continuous ambulatory peritoneal dialysis (CAPD) or automated peritoneal dialysis using a cycler machine (APD). Outcomes studies show no difference in survival between CAPD and APD modalities. Patients may have a preference for one modality over the other and should be fully presented with their options. Some may prefer the simplicity of gravity driven, manual exchanges of CAPD. Some patients may prefer the liberation of their daytime hours by using an automated cycler device to perform dialysis exchanges during sleep. It is preferable to allow the patient to "own" this decision, as a means of patient empowerment.

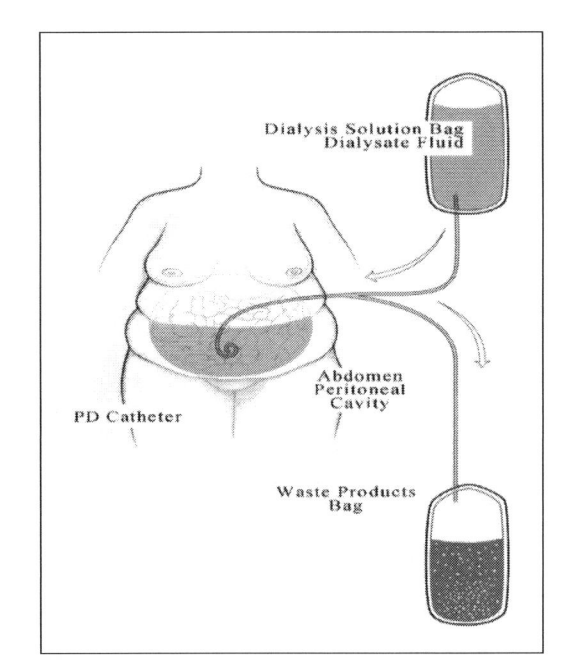

Fill

Manual, gravity driven CAPD

Dwell

Drain

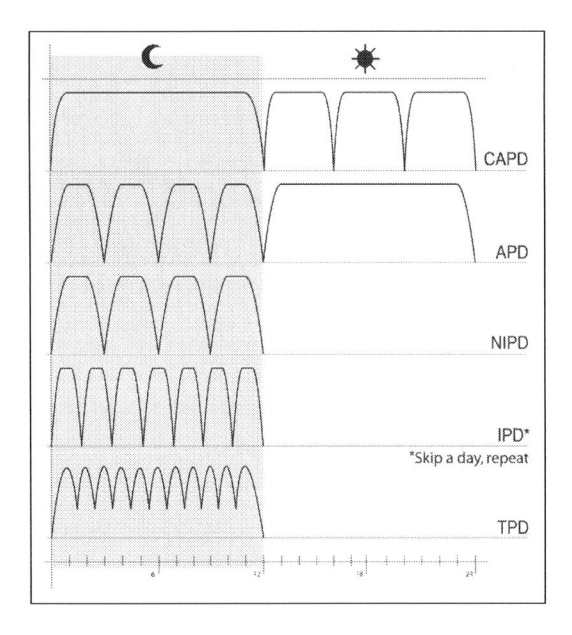

Different modality options for manual or automated PD

The various treatment options in PD therapy are illustrated here. As mentioned, they vary from manual exchanges to a variety of automated options including cycler therapy at night followed by either a wet (APD) or dry day (nightly intermittent PD- NIPD). Additional regimens include PD performed on an intermittent schedule (IPD) or regimens in which the full drain phase is interrupted by a re-infusion (Tidal PD, TPD).

Initial Empiric Prescription

After the modality has been selected, the initial chronic PD prescription is largely empiric, as the practitioner does not have the benefit of a PET to characterize membrane transport and may not have recent quantification of residual kidney function. Most patients initiating chronic PD have significant RKF and the contribution of this RKF to total small solute clearance is substantial - often representing more weekly clearance than the peritoneal component. This allows for more leeway in the initial prescription as a wide range of empiric prescriptions have been found to meet clearance targets. The empiric PD prescription should aim to prescribe sufficient total small solute clearance to meet recommended targets (presently set at a total Kt/V of 1.7 by K/DOQI in the USA).

Reasonable empiric prescriptions are:

CAPD- 8 liters per day as 4 exchanges of 2 liters

APD- 10 liters per day as 4 exchanges per night with 2 liter fill volumes and a 2 liter day exchange.

Patients with significant RKF may be able to use less volume or exchanges and those patients who have reached anuria can be increased to greater volumes. The ultrafiltration requirements determine which dextrose concentrations are used for the exchanges. To avoid unnecessary dextrose exposure, attempts should be made to reach ultrafiltration targets with solutions of lowest osmolality. The time on the cycler is typically dictated by how long a patient sleeps, with attempts made to match cycler time to the patient's typical bedtime schedule.

This empiric prescription should be adequate and continued for the first month of therapy. During the first month, preferably toward the end of the month (to allow for peritoneal accommodation/adjustment to the dialysate) a formal clearance determination should be made. The details of this collection were reviewed in Chapter 4. This Kt/V determination will indicate whether changes are needed to the empiric prescription.

Tailoring the Empiric Prescription

Between weeks 4 to 8 a formal PET should be determined. This PET allows for classification of peritoneal membrane function into one of 4 transport types. The details of the PET collection were reviewed in Chapter 3. The 4-hour dialysate-to-plasma creatinine ratio (D/P Cr) will allow for categorization of transport status as high, high-average, low-average, low.

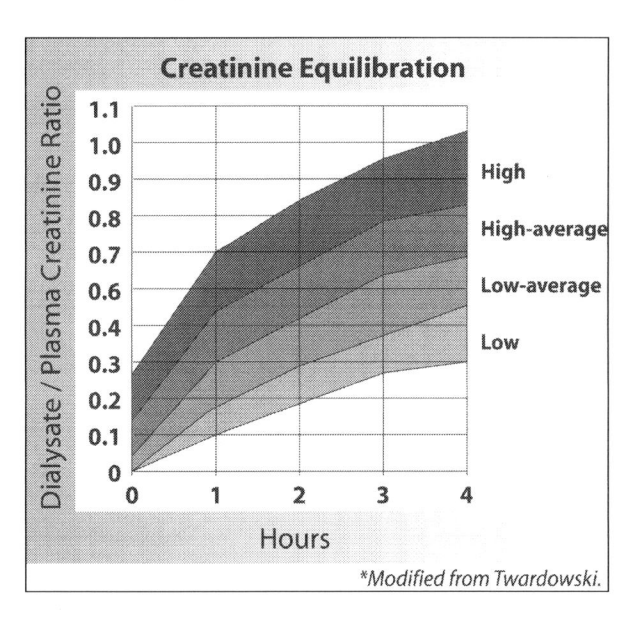

Based on this information, the empiric PD prescription can be tailored to the individual patient. It must be emphasized that if the empiric prescription meets clearance targets and has been felt to be otherwise acceptable there is no need to change the prescription solely based on the PET. Changing a patient's prescription too frequently risks making the therapy appear onerous and risks burn out.

The information derived from the PET is most useful in addressing *inadequate* clearance or ultrafiltration concerns – but, as mentioned, does not dictate that changes should be made to a prescription that has otherwise been deemed acceptable. If changes are made, patients with high transport status may benefit from shorter dwell times on the cycler and an increase in nightly cycler number to 5 exchanges. Patients on APD that are lower transporters may benefit from slowing the cycler exchanges to prolong the dwell time.

Over time, as RKF declines, it is important to ensure that the PD prescription delivers a full dose of dialysis to meet adequacy targets. CAPD patients should continue up to 4 exchanges a day and APD regimens should have the appropriate number of cycles (based on the membrane transport type) and the daytime should be used for longer dwells. It is the long dwells that allow for the greatest middle molecule clearance and additional sodium removal that may not have occurred during the shorter APD cycles.

To assist in designing the ideal prescription, it is perhaps easiest to employ computer simulation programs available from some dialysis solution providers. These computer simulations model peritoneal clearance and ultrafiltration based on the three pore model of membrane physiology. Inputs required include the patient's total body water estimation (V), D/P Cr, dwell volume and % dextrose concentration. After entering this data, different prescriptions can be tested to determine if they meet required clearance and ultrafiltration targets. These simulations can assist the practitioner in predicting what changes to the prescription would have the desired outcome. The effects of changing cycle number, dwell volume, or dwell time can be simulated with these programs, allowing the clinician to choose the regimen that achieves the desired targets with the least disruption in lifestyle or comfort.

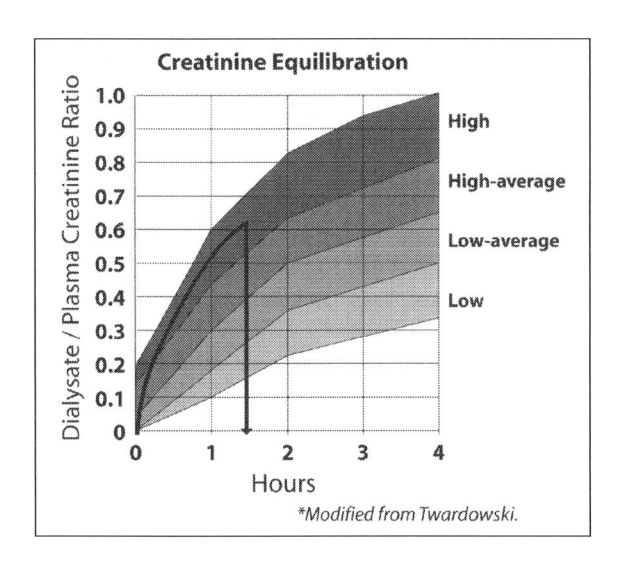

For practitioners who do not have access to simulation software, the PET can be analyzed to determine the ideal dwell time for APD overnight cycles. By analyzing the PET, the practitioner can estimate when "peak efficiency" of diffusion and ultrafiltration has occurred. The ideal dwell time takes advantage of

Higher transporters reach equilibration more rapidly and therefore shorter dwell times maximize peak clearance rates

Creatinine Equilibration

Modified from Twardowski.

the peak removal of toxins and fluid and then drains the fluid before the osmotic gradient begins to dissipate and diffusion slows to approach equilibrium. As can be predicted from the below PET diagrams, the arrow designates the end of the peak in toxin removal and indicates when the cycle could be terminated and drained, to allow for fresh dialysate to be re-infused.

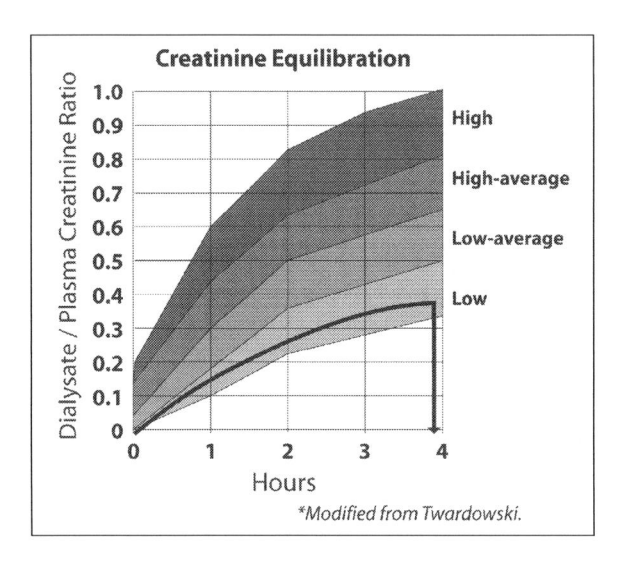

Lower transporters take longer to reach equilibrium therefore longer dwell times are required

Low to low-average transporters would require longer dwell times to reach efficient clearance per dwell time.

Therefore, a basic understanding of the PET helps practitioners tailor the prescription. High and high-average transporters benefit from cycles at night that are more frequent. A lower transporter would benefit from longer dwell times on a cycler or may require CAPD.

Understanding the implications of underlying peritoneal membrane transport properties and designing an appropriate dwell time is a critical step in individualizing the PD prescription. This basic but fundamental step can ensure long-term adequacy clearance targets are met as well as enhance ultrafiltration to maintain fluid balance.

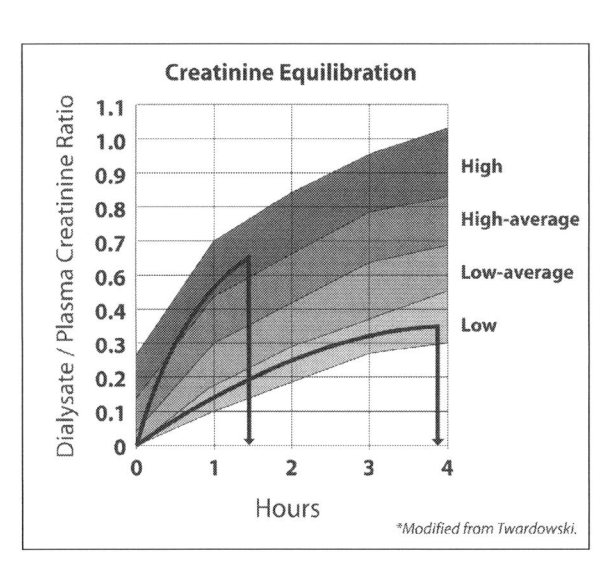

In patients requiring increased dialysis, the most predictable method to increase clearance is to increase the dwell volume. Many practitioners recommend simply

During cycler therapy dwell times should be prescribed to allow for efficient solute clearance per time infused. For high transporters, the first several hours represent peak efficiency, for lower transporters and longer dwell time will be required

increasing the dwell volumes, if possible, before making any other changes to the dialysis time or cycle number. Increasing dwell volume adds more dialysate to contact the peritoneal membrane, the dialyzer, and increases the total surface area of contact between fluid and peritoneum. This increases the effective surface area of the "dialyzer" and results in increased diffusion of solute from plasma to dialysate. Dwell volumes increased to 2.5 liters can be tolerated by most patients and larger patients may accommodate 3 liter exchanges.

Optimization of the Long Dwell

The nighttime exchange in CAPD and the day exchange in APD are referred to as the "long dwells". The long dwell represents the most inefficient exchange in the PD prescription and may adversely affect the desired clearance and ultrafiltration. Dextrose-based dialysate solutions result in early ultrafiltration that peaks and then is gradually reabsorbed over the long exchange.

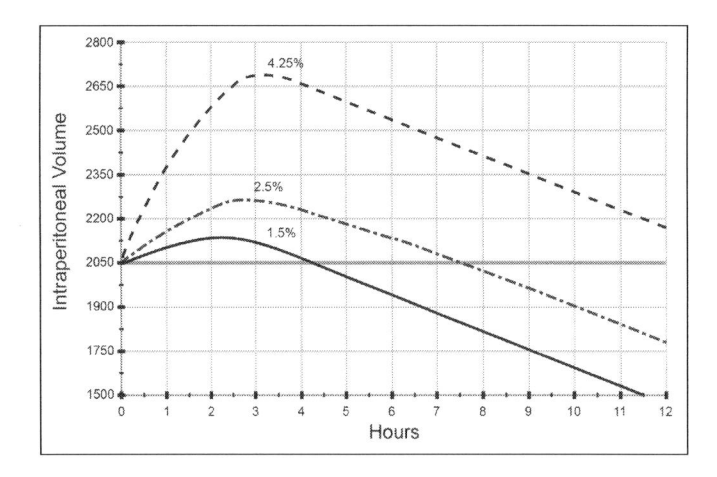

Profiles of dextrose-based solutions show temporal loss of peak ultrafiltration

The long dwell can be optimized by one of three possible prescription alterations. The long dwell tonicity can be increased in an attempt to improve ultrafiltration. For example, a 2.5% dextrose exchange can be substituted for a 4.25% exchange but at the metabolic cost of exposing the peritoneal membrane and patient to the increased glucose load. A second option in APD is termed the "midday exchange". This option results in the long day exchange in APD to be broken into two exchanges. This results in a long exchange being substituted by two exchanges of shorter duration. By reducing the length of the long exchange there may be enhanced total ultrafiltration. The addition of the midday exchange may also increase total daily solute clearance. The midday exchange, therefore, may be indicated in any patient requiring an improved Kt/V or enhanced ultrafiltration.

The midday exchange, however, has significant impact on patient lifestyle and freedom. PD as a modality was often chosen by the patient due to the APD option that allowed for the day time period to be free of dialysis procedures. The midday day exchange

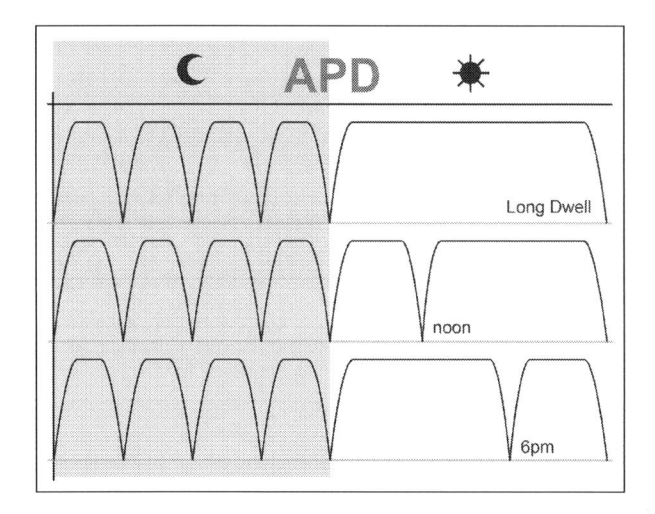

The long dwell in APD can be interrupted with a midday exchange to reduce the dwell length and prevent reabsorption

requires the patient perform an exchange in this day period and negatively impacts quality of life. If a midday exchange is required clinicians should attempt to introduce the midday exchange at the most convenient time in the patients schedule. Some patients may prefer to perform the short day exchange at noon while others may prefer to perform the exchange in the early evening, after returning from a day's activities.

Either option can result in the same desired result- a shortening of the long exchange with the improved clearance and ultrafiltration with the most minimal impact on quality of life.

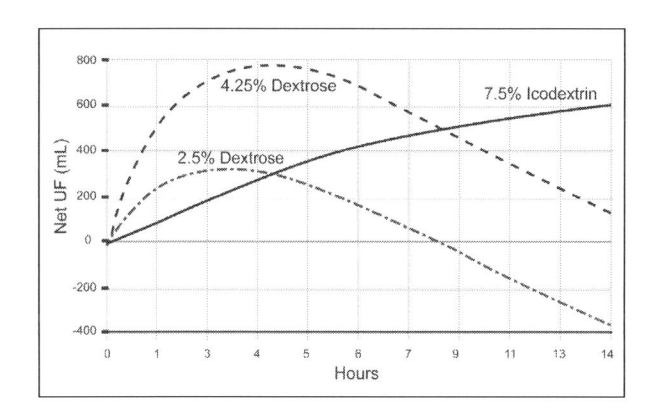

Colloidal ultrafiltration profile of icodextrin versus dextrose-based solutions

A third option is to change the osmotic agent used for the long dwell. As mentioned, glucose-based solutions may not result in the desired ultrafiltration due to absorption over the long dwell. Colloidal-based solutions, icodextrin, have unique ultrafiltration profiles with a more gradual increase in the ultrafiltration volume over time. These solutions are, therefore, less impacted by the longer exchange and are indicated for only the long exchange.

These three options allow the clinician to optimize the long dwell in patients requiring increased clearance or ultrafiltration. The patients most at risk of inadequate dialysis during the long dwell are those with higher membrane transport and more rapid reabsorption of glucose. Patients with high-average or high membrane transport categories on the PET should have careful assessment of the long dwell as a critical component of their longitudinal follow-up.

Tidal Peritoneal Dialysis

Tidal PD (TPD) is a type of APD in which the dwell volume is not completely drained before the next fill cycle is initiated. Typical TPD regimens are programmed to leave 250, 500 or 1000 mL as a "reservoir" and then subsequent infusions/drains occur into the reservoir. TPD can be used in patients with pain at the beginning or end of the infusion or in those who typically drain very slowly and inefficiently at the end of the drain. By not completely draining the abdomen dry, the efficiency of the dialysis can often be improved by re-infusing dialysate at the transition point of slow draining.

In TPD regimens, care must be taken to avoid overfill by programming in the necessary ultrafiltration target for each exchange and ensuring that the reservoir volume plus subsequent fill volumes do not exceed the desired total dwell volume.

Incremental Peritoneal Dialysis

There remains a debate on whether a patient starting PD requires a full dose of PD seven days a week or whether the patient with significant residual kidney function can be started on lower total volumes of PD. This lower volume initiation has been termed "incremental PD" and is used by some centers to allow for a more simplified initiation of dialysis. Depending on degree of RKF, patients can be started on incremental regimens of 1-2 manual exchanges a day, that can be increased to 3 or full dose PD as RKF declines. Incremental PD may be a more acceptable method to initiate dialysis for many patients and can help ease the initial fear that many patients may have about training on a cycler device. Proponents of an incremental start to dialysis believe this approach can improve the acceptance of PD as the initial dialysis modality, offers a better quality of life, lower number of exchanges and therefore lower peritonitis risk and lower initial glucose exposure to the peritoneal membrane.

Foggensteiner and colleagues described initiating PD in 39 patients with a single overnight exchange a day. Clinical and adequacy parameters were followed and the prescription adjusted to maintain a combined renal and peritoneal Kt/V over 2.0. Only after a median of 297 days did the patients require an incremental increase in the PD exchanges. The authors concluded that the timely initiation of PD with a single exchange in patients with significant RKF was well tolerated.

Starting NIPD with a dry day is considered incremental PD as the daytime exchange is initially omitted. The day exchange is started later in the patients course when full-dose PD is required.

Incremental PD would be less indicated in the patient with significant ultrafiltration requirements. In centers practicing an incremental policy, caregivers must insure that the total Kt/V delivered (pKt/V and rKt/V) meets the minimum target total Kt/V of 1.7.

Intermittent Peritoneal Dialysis

Intermittent PD (IPD) is an older regimen in which patients are dialyzed intermittently on a 3 or 4 times a week schedule. In some countries, patients who cannot perform PD themselves are dialyzed in-center with IPD regimens. Patients with new catheters can initiate PD with lower volume, recumbent IPD regimens until the new catheter has fully matured and home training can begin. Many existing PD patients who undergo subsequent hernia repair can use recumbent IPD regimens and continue PD in the post-operative period, thereby avoiding temporary conversion to HD.

Recent interest in the USA in "urgent-start PD" has resulted in an increase in in-center IPD regimens for the late-referred patient whom requires urgent catheter placement followed by early initiation of PD. These urgent-start PD programs can enable patients to avoid temporary vascular catheters and subsequent vascular access surgeries and elect to initiate dialysis with a single PD catheter procedure-the only access procedure that would be required, for both the acute and chronic setting. Until the new catheter has fully matured, the patient receives IPD with lower volumes, in the recumbent position (see below).

Urgent-Start PD Prescription for the Late-Presenting Patient

Many patients present late in the course of their disease or have unexpected deterioration in their CKD and require the urgent initiation of dialysis. In many countries these patients are not felt to be PD candidates due to the lack of a catheter. Instead, the patient is treated with a temporary vascular access and initiated on HD. These temporary catheters increase the risk of bacteremia and sepsis and have been associated with increased mortality.

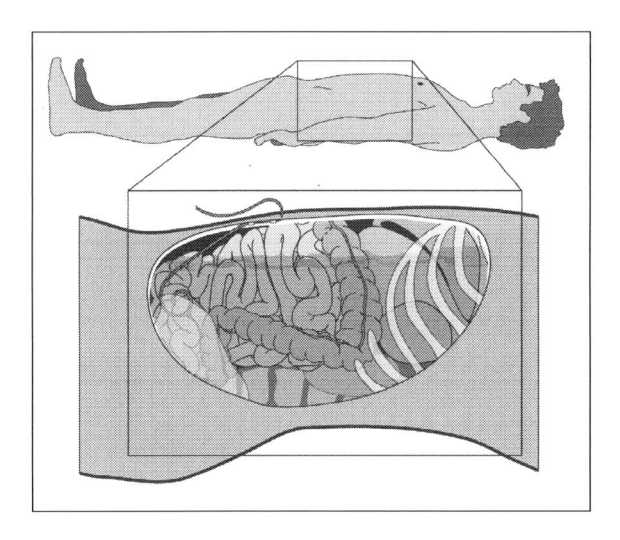

Recent reports in the USA, Asia, and Europe have re-emphasized that PD can be initiated urgently in the late-referred patient. Urgent-start PD programs require certain infrastructure and prescription modifications and have established protocols

Chronic PD can be initiated urgently in the late-presenting patient by using lower volume exchanges in the recumbent position soon after catheter placement

to achieve urgent cuffed PD catheter placement by either a surgeon or interventionalist. Publications by Ghaffari and Casaretto et al. in the USA and Koch, Lobbedez, and Povlsen in Europe have described urgent-start PD experiences and documented successful initiation of urgent PD using lower volume dwells in the recumbent position.

With these publications there has been recent interest in the use of IPD as a bridge therapy for the patient with a newly placed catheter whom needs to initiate PD more urgently. Typically PD is started after catheter maturation to allow for the cuffs and exit-site to have fully healed. Using the catheter early may increase the risk of leak. However, recent reports of IPD treatments using low-volume dwells in the supine position have documented success in initiating urgent or acute PD. These reports by Ghaffari, Casaretto, and others have described IPD programs for the initiation of urgent-start PD.

Urea kinetic modeling of various IPD regimens has recently been described by Guest and colleagues. To meet current clearance goals, IPD regimens themselves are unlikely to provide long-term adequate urea clearance in most patients. Therefore, the contribution of residual kidney function must be considered and, in patients with substantial residual function, IPD regimens may deliver adequate clearance and allow for a bridge therapy until fuller dose PD is initiated.

Conclusions

Due to significant residual kidney function present at the start of PD, in most patients, the initial prescription can be empiric and will allow for achievement of an acceptable total Kt/V. It is reasonable to prescribe 8 liters a day for patients on CAPD and APD patients can employ 10 liters per day. As adequacy targets are usually easily achievable, the initial prescription should be directed toward the osmolality of the solutions required to meet ultrafiltration goals. Once PET information is known, the chronic PD prescription can be individualized and the practitioner can design a tailored prescription that meets adequacy targets and maintains euvolemia. With these steps: (1) prescribing appropriate dwell volumes for the exchanges, (2) establishing a dwell time based on the PET that takes advantage of peak efficiency, and (3) using appropriate number of exchanges and time on the therapy, the appropriate prescription can be achieved and ensure long-term success on PD.

References:

Blake P, Burkart JM, Churchill DN, et al. Recommended clinical practices for maximizing peritoneal dialysis clearances. Perit Dial Int 1996;16:448-456.

Durand PY. APD schedules and clinical results. Contrib Nephrol 2006;150:285-290.

Foggensteiner L, Baylis J, Moss H, Williams P. Timely initiation of dialysis- single-exchange experience in 39 patients starting peritoneal dialysis. Perit Dial Int 2002;22:471-478.

Fourtounas C, Hardalias A, Dousdampanis P, et al. Intermittent peritoneal dialysis (IPD): an old but still effective modality for severely disabled ESRD patients. Nephrol Dial Transplant 2009;24:3215-3218.

Harty J, Boulton H, Venning M, Gokal R. Impact of increasing dialysis volume on adequacy targets: a prospective study. J Am Soc Nephol 1997;8:1304-1310.

Mehrotra R, Chiu YW, Kalantar-Zadeh K, Vonesh E. The outcomes of continuous ambulatory and automated peritoneal dialysis are similar. Kidney Int 2009;76:97-107.

Nakayama M, Nakano H, Nakayama M. Novel therapeutic option for refractory heart failure in elderly patients with chronic kidney disease by incremental peritoneal dialysis. J Cardiology 2010;55:49-54.

NKF-KDOQI Clinical Practice Guidelines for Peritoneal Dialysis Adequacy. Am J Kidney Dis 2006;48[Suppl1]:S91-S158.

Perez RA, Blake PG, McMurray S, et al. What is the optimal frequency of cycling in automated peritoneal dialysis? Perit Dial Int 2000;20:548-556.

Rodriguez-Carmona A, Perez-Fontan M, Garcia-Naveiro R, et al. Compared time profiles of ultrafiltration, sodium removal, and renal function in incident CAPD and automated peritoneal dialysis patients. Am J Kidney Dis 2004;44:132-145.

Sarkar S, Bernardini J, Fried L, et al. Tolerance of large exchange volumes by peritoneal dialysis patients. Am J Kidney Dis 1999;33:1136-1141.

Tzamaloukas AH, Raj DS, Onime A, et al. The prescription of peritoneal dialysis. Semin Dial 2008;21:250-257

Viglino G, Neri L, Barbieri S. Incremental peritoneal dialysis: effects on the choice of dialysis modality, residual renal function and adequacy. Kidney Int 2008;108:S52-S55.

Vychytil A, Horl WH. The role of tidal peritoneal dialysis in modern practice: a European perspective. Kidney Int 2006;70:S96-S103.

Urgent-start PD prescription in the late-referred patient

Casaretto A, Rosario R, Kotzker WR, et al. Urgent-start peritoneal dialysis: report from a U.S. private nephrology practice. Adv Perit Dial 2012;28:102-105.

Ghaffari A. Urgent-start peritoneal dialysis: a quality improvement report. Am J Kidney Dis 2012;59:400-408.

Guest S, Akonur A, Ghaffari A, et al. Intermittent peritoneal dialysis: urea kinetic modeling and implications of residual kidney function. Perit Dial Int 2012;32:142-148.

Koch M, Kohnle M, Trapp R, et al. Comparable outcome of acute unplanned peritoneal dialysis and haemodialysis. Nephrol Dial Transplant 2012;27:375-380.

Lobbedez T, Lecouf A, Ficheux M, et al. Is rapid initiation of peritoneal dialysis feasible in unplanned dialysis patients? A single-center experience. Nephrol Dial Transplant 2008;23:3290-3294.

Povlsen JV, Ivarsen P. How to start the late referred ESRD patient urgently on chronic APD. Nephrol Dial Transplant 2006;21[Suppl 2]:ii56-ii59.

Chapter 11:
Infectious Complications

ALL RENAL REPLACEMENT THERAPIES expose the patient to the risk of infection. Hemodialysis is associated with vascular access infections and a higher rate of sepsis. Peritoneal dialysis is associated with infection at the catheter exit site, tunnel and/or peritonitis. The PD clinician should take prudent measures to reduce the risk of infection and have established protocols for the diagnosis and management of PD-related infections. These issues will be addressed in this chapter.

As PD is a home-based therapy, the initial indication that infection may be present is typically made by the patient. Therefore, it is important that patients be educated about symptoms and signs of infection. The patient should be taught to examine, clean and dress the exit site daily, report any discomfort at the catheter or tunnel location, and be able to recognize the earliest presentation of peritonitis to aid the clinicians in early diagnosis and treatment.

Fortunately, advances in PD therapy such as the concept of "flush before fill", connect assist devices and exit site prophylaxis have reduced infections dramatically. According to recent USRDS data, most PD-related infections are managed on an outpatient basis, with only a third or less of peritonitis cases requiring hospitalization.

In 2005 and 2010, the Ad Hoc Advisory Committee of the International Society of Peritoneal Dialysis (ISPD) updated recommendations for management of peritoneal dialysis related infections in adults. The guidelines were originally published in 1983. The committee has presented evidence-based recommendations, where evidence exists, and issues "opinions" based on experience if sufficient randomized, controlled trials are not available. It is recommended that PD units have access to these publications as a reference. Many of these recommendations will be reviewed in this chapter.

Prevention of Exit Site Infections

The PD catheter must exit the body and this catheter/skin interface is termed the "exit site". Proper initial placement of the PD catheter is the most critical component in a preventive strategy to avoid a subsequent exit site infection (ESI). The exit site should be chosen so that it avoids the abdominal pannus or skin fold creases in the obese patient. The exit site should be planned in advance, so that it avoids the beltline ensuring that clothing does not put undue friction on the site. The tunnel and exit site should be positioned in a downward and lateral orientation so that, during showering, water falls away from the exit site and naturally cleanses the site, without the risk that non-sterile shower water or sweat collects within the exit site. Keeping the catheter bandaged and relatively immobile may reduce shear stress on the catheter exit site.

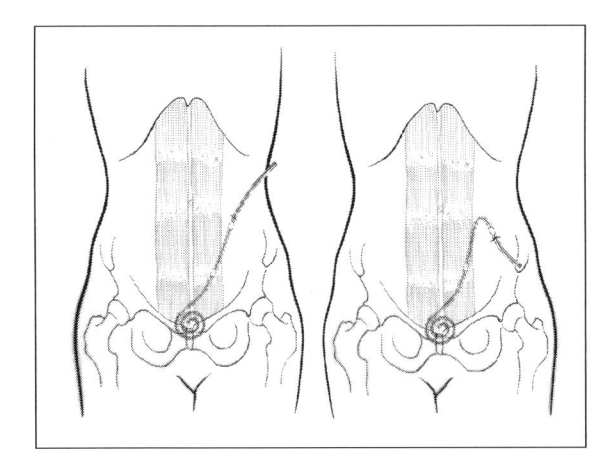

Suboptimal, upward oriented exit site on left allows for the collection of sweat, water, and cellular debris in the catheter-skin interface. The recommended downward oriented exit site is illustrated on the right

Because the Staphylococcus aureus organism can colonize the nares, this colonization was considered a risk factor for S. aureus exit site infections. To attempt to eradicate nasal carriage, a European trial compared intranasal mupirocin cream to placebo. Intranasal mupirocin significantly reduced the exit site infections from all organisms and specifically those due to S. aureus. Concurrently with this European trial, a Pittsburgh study compared cyclical oral rifampin therapy with mupirocin applied daily to the exit site directly. There was a reduction in ESI's in both arms.

After reviewing all available data and registering the concerns that intermittent rifampin may lead to resistance of this important anti-tuberculous agent, combined with the difficulties applying intranasal creams, the PD community widely adopted the strategy of applying mupirocin cream to the exit site. To further support direct exit site application of mupirocin versus intranasal application, genomic testing revealed that staphylococcal organisms causing ESI's were found in other sites than the nose.

A subsequent study by Bernardini and the Pittsburgh group compared mupirocin cream applied to the exit site versus gentamicin cream. Gentamicin cream had been noted to have anti-staphylococcal activity as well as gram-negative coverage. This trial showed that both creams reduced S. aureus ESI's. An additional observation was that the mupirocin cream had no effect on pseudomonal ESI's whereas the gentamicin cream reduced these infections significantly. The gentamicin group also had less peritonitis rates overall mainly due to a reduction in gram-negative infections. Based on this data many PD units adopted this gentamicin regimen to prevent ESI's.

In the MP^3 study, a polysporin ointment containing bacitracin, gramicidin, and polymyxin B was placed on the exit site daily and compared to mupirocin. The primary outcome of the study was time to first catheter-related infection. While bacterial infection rates were the same in both groups, the polysporin cohort had increased rates of fungal exit site infections and fungal peritonitis. The authors concluded that use of this broader spectrum topical antibiotic was contraindicated. An additional study, the Honeypot study, will assess the ability of honey to prevent ESI. Honey has antimicrobial properties against a variety of bacterial and fungal species, including methicillin resistant S. aureus and vancomycin resistant enterococci. The antimicrobial properties of honey are based on its low pH, high osmolality, content of defensin-1, and production of hydrogen peroxide and phenolic acids on dilution. The Honeypot Study will compare honey (Medihoney Antibacterial Wound Gel: Comvita, Te Puke, New Zealand) versus nasal application of mupirocin.

Sodium hypochlorite is a topical solution with broad activity against bacterial, fungal and mycobacterial organisms. Also termed "Dakin's solution", after chemist Henry Dakin, it was originally developed as a antibacterial wash to treat wound infections in World War I. In the PD literature, publications have described using dilute sodium hypochlorite directly on the exit site during daily care as well as for wiping the catheter cap and transfer set just prior to an exchange. In a limited number of publications, use of this solution has been shown to lower not only exit site infection rates but also peritonitis rates. Sodium hypochlorite solutions are available in two concentrations - 0.55% (Alcavis 50, Alcavis HDC, LLC, Gaithersburg, MD) for application on the transfer set and 0.114% (ExSept Plus, Alcavis HDC, LLC, Gaithersburg, MD) for the exit site.

Daily exit site care should be performed in a clean environment, with doors and windows closed, fans turned off, masks worn. Sterile or non-sterile gloves are not required. Prior to cleaning the exit site, hands should be thoroughly washed with clean water and soap, followed by toweling completely dry with clean disposable towels and an alcohol hand rub, if available.

During daily care, the exit site should be inspected for any evidence of infection. There should be no redness, pain, or purulence. During showering, the exit site can be cleaned with a washcloth applying gentle application of soap and water, thoroughly rinsed, and dried. Then a small amount of an antibacterial cream or ointment is applied to the site with a Q-tip or gauze, covered with a bandage, taped, and the catheter immobilized with tape. Securing the catheter helps avoid mechanical trauma and is especially important in newly placed catheters.

Treatment of Exit Site Infections

An ESI may present as new tenderness at the catheter exit site. The patient may notice some new drainage or erythema at the site and should be instructed to report this concern to the PD clinician. On presentation, the exit site should be carefully examined and an attempt made to express any purulence for culturing.

In cases of possible early ESI, when the signs are equivocal, clinicians could elect to not start oral antibiotics but increase the local exit site cleaning regimen with careful following of the exam. Locally applied antiseptics such as hypertonic saline soaks, antibacterial soaks, dilute sodium hypochlorite or hydrogen peroxide, and topical antibacterial creams could be used initially to attempt to avoid a course of oral antibiotics. The soaks can be administered 2 to 4 times a day.

Anti-Septic Topical Regimens

Hypertonic saline soaks	Use 3% saline or add one tablespoon of salt to 0.5L of sterile water and use solution to soak gauze wrapped around the exit site. Soak for 10 minutes twice a day
Sodium hypochlorite 0.144%	Applied to exit site as soak or spray and let to dry for 1 minute
Hydrogen peroxide	To clean surrounding skin
Topical antibiotic agents	Mupirocin ointment or cream -1 % applied daily Gentamicin 0.1% cream daily
Chlorhexidine	To clean site and surrounding skin
Povidone iodine solution	To clean surrounding skin

An obvious ESI should be treated with increased local care and oral antibiotics. Concurrently, clinicians should consider advising the patient to increase the exit site care from daily to twice a day. If indurated "proud flesh" is noted at the exit site, this flesh can be carefully cauterized with a silver nitrate stick, to discourage outward granulation of tissue and speed healing and epithelialization. Empiric oral antibiotics should be started to cover gram-positive skin organisms. Oral penicillins or first generation cephalosporins are typically recommended.

Empiric oral antibiotic regimens have been recommended and the medication doses have been adjusted for the reduced GFR of a PD patient. Most recommendations are to treat for a total of 14 days and then reassess.

Dicloxacillin	500 mg four times a day
Cephalexin	500 mg twice to three times a dy
Trimethoprim/sulfamethoxazole	80/400 mg daily
Erythromycin	500 mg four times a day
Metronidazole	400 mg three times a day
Linezolid	400 - 600 mg twice a day

Source: Perit Dial Int 2010;30:393-423. This reference also lists additional treatment regimens.

If the ESI is due to methicillin resistant S. aureus (MRSA), vancomycin or linezolid may be required. If the exit site culture implicates a gram-negative organism empiric oral antibiotic therapy can be changed to a quinolone. Pseudomonal ESIs can be particularly difficult to eradicate and 2 antibacterial agents should be used, such as an oral quinolone and intraperitoneal ceftazadime. The pseudomonal organisms may invade the catheter's siliconized rubber and be difficult to eradicate. If treatment of a pseudomonal ESI is not considered successful, the PD catheter should be removed to eliminate the infected foreign body. If this is done, clinicians could consider simultaneous replacement of a new catheter with different exit site during the procedure, with institution of temporary low volume PD, to avoid the need for temporary HD.

Fungal Exit Site Infections

Fungal exit site infections may occur as a consequence of general debilitation or, more commonly, a sequelae of broader antibiotic use for a bacterial exit site infection. Fungal infections at the exit site are rare- estimated by Frietas and colleagues to be 0.004 episodes per patient-year. Treatment measures include increased local care of the exit site, discontinuation of antibiotics once process identified as fungal and not bacterial, and oral antifungal agents. ISPD recommendations (2010) for treatment of fungal exit sites include fluconazole 200 mg a day for 2 days followed by 100 mg a day until resolved. Flucytosine is an alternative agent but requires measurement and titration of serum levels. As with bacterial exit site infections, if the process appears refractory to treatment or there is suspicion that the catheter superficial cuff may be infected, catheter removal may need to be considered.

Tunnel Infection

An ESI can extend along the catheter track and result in a so called "tunnel" infection. Tunnel infections rarely occur without a concurrent ESI and, when present, are diagnosed by tenderness on palpation of the catheter's subcutaneous track and boggy induration of the area. However, tunnel site infections can be somewhat occult and notable only by imaging techniques, such as ultrasound or CT. The image below illustrates abnormalities along the tunnel's subcutaneous tissue, assisting in making the diagnosis of an occult tunnel infection.

At presentation with a suspected ESI, it is not necessary to obtain CT or ultrasound imaging in all cases but careful examination of the tunnel is important and in refractory or worsening cases of ESI further imaging may assist in diagnosis of a tunnel infection. In cases of tunnel infection, intravenous or intraperitoneal antibiotics may be more indicated, compared to oral agents alone, based on clinical judgment. If the deep cuff is also felt to be infected, the catheter should be removed. If the tunnel infection is associated with subcutaneous cuff involvement, the cuff can often be externalized with a minor surgical debridement and then removed by shaving to allow the exit site to re-heal. This procedure should be done while the patient is on antibiotics.

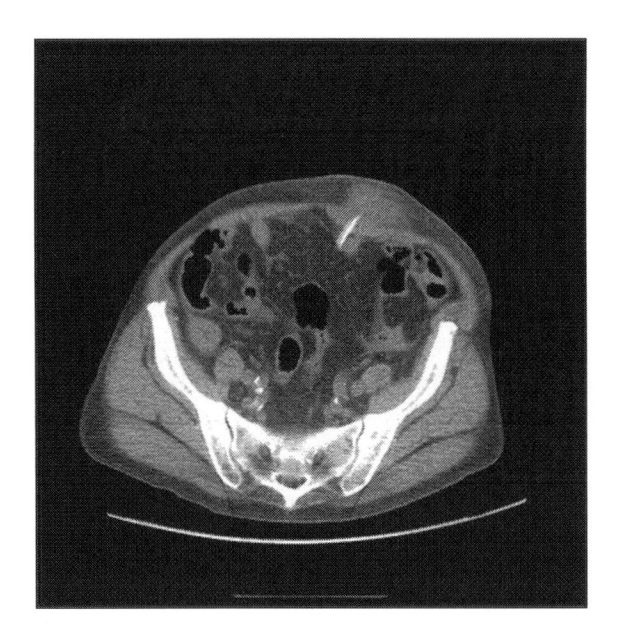

Subcutaneous tunnel infection detected on CT scan

Peritonitis

Peritonitis is the most serious infectious complication associated with PD therapy. As mentioned, peritonitis rates, overall, have declined during the last decades. Improvements in catheter materials, connectology, and placement techniques have reduced peritonitis rates. Strategies to improve the location of the exit site to avoid abdominal creases or a large pannus, and antibiotic cream application to the exit site have reduced peritonitis rates. Additionally, improvements in patient education have led to reductions in this complication.

Peritonitis rates vary around the world. In the USA, most recent estimates suggest a national average of one episode of peritonitis every 24 patient-months. Some centers have rates of one episode at 60 patient-months (1 episode at 5 years of treatment). PD centers should be knowledgeable of their peritonitis rates and routinely follow this quality indicator. If peritonitis rates are felt to be suboptimal, increased adherence to best demonstrated practices is advised.

Preventive Strategies

Patient education is the key to reducing the risk of peritonitis. Most episodes of peritonitis are due to touch contamination with some break in proper technique. Training of patients must take place at a pace that allows sufficient time for the patient to learn and retain proper exchange techniques. It should be emphasized in the training that exchanges are performed in a room where windows and doors are closed to prevent any cross drafts. Pets should not be in the room during an exchange nor be allowed to play with the drainage lines or equipment. For example, many descriptions of Pasteurella peritonitis have been attributed to cats biting the PD catheter, solution lines, or PD bags.

Patients should be fully instructed to perform exchanges after hand washing and while wearing a mask. It is not necessary to have patient's use sterile gloves for exchanges but, rather, wash hands with soap and water and/or clean hands with an antibacterial gel. Patients must allow the hands to completely dry, as water droplets on the hands are not sterile, and may lead to contamination during the exchange.

In a closed room, after cleaning and thoroughly drying the hands and while wearing a mask, a connection or disconnection is made. At an exchange connection, the concept of "flush before fill" is critical to reducing peritonitis rates. In this procedure, the patient is instructed to drain any indwelling dialysate into the drain bag, thus flushing any contaminating bacteria away from the peritoneum, before any infusion of dialysate enters the body. Again, only after this flushing of any possible contaminating bacteria into the drainage bag is new solution infused into the peritoneum. PD practitioners believe this simple procedure has dramatically reduced peritonitis risk.

As mentioned above, ESIs can increase the risk that bacteria track along the catheter and enter the peritoneum. The procedures to properly care for the exit site, therefore, are also methods of reducing peritonitis risk. Studies employing topical antibiotics at the exit site showed reductions in peritonitis, as well as ESIs.

Procedural Prophylaxis

Antibiotic prophylaxis is recommended before a variety of procedures. Care should be given to questioning patients about any upcoming procedures so that pre-treatment prophylaxis can be administered. In general, any oral, abdominal, or gynecologic procedure should be considered for antibiotic prophylaxis.

Dental prophylaxis for PD Patients

Periodontal disease has been associated with chronic inflammation, accelerated atherosclerosis and cardiovascular disease. Antibiotic prophylaxis before extensive dental work is recommended in patients on peritoneal dialysis. The rationale for prophylaxis is to reduce the likelihood that any transient bacteremia created during the procedure would seed other locations including the peritoneum, resulting in peritonitis. Proponents argue that the ESRD population is immunocompromised and that preventing any bacteremia would be prudent. Antibiotic use before dental work is not, however, consistently employed and surveys of nephrologists have indicated less than 50% felt that prophylaxis was indicated.

There are no randomized controlled trials showing benefit of dental prophylaxis in PD patients. There are, however, observational reports of streptococcal peritonitis in which an oral source was suspected. The ISPD treatment guidelines for PD related infections issued in 2005 simply states "a single dose of amoxicillin (2 gm) 2 hours before extensive dental procedures is reasonable, although there are no studies to support this approach (opinion)".

Prophylaxis before colonoscopy

Colonoscopy can lead to transient bacteremia and colonoscopy with and without polypectomy can result in peritonitis. Estimates are that 6% of colonoscopy procedures in PD patients result in peritonitis. Therefore, it is reasonable to consider special measures for the PD patient who is to undergo colonoscopy.

A general recommendation is to drain all dialysate from the abdomen prior to the procedure to lessen the risk that bacteria escape from the enteric space and enter the glucose-rich dialysate. Antibiotic prophylaxis should be considered employing 2 to 3 agents to fully treat enteric organisms. The ISPD treatment guidelines state that antibiotic administration may lessen the risk of peritonitis after colonoscopy. This advisory document suggests using ampicillin 1 gram intravenously before the procedure with a single dose of an aminoglycoside, with or without metronidazole.

Prophylaxis for gynecologic procedures

Whether antibiotic prophylaxis should be routinely given prior to gynecologic procedures has been somewhat unclear. However, peritonitis has been described after gynecological examinations and procedures such as hysteroscopy. The ISPD recommends that the abdomen be emptied before invasive gynecological procedures such as endometrial biopsy. A recent review of the impact of prophylactic antibiotics before a variety of gynecological procedures, such as IUD implantation, showed significant protection with pre-procedure antibiotics. This report by Wu and colleagues would suggest that antibiotics may play a significant role in preventing peritonitis before gynecologic procedures.

Hand Hygiene

Maintaining reasonable hand hygiene is an important part of patient training and combined with proper connection technique can reduce the likelihood of touch contamination and peritonitis. Hand washing recommendations have been published and these are to perform hand washing in alignment with hand washing recommendations for health care workers published by the World Health Organization. These recommendations include a general hand wash to remove the major surface grim followed by a more focused wash that concentrates on the fingernails, skin web between the thumb and index finger, and webs between the fingers. Hand washing alone will not sterilize the hands and many centers augment hand washing with subsequent application of an alcohol-based gel or foam. Additional recommendations are to avoid nail polish or artificial nails, avoid rings if possible, keep the fingernails trimmed closely, and to assure that the hands are completely dry before making a connection- as tap water itself is not sterile. These recommendations were recently summarized in a review article by Firanek et al.

Additional Preventive Strategies

A recent publication identified hypokalemia as an independent risk factor for gram-negative peritonitis. These authors speculated that chronic hypokalemia reduces bowel motility and allows for bacterial overgrowth. This increases the possibility of translocation of bowel organisms into the peritoneal cavity. Additionally, hypokalemia may contribute to constipation and aggressive laxative therapy may precipitate peritonitis. Therefore, hypokalemia should be treated in all PD patients to reduce this possible infectious complication. Chronic hypokalemia may be a marker of general malnutrition, as it has been associated with lower serum albumin, phosphorus, and fasting total cholesterol levels. Malnourished patients with hypoalbuminemia may have diminished cell-mediated and humoral immunity and be at greater risk of peritonitis. Aggressive nutritional interventions are indicated in this patient population.

A recent small report described lower peritonitis rates in patients using daily lactulose therapy. Lactulose is a non-absorbable disaccharide used as a stool softener. Lactulose is degraded by intestinal bacteria into lactic and pyruvic acid thus acidifying the stool which reduces bacterial colonization and increases colonic motility. Regular use of lactulose was associated with a lower peritonitis rate. Additional studies are needed to confirm this observation.

Strategies to Reduce the Risk of Peritonitis

1. Proper initial training on handwashing, proper drying of hands, wearing mask, and exchange technique

2. Exchanges should be done in controlled settings with no pets in the room, the windows and doors closed

3. Inspection of the dialysate bags and tubing to assess for any damage or contamination

4. After connection is made, dialysate is flushed away from the patient first - the concept of flush before fill

5. Consideration of topical antibacterial agent for daily exit site care

6. Patients at risk of touch contamination should be instructed on use of connection assist devices if available

7. Avoid hypokalemia and resultant bowel stasis

8. Antibiotic prophylaxis before dental work, colonoscopy, and gynecological procedures

9. If frequent laxative required, consider lactulose

Diagnosis of Peritonitis

The clinical presentation of peritonitis usually includes diffuse abdominal pain. The discomfort is mild and intermittent at the early stages but more persistent and painful with delays in treatment. The patient may note anorexia, nausea, or vomiting. Fever may or may not be present. As peritonitis rarely leads to active bacteremia, chills and rigors are noted less often. Occasionally loose stools or constipation are described.

Patients should be advised that with any of the above symptoms the PD fluid should be checked for evidence of infection. The patient who is at home can be instructed to perform an exchange and bring this freshly drained solution into the PD unit or emergency room, for visual inspection and for laboratory analysis.

The drained PD fluid should be sent for peritoneal total cell count with cell count differential and culturing. It is critical to obtain a positive culture result so that the infecting organism is identified and appropriate therapy can be determined. To assure organism identification, a 50 mL sample of dialysate is obtained and centrifuged at 3000 g for 15 minutes to a pellet. The pellet is then re-suspended in up to 5 mL of sterile saline and inoculated into standard blood culture bottle as well as microbiological culture plates.

PD units should select their preferred culture technique and be consistent, to minimize chances of protocol deviations, mishandling of the fluid, or other errors.

The diagnosis of peritonitis is confirmed by the symptomatology described above with a total PD fluid cell count of > 100 WBC's/microliter, with > 50% polymorphonuclear cells. Some centers advocate gram staining of the PD fluid, in an attempt to identify a possible bacterial species and to rule out fungal elements. Other centers believe that the drained dialysate is too dilute and that the yield in gram stain procedures is too low to warrant the time and effort. It seems reasonable, however, to recommend that if laboratory facilities are readily available and the procedure does not result in any delays in treatment, gram staining of dialysate can be attempted.

Diagnosis of Peritonitis

1. Patient presents with clinical symptomatology that could be consistent with peritoneal inflammation such as diffuse abdominal pain, nausea, vomiting, change in bowel pattern

2. Drained PD fluid appears cloudy - in subtle early cases the drained bag can be placed on a newspaper and if it is difficult to read the newspaper print through the fluid it suggests that the fluid is not clear

3. PD fluid is sent for total WBC count, differential, bacterial and fungal culturing

4. Diagnosis confirmed if dialysate total WBC count > 100 cells/microliter with at least 50% polymorphonuclear neutrophil cells

It is recommended that PD centers have established protocols for the diagnosis and treatment of peritonitis. These established protocols are agreed upon by the medical team and provide a unified, consistent response to this complication reducing the impact that this event has on the patient and unit. These protocols can be followed by the nursing staff so that initial diagnosis and treatment of peritonitis is begun per protocol and prior to notification of the nephrologist. This reduces the risk of delays in treatment. On notification of a possible peritonitis presentation, the PD staff should have an organized and consistent response that reduces chances of erratic fluid sampling, culturing, and delays in treatment.

As mentioned, on a monthly to quarterly basis it is advised that the PD staff review the peritonitis cases and calculate a monthly peritonitis rate. For example, if the unit has 100 PD patients in its census in the month of August and had 2 episodes of peritonitis, the peritonitis rate for August would be 1 episode every 50 patient-months. This peritonitis rate can be followed monthly so that any unusual trends in peritonitis rates can be addressed by the unit. A PD unit that does not readily know its own peritonitis rates is like a ship at sea without a map. Only when peritonitis rates are monitored by the unit can the unit have a broad understanding of this complication and its impact.

For each case of peritonitis, an attempt should be made to identify a possible root cause to attempt to correct. Was there an obvious break in technique, is a re-training necessary, are pets in the home, was there a break in the hand-washing procedure, were the doors or windows open, a new caregiver assisting the procedure, etc? A PD unit that monitors the overall rate of peritonitis, understands the factors that possibly led to the infections, takes measures to correct what factors are remediable and maintains a pro-active approach with this complication feels empowered and more confident that this complication is manageable and being closely monitored. This pro-active response to this serious complication adds confidence to the patient and staff's belief in their ability to manage this complication. Large PD units abroad and some US centers are now reporting peritonitis rates of one episode every 5 years. Managing a dialysis complication to this degree can prolong the therapy, reduce drop out, and improve overall clinical outcomes.

Peritonitis Treatment

Treatment of peritonitis should initially be empiric based on a high level of clinical suspicion. It is recommended that antibiotic therapy be started empirically, before laboratory confirmation of peritonitis to avoid delays in treatment. As the peritonitis may have occurred due to contamination of the transfer set, the transfer set should be changed. Prior to administering IP antibiotics, some centers prefer 2 rapid in-and-out flushes to remove inflammatory mediators and reduce pain, but this intervention has not been rigorously evaluated.

Only in the most equivocal presentations should therapy be withheld pending laboratory confirmation. Empiric therapy should be directed at both gram-positive and negative bacterial species. Due to concerns over the development of vancomycin resistant enterococcus (VRE), empiric vancomycin should be limited, if possible. In PD centers with higher rates of MRSA infections, empiric vancomycin may be justified. Alternatives for empiric gram-positive coverage include first generation cephalosporins or penicillins such as nafcillin. Empiric gram-negative coverage could include gentamicin, tobramycin or a third generation cephalosporin such as ceftazadime.

Intraperitoneal dosing strategies are recommended, as they lead to rapid intraperitoneal therapeutic drug levels. However, if emergency room staff or clinics are less familiar with intraperitoneal administration of antibiotics, the traditional IV dosing should be employed to avoid delays in treatment or additional risks of contamination by untrained staff, unfamiliar with intraperitoneal administration. If the patient appears quite toxic and possibly even with early sepsis, the intravenous route of delivery may be more prudent to ensure rapid serum levels of antibiotics. It must be emphasized again that if peritonitis is suspected there should not be undue delays in treatment. Control of the patient's symptoms, intra-abdominal inflammatory reaction, risk of peritoneal membrane damage, and rapid bacterial doubling time all dictate that antibiotic therapy should be started as soon as possible. Peritonitis is usually managed in the outpatient setting, but delays in diagnosis and treatment can lead to hospitalization, increase overall morbidity and, rarely, result in death. Patients that live in remote locations may be given antibiotic vials to keep at home, to self administer empiric therapy, after they have collected samples of drained PD fluid for laboratory analysis.

After empiric therapy has been initiated, the dialysate culture results should be obtained to determine whether alterations in antibiotics are warranted. If gram-positive species such as S. epidermidis or aureus are isolated, the empiric gram-negative coverage can be discontinued. Similarly, if gram-negative organisms are identified the empiric gram-positive therapy can be held.

Intraperitoneal Heparin

Intraperitoneal heparin has been used during episodes of peritonitis. Heparin down-regulates intraperitoneal fibrinogen-fibrin turnover and has been noted to reduce IL-6 production. As thrombin stimulates monocyte cytokine production, inhibiting thrombin during peritonitis has been speculated to diminish cytokine release and reduce inflammation. Heparin also reduces fibrin formation that may be increased during peritonitis.

ISPD Dosing Recommendations

Below are the antibiotic dosing recommendations derived from 2010 ISPD guidelines / recommendations for peritoneal dialysis-related infections. These dosages should be increased by 25 % in patients with residual kidney function manifested by greater than 100 mL/day urine output.

Antibiotic Regimens

Intraperitoneal Antibiotic Medication Added Daily to One Exchange in CAPD

CAPD

Antibiotic	Dose added to one exchange
Cefazolin	15 mg/kg
Cefepime	1000 mg
Ceftazadime	1000-1500 mg
Cephalothin	15 mg/kg
Cephradine	15 mg/kg
Ceftizoxime	1000 mg
Gentamicin	0.6 mg/kg
Tobramycin	0.6 mg/kg
Vancomycin	15-30 mg/kg (repeated in 5-7 d)*
Antibiotic	**Dose added twice a day**
Ampicillin/sulbactam	2 grams but requires q12 hr dosing
Imipenem/cilistatin	1000 mg twice a day

No firm data exist for intermittent dosing of simple penicillins or quinolones.
The above recommendations are from the Ad Hoc Advisory Committee on Peritoneal Dialysis Related Infections under the auspices of the International Society of Peritoneal Dialysis. Additional antibiotics are mentioned in this original publication.

*In patients with UOP greater than 500 mL/day IP vancomycin should be redosed at 2-3 day intervals. If UOP is less than 500 mls per day dosage repeated at 5-7d. Vancomycin serum levels can be obtained to guide the dosing interval with redosing if serum levels reach 15 mcg/mL.

Continuous Antibiotic Dosing in CAPD
(Intraperitoneal medication added to each exchange)

CAPD

Antibiotic	Initial Loading Dose To First Bag	Subsequent Doses To Each Bag
Ampicillin	125 mg/Liter	125 mg/Liter
Ampicillin/sulbactam	1000 mg/Liter	100 mg/Liter
Aztreonam	1000 mg/Liter	250 mg/Liter
Cefazolin	500 mg/Liter	125 mg/Liter
Cefepime	500 mg/Liter	125 mg/Liter
Ceftazadime	500 mg/Liter	125 mg/Liter
Ceftizoxime	250 mg/Liter	125 mg/Liter
Cephalothin	500 mg/Liter	125 mg/Liter
Cephradine	500 mg/Liter	125 mg/Liter
Ciprofloxacin	50 mg/Liter	25 mg/Liter
Daptomycin	100 mg/Liter	20 mg/Liter
Gentamicin	8 mg/Liter	4 mg/Liter
Imipenem/cilistatin	250 mg/Liter	50 mg/Liter
Nafcillin	125 mg/Liter	125 mg/Liter
Tobramycin	8 mg/Liter	4 mg/Liter
Vancomycin	1000 mg/Liter	25 mg/Liter

Continuous antibiotic dosing is not recommended in APD due to variations in the short and long dwell times and resultant fluctuations in therapeutic drug levels.

Intraperitoneal Antibiotic Dosing in APD

APD

Antibiotic	Loading Dose	Subsequent Doses
Cefazolin	20 mg/kg in initial long dwell	Continue with 20 mg/kg daily in each long dwell

Cefepime	1000 mg total in the initial long dwell	1000 mg daily in the long dwell
Tobramycin	1.5 mg/kg in initial long dwell	0.5 mg/kg daily in each long dwell
Vancomycin	30 mg/kg in initial long dwell	Repeat dosing at 15 mg/kg every 3-5 days*

*For patients with significant residual kidney function (urine output over 500 L/day) on APD, many authors recommend redosing of vancomycin every 3 days based on serum levels, with redosing indicated if the serum random level is < 15 mg/dl.

Fungal Peritonitis Treatment Recommendations

Anti-Fungal Agent	Recommended Doses
Fluconazole	100 mg - 200 mg daily Can be given IP in one exchange a day every 24-48 hours, or as intravenous or oral dose
Flucytosine	500 mg oral bid
Caspofungin	70 mg IV loading followed by 50 mg IV daily
Voriconazole	200 mg IV twice daily

As a quick reference, specific comments can be made for various peritonitis presentations:

Staphylococcus epidermidis

Staphylococcus epidermidis (coagulase negative staph [CNS]) is a more common cause of peritonitis and recommended treatment is with intraperitoneal first generation cephalosporin or vancomycin for 14 days.

Staphylococcus aureus

Staphylococcus aureus peritonitis is less frequent (6-8%) but typically more severe than S. epidermidis peritonitis and is associated with higher rates of hospitalization, catheter removal, and relapse. ISPD guidelines suggest that antibiotics alone may be insufficient to eradicate the infection and catheter removal may be required.

Treatment of S. aureas peritonitis is with a first generation cephalosporin antibiotic or vancomycin, depending on local sensitivity patterns. Intraperitoneal antibiotic delivery is recommended and several initial days of intraperitoneal gentamicin, and/or oral rifampin can be added for synergy.

Methicillin sensitive S. aureus (MSSA) can be treated with either a first generation cephalosporin or vancomycin but methicillin resistant S. aureus (MRSA) should be treated with vancomycin, quinupristin/dalfopristin, linezolid, or daptomycin. ISPD guidelines recommend treating all S. aureus peritonitis episodes with 21 days of antibiotics.

Non-pseudomonal gram-negative peritonitis

Gram-negative organisms may colonize the exit site but the predominant location is within the gastrointestinal lumen. Peritonitis from intestinal gram-negative organisms may be due to transmural migration from micro-perforations, diverticulosis, or the presence and treatment of constipation.

After culture results suggest gram-negative peritonitis, the empiric gram-positive antibiotic treatment can be discontinued. Treatment for the non-pseudomonal gram-negative organism is for 14-21 days. As mentioned, use of exit site prophylaxis with gentamicin cream reduced subsequent gram-negative peritonitis.

Polymicrobial peritonitis

Polymicrobial peritonitis with multiple enteric organisms is suspicious of intra-abdominal catastrophe and broad spectrum antibiotic coverage, including anaerobic organisms, is recommended. Surgical consultation should be obtained as multiple enteric organisms suggest intestinal perforation or other visceral injury may have occurred. Polymicrobial peritonitis has been reported in cases of colon carcinoma with perforation, necrotic cholecystitis, intestinal ischemia, and incarcerated hernias.

Pseudomonal peritonitis

Pseudomonas species are virulent organisms often associated with severe peritonitis, poor response to treatment with single antibiotics, and the ability to invade catheter materials and create biofilms necessitating catheter removal. ISPD guidelines recommend that pseudomonal peritonitis be treated with dual antibiotic therapy including combinations of aminoglycosides, quinolones, or a third generation cephalosporin, such as ceftazadime. Failure to promptly respond to antibiotics within 3-4 days should be an indication for urgent catheter removal. Even if the patient is responding and the catheter is left in place, treatment should be prolonged to 21 days. If the catheter is removed, treatment should continue for 2 weeks after catheter removal.

Enterococcal peritonitis

Enterococci are anaerobic, gram-positive cocci that play prominent roles in nosocomial infections. The two most common species are Enterococcus faecalis and Enterococcus faecium and both can cause peritonitis by migrating hematogenously or by translocation from bowel. Estimates are that from 2 to 4% of peritonitis episodes may be due to enterococcal species. Approximately half of enterococcal peritonitis episodes are associated with other organisms, usually gram-negative organisms suggesting bowel pathology.

ISPD Guidelines recommend that treatment of enterococcal peritonitis is IP ampicillin with possible addition of aminoglyosides for synergy. Use of vancomycin, in susceptible species, has been successful but increases risk of development of vancomycin-resistant enterococcus (discussed below). Recommended treatment is for 3 weeks.

Vancomycin-resistant enterococcus (VRE) peritonitis

VRE peritonitis typically occurs in patients with underlying VRE stool colonization from recent hospitalization and exposure to broad spectrum antibiotics. The antibiotic resistance pattern of VRE organisms makes treatment problematic. Various intravenous regimens have documented success in treating VRE peritonitis including IV gentamicin, chloramphenicol, ampicillin, oral and IV linezolid, quinupristin/dalfopristin and higher dose IP vancomycin that apparently exceeded the minimal inhibitory concentration. These cases required both catheter removal and antibiotics to resolve to completion.

Daptomycin is a newer cyclic lipopeptide with bactericidal activity against gram-positive organisms. It is strongly protein bound making IV dosing problematic for the treatment of peritonitis. Recent reports of intraperitoneal daptomycin demonstrated successful eradication of VRE peritonitis without catheter removal. Daptomycin is relatively unstable in dextrose solutions, so the antibiotic must be injected into the dialysate just prior to infusion and the dwell time is 4 to 6 hours during CAPD. The daptomycin dose was IP 15 mg/kg once weekly in one report. In another report the administered dose was 20 mg/L in each exchange, repeated every 4 hours. Both 10 day and 14 day antibiotic courses were successful in eradicating the peritonitis. No APD dosing strategy for daptomycin has been published to date.

Culture-negative peritonitis

This presentation is defined as patients with abdominal pain and laboratory evidence of peritonitis yet remain culture negative at 72 hours. This presentation usually suggests that suboptimal culturing techniques may have occurred. As mentioned, the ISPD has recommended centers not have culture negative peritonitis rates of greater that 20%. To increase the yield of positive cultures, the ISPD recommends removing a 50 mL sample of dialysate, collected in sterile fashion, centrifuged at 3000 g for 15 minutes with the centrifuged pellet resuspended in 3 to 5 mL of sterile saline and used to inoculate on solid culture plates as well as injected into blood culture media. Culture negative bacterial peritonitis episodes have been associated with higher antibiotic cure rates and lower rates of hospitalization and catheter removal.

In culture negative peritonitis, treatment decisions are hampered by the failure to identify the pathogen. The treatment options are to continue empiric coverage for both gram-positive and negative organisms for 2 weeks or simplify to gram-positive coverage only for 2 weeks with the realization that most infectious cases are from gram-positive organisms.

Culture-negative peritonitis may also occur in patients with recent exposure to antibiotics, unusual fastidious organisms, or fungal/mycobacterial infections, represent non-infectious chemical peritonitis, or falsely diagnosed cloudy fluid that was due to chlyous ascites or eosinophilic peritonitis. Culture negative peritonitis has recently been described in a patient whom presented with left upper quandrant pain due to a splenic infarction.

Pasteurella multocida peritonitis

Pasteurella (named after Louis Pasteur) multocida is a zoonotic organism found in the mouths of dogs, cats, and other wild and domestic animals. This organism is a gram-negative coccobacillus and has been a rare cause of peritonitis in patients who allow pets to come in contact with the dialysis supplies, solutions, tubing, or be in the room during exchanges. Contact with cats has been the most common link and descriptions of cats playing with and biting the tubing are most common. Other reports of cat scratches on the hands and cat fur caught in the tape used at the exit site have been associated with pasteurella infections. The most recent case reported by Sol et al in 2013 noted that a domestic cat was suspected as the source and that the cat preferred to nap on the cycler heating tray- an understandable attraction for a cat. Precautions should be given to patients that have pets at home- to assure that the pets do not come into contact with the PD supplies and should not be in the room during exchanges. Prior to exchanges, the need for strict hand washing, after handling pets, should be emphasized.

Pasteurella peritonitis can be treated with a variety of antibiotics and the organisms tend to be sensitive to penicillins, cephalosporins, fluoroquinolones, trimethoprim/sulfamethozaxole, aminoglycosides and clindamycin with antibiotic sensitivity guiding the treatment decision. Treatment should be for at least 2 weeks.

Corynebacterium

Corynebacteria are anaerobic gram-positive rods that exist as normal skin flora. Specimen samples containing corynebacterium were originally felt to have skin touch contamination and not represent true virulent organisms. However, recent reports show a wide variety of true infectious complications from this organism, including cases of peritonitis. Most, but not all, infections with corynebacterium involve immunocompromised hosts. ISPD guidelines make no mention of this bacterial species and the recommended treatments. A recent report of 82 cases of corynebacterium peritonitis was published from an Australian database - these cases represented 2.3% of all peritonitis episodes. Treatment was successful with a first-generation cephalosporin or vancomycin and a 2 week treatment course appeared sufficient.

Recurrent peritonitis

Recurrent peritonitis is defined as a peritonitis episode that occurs within 4 weeks of a prior episode, but with a different organism. The implications of recurrent peritonitis are lapses in sterile technique, or a compromised immune system. Recurrent peritonitis from enteric organisms raises the concern of occult gastrointestinal lesions and may indicate that screening for benign and malignant polyps, or other intestinal lesions may be indicated. Enteric peritonitis that does not improve with typical antibiotic administration may suggest intra-abdominal perforation and surgical consultation may be indicated.

Relapsing peritonitis

Relapsing peritonitis is defined as an episode of peritonitis that again occurs, with the same organism, within 4 weeks after the appropriate treatment of a prior episode. The implications of relapsing peritonitis are that the offending organism may have developed antimicrobial resistance contributing to the treatment relapse. Alternatively, relapsing peritonitis may suggest that the original organism has harbored underneath a protective biofilm, within the catheter lumen, and evaded eradication. Consideration will need to be given to catheter removal or attempts to eradicate catheter biofim with intra-catheter thrombolytics followed by re-treatment of appropriate antibiotics.

Mycobacterial peritonitis

Peritonitis with tuberculous and non-tuberculous mycobacterial organisms has been reported. The presenting cell count has either a predominance of polymorphonuclear cells or lymphocytes. Initial bacterial cultures are negative, triggering the broader culturing for fungal and mycobacterial species. Culture yield can be increased by centrifuging 50 to 150 mL of dialysate and culturing the pellet on solid and fluid media. Tuberculous peritonitis is more common in endemic areas and non-tuberculous infection has been attributed to immune deficiencies, nutritional factors, or environmental exposures to contaminated water or soil. Municipal water supplies used for showering and tap water can contain these organisms and exposure to water harboring these organisms has been been associated with exit site infections.

Treatment of mycobacterial peritonitis should include multiple medications. For tuberculous peritonitis, the recommended initial treatment is a four drug regimen of isoniazid, rifampin, pyrazinamide, and ofloxacin. Pyrazinamide and ofloxacin are stopped after 3 months - isonizid and rifampin are continued for one year. For non-tuberculous species such as Mycobacterium chelonae or fortuitum treatment is guided by microbial sensitivity testing. For tuberculous and non-tuberculous peritonitis there is no consensus on whether the catheter should be removed, as successful responses have been described in both situations. If exit site and tunnel involvement is also noted it seems prudent to remove the catheter.

Fungal peritonitis

In patients presenting with fungal peritonitis, strong consideration should be given to timely catheter removal. Fungal organisms can invade the catheter material and set up a nidus that is refractory to treatment. Expeditious removal of the foreign body can have a significant impact on the prognosis of this serious infection.

Amphotericin B administration is possible yet intraperitoneal administration causes significant abdominal pain. Given intravenously, amphotericin is 90% protein bound and diffuses poorly into the peritoneum. Amphotericin B is nephrotoxic and caution must be used to protect residual renal function. Given these limitations, amphotericin B may be most justified in patients with severe non-candida species or in cases refractory to oral treatments.

Fluconazole may be given orally, intravenously, or intraperitoneally. Fluconazole is well absorbed from the gastrointestinal tract and has good penetration into the peritoneal cavity. Fluconazole is most indicated for candida species and may be less ideal for non-candida organisms. Some centers add oral Flucytosine for synergy. Flucytosine is not used as monotherapy due to concerns of the rapid development of resistance. Flucytosine has both liver and bone marrow toxicity, so caution should be used to avoid this agent in any patient taking other medications that may suppress the bone marrow, or with other risks of hepatotoxicity.

For fungal peritonitis, the 2010 ISPD guidelines recommend immediate catheter removal after diagnosis of fungal peritonitis. In general, there is no consensus on the treatment of fungal peritonitis and a variety of medications and lengths of treatment have been published. It would be prudent to remove the PD catheter as soon as possible and continue anti-fungal therapy for at least 10 days, although some literature suggests therapy should be continued for 4 to 6 weeks. In PD-related fungal peritonitis, there is emerging experience with the newer azoles such as voricanazole or itraconazole. Voriconazole doses of 200 mg IV twice a day for 5 weeks after catheter removal have been described.

For fungal prophylaxis during treatment of bacterial peritonitis, some centers employ oral fluconazole or nystatin. Reports in the literature have not consistently confirmed the benefit of oral fungal prophylaxis.

Eosinophilic peritonitis

Bacterial and fungal peritonitis may rarely present with an eosinophilic predominance to the cell count. Infectious etiologies should always be ruled out in a patient presenting with eosinophilic peritonitis. However, most cases of eosinophilic peritonitis are culture negative and felt not to be infectious in etiology. For additional information on eosinophilic peritonitis refer to Chapter 12.

Gynecologic Causes of Peritonitis

There are a variety of special considerations in the female patient in regards to potential causes of peritonitis. Specific factors increase the differential diagnosis of a peritonitis presentation such as open and patent fallopian tubes, reflux menstruation, and foreign bodies such as tampons and intrauterine devices. Ascending infection from pelvic inflammatory disease, a tubo-ovarian abscess, pelvic examination, or septic abortion may be associated with a secondary peritonitis presentation. These factors should be considered in the female patient presenting with peritonitis with the intake history and physical exam directed at excluding these risk factors as the cause. If suspected the empiric treatment of peritonitis should be broad spectrum and potentially include concurrent anti-fungal therapy followed by gynecologic consultation.

Gynecologic Causes of Peritonitis

1. Pelvic examination

2. Migrated intrauterine device

3. Infected tampon

4. Septic abortion

5. Vaginal or uterine perforation secondary to catheter trauma

6. Tubo-ovarian abscess

7. Pelvic inflammatory disease

8. Post-partum peritonitis

9. Retrograde menstruation

Expected Clinical Response to Treatment of Bacterial Peritonitis

After initiation of appropriate antibiotics, the peritoneal fluid should gradually clear with clinical improvement over the initial 72 hours. ISPD guidelines recommend that if symptoms and cloudy fluid persist after 4 to 5 days the peritonitis is refractory to treatment and the foreign body (catheter) should be removed.

An interesting study by Chow and colleagues determined the predictive value of dialysate cell counts in peritonitis. They determined that on day three of peritonitis treatment, a persistent dialysate cell count of > 1090/mm^3 carried a 9-fold greater risk of treatment failure. Therefore, clinicians could initiate peritonitis treatment on day 1, follow the dialysate cell count on day 3 and have an early indication of which patients may indeed be non-responders by the 4-5 day interval. This early indication may allow for the necessary communications to surgeons of the need to remove the catheter by day 5. If catheter removal is required in refractory peritonitis, antibiotics should be continued for at least an additional week.

Overview References:

Bender FH, Bernardini J, and Piraino B. Prevention of infectious complications in peritoneal dialysis: best demonstrated practices. Kidney Int 2006;70[suppl 103]:S44-54.

Li PKT, Szeto CC, Piraino B, et al. Peritoneal dialysis-related infections recommendations: 2010 update. Perit Dial Int 2010;30:393-423.

Nessim SJ. Prevention of peritoneal dialysis-related infections. Semin Nephrol 2011;31:199-212.

Piraino B, Bernardini J, Brown E, et al. ISPD position statement on reducing the risks of peritoneal dialysis-related infections. Perit Dial Int 2011; 31:614-630.

Piraino B, Bailie G, Bernardini J, et al. Peritoneal dialysis-related infections recommendations: 2005 update. Perit Dial Int 2005;25:107-131.

General References:

Afsar B, Elsurer R, Bilgic A, et al. Regular lactulose use is associated with lower peritonitis rates: an observational study. Perit Dial Int 2010;30:243-246.

Akpolat T. Tuberculous peritonitis. Perit Dial Int 2009;29[Suppl 2]:S166-169.

Antony SJ, Oglesby KA. Peritonitis associated with pasteurella multocida in peritoneal dialysis patients- case report and review of the literature. Clin Nephrol 2007;68:52-56.

Bailey EM, Faber M, Nafziger DA. Linezolid for treatment of vancomycin-resistant enterococcal peritonitis. Am J Kidney Dis 2001;38:E20.

Barraclough K, Hawley CM, McDonald SP, et al. Corynebacterium peritonitis in Australian peritoneal dialysis patients: predictors, treatment and outcomes in 82 cases. Nephrol Dial Transplant 2009;24:3834-3839.

Bernardini J, Bender F, Florio T, et al. Randomized, double-blind trial of antibiotic exit site cream for prevention of exit site infection in peritoneal dialysis patients. J Am Soc Nephrol 2005;16:539-545.

Choi P, Nemati E, Banerjee A, et al. Peritoneal dialysis catheter removal for acute peritonitis: a retrospective analysis of factors associated with catheter removal and prolonged postoperative hospitalization. Am J Kidney Dis 2004;43:103-111.

Chow KM, Szeto CC, Cheung K, et al. Predictive value of dialysate cell counts in peritonitis complicating peritoneal dialysis. Clin J Am Soc Nephrol 2006;1:768-773.

Chua AN, Goldstein SL, Bell D, Brewer ED. Topical mupirocin/sodium hypochlorite reduces peritonitis and exit-site infection rates in children. Clin J Am Soc Nephrol 2009;4:1939-1943.

Chuang YW, Shu KH, Yu TM, et al. Hypokalaemia: an independent risk factor of enterobacteriaceae peritonitis in CAPD patients. Nephrol Dial Transplant 2009;24:1603-1608.

Chu KH, Choy WY, Cheung CC, et al. A prospective study of the efficacy of local application of gentamicin versus mupirocin in the prevention of peritoneal dialysis catheter-related infections. Perit Dial Int 2008;28:505-508.

Cox SD, Walsh SB, Yaqoob MM, Fan SLS. Predictors of survival and technique success after reinsertion of peritoneal dialysis catheter following severe peritonitis. Perit Dial Int 2007;27:67-73.

Demoulin N, Goffin E. Intraperitoneal urokinase and oral rifampicin for persisting asymptomatic dialysate infection following acute coagulase-negative staphylococcus peritonitis. Perit Dial Int 2009;29:548-553.

De Vin F, Rutherford P, Faict D. Intraperitoneal administration of drugs in peritoneal dialysis patients: a review of compatibility and guidance for clinical use. Perit Dial Int 2009;29:5-15.

Edey M, Hawley CM, McDonald SP, et al. Enterococcal peritonitis in Australian peritoneal dialysis patients: predictors, treatment and outcomes in 116 cases. Nephrol Dial Transplant 2010;25:1272-1278.

Fahim M, Hawley CM, McDonald SP, et al. Culture-negative peritonitis in peritoneal dialysis patients in Australia: predictors, treatment, and outcomes in 435 cases. Am J Kidney Dis 2010;55:690-697.

Firanek C, Guest S. Hand hygiene in peritoneal dialysis. Perit Dial Int 2011;31:399-408.

Fontan MP, Rodriguez-Carmona A, Galed I, et al. Incidence and significance of peritoneal eosinophilia during peritoneal dialysis-related peritonitis. Perit Dial Int 2003;23:460-464.

Freitas C, Rodrigues A, Carvalho MJ, Cabrita A. Exit site infections: systematic microbiologic and quality control are needed. Adv Perit Dial 2009;25:26-31.

Govindarajulu S, Hawley CM, McDonald SP, et al. Staphylococcus aureus peritonitis in Australian peritoneal dialysis patients: predictors, treatment, and outcomes in 503 cases. Perit Dial Int 2010;30:311-319.

Hassoun AA, Coomer RW, Mendez-Vigo L. Intraperitoneal daptomycin used to successfully treat vancomycin-resistant enterococcus peritonitis. Perit Dial Int 2009;29:671-673.

Huen SC, Hall I, Topal J, et al. Successful use of intraperitoneal daptomycin in the treatment of vancomycin-resistant enterococcus peritonitis. Am J Kidney Dis 2009;54:538-541.

Johnson DW, Clark C, Isbel NM, et al. The honeypot study protocol: a randomized controlled trial of exit-site application of medihoney antibacterial wound gel for the prevention of catheter-associated infections in peritoneal dialysis patients. Perit Dial Int 2009;29:303-309.

Matuszkiewicz-Rowinska J. Update on fungal peritonitis and its treatment. Perit Dial Int 2009;29[Suppl 2];S161-S165.

Majkowski NL, Mendley SR. Simultaneous removal and replacement of infected peritoneal dialysis catheters. Am J Kidney Dis 1997;29:706-711.

McQuillan RF, Chiu E, Nessim S, et al. A randomized controlled trial comparing mupirocin and polysporin triple ointments in peritoneal dialysis patients: the MP^3 study. Clin J Am Soc Nephrol 2012;7:297-303.

Mujais S. Microbiology and outcomes of peritonitis in North America. Kidney Int 2006;70[Suppl 103]:S55-S62.

Nessim SJ, Bargman JM, Austin PC, et al. Predictors of peritonitis in patients on peritoneal dialysis: results of a large, prospective Canadian database. Clin J Am Soc Nephrol 2009;4:1195-1200.

Piraino B. Mupirocin for preventing exit-site infection and peritonitis in patients undergoing peritoneal dialysis. Was it effective? Nephrol Dial Transplant 2010;25:349-352.

Piraino B, Bernardini J, Bender FH. An analysis of methods to prevent peritoneal dialysis catheter infections. Perit Dial Int 2008;28:437-443.

Prasad N, Gupta A. Fungal peritonitis in peritoneal dialysis patients. Perit Dial Int 2005;25:207-222.

Rho M, Bia F, Brewster UC. Nontuberculous mycobacterial peritonitis in peritoneal dialysis patients. Semin Dial 2006;20:271-276.

Salzer W. Antimicrobial-resistant gram-positive bacteria in PD peritonitis and the newer antibiotics used to treat them. Perit Dial Int 2005;25:313-319.

Schweinburg FB, Seligman AM, Fine J. Transmural migration of intestinal bacteria: a study based on the use of radioactive Escherichia coli. N Eng J Med 1950;242:747-751.

Siva B, Hawley CM, McDonald SP, et al. Pseudomonas peritonitis in Australia: predictors, treatment, and outcomes in 191 cases. Clin J Am Soc Nephrol 2009;4:957-964.

Sjoland JA, Smith Pedersen R, Jespersen J, Gram J. Intraperitoneal heparin reduces peritoneal permeability and increases ultrafiltration in peritoneal dialysis patients. Nephrol Dial Transplant 2004;19:1264-1268.

Sjoland JA, Pedersen RS, Jespersen J, Gram J. Intraperitoneal heparin ameliorates the systemic inflammatory response in PD patients. Nephron Clin Pract 2005;100:c105-c110.

Sol PM, van de Kar NC, Schreuder MF. Cat induced pasteurella multocida peritonitis in peritoneal dialysis: a case report and review of the literature. Int J Hyg Environ Health 2013;216:211-213.

Szeto CC, Kwan BC, Chow K, et al. Coagulase negative staphylococcal peritonitis in peritoneal dialysis patients: review of 232 consecutive cases. Clin J Am Soc Nephrol 2008;3:91-97.

Szeto CC, Kwan BC, Chow K, et al. Recurrent and relapsing peritonitis: causative organisms and response to treatment. Am J Kidney Dis 2009;54:702-710.

Teitelbaum I. Cloudy peritoneal dialysate: it's not always infection. Contrib Nephrol 2006;150:187-194.

Tong DC, Walker RJ. Antibiotic prophylaxis in dialysis patients undergoing invasive dental treatment. Nephrology 2004;9:167-170.

Yap DY, Tse KC, Lam MF, et al. Polymicrobial CAPD peritonitis after hysteroscopy. Perit Dial Int 2009;29:237-238.

Yip T, Tse KC, Lam MF, et al. Risks and outcomes of peritonitis after flexible colonoscopy in CAPD patients. Perit Dial Int 2007;27:560-564.

Wu HH, Li IJ, Weng CH, et al. Prophylactic antibiotics for endoscopy-associated peritonitis in peritoneal dialysis patients. PLos One 2013;8:e71532.

Antibiotic pharmacokinetics

Cardone KE, Grabe DW, Kulawy RW, et al. Ertapenem pharmacokinetics and pharmacodynamics during continuous ambulatory peritoneal dialysis. Antimicrob Agents Chemother 2012;56:725-730.

Cardone KE, Lodise TP, Patel N, et al. Pharmacokinetics and pharmacodynamics of intravenous daptomycin during continuous ambulatory peritoneal dialysis. Clin J Am Soc Nephrol 2011;6:1081-1088.

Montanes Pauls B, Alminana MA, Casabo Alos VG. Vancomycin pharmacokinetics during continuous ambulatory peritoneal dialysis in patients with peritonitis. Eur J Pharm Sci 2011;43:212-216.

Varghese JM, Roberts JA, Wallis SC, et al. Pharmacokinetics of intraperitoneal gentamicin in peritoneal dialysis patients with peritonitis (GIPD Study). Clin J Am Soc Nephrol 2012;7:1249-1256.

Chapter 12:
Non-Infectious Complications

THIS CHAPTER WILL REVIEW a variety of non-infectious complications that can present during PD therapy. Knowledge of these complications and their management can give added confidence to the PD practitioner. Recognition of the complication, with a strategy to rectify, if possible, can reduce unnecessary patient morbidity and increase long term technique success.

Hernias

Hernias are one of the more frequent non-infectious complications of PD. Increased intra-abdominal pressure due to the dialysate can create or exacerbate pre-existing weaknesses in the supporting abdominal wall structures, leading to hernia formation. The prevalence of hernias in the PD population is reported to be 9% or greater. Umbilical and inguinal hernias are most common. Some, but not all, studies have reported no association between hernias and size of dialysate dwell volume, patient age, catheter type, or body surface area. The majority of hernias presenting during therapy were present before initiating PD. This high incidence of pre-existing hernias suggests that efforts should be made by the surgeon implanting the catheter to consider hernia repair at the time of catheter placement. During the original catheter insertion an intentional inspection of the peritoneal cavity should be performed to detect a patent processus vaginalis or other potential source of hernia with the patient consented for any needed repair at the time of catheter placement.

There are many clinical factors that contribute to the higher risk of hernias in PD patients. The processus vaginalis is a peritoneal diverticulum in the embryonic lower abdominal wall that traverses the inguinal ligament and should normally fuse during fetal development. A patent processus vaginalis, possible in males and females, is felt to be the single most common source of a PD-related hernia. Recurrent direct hernias and incisional hernias can be worsened by the pressure of indwelling PD fluid. Mid-line catheters have a higher incidence of subsequent incisional hernia formation so placement of the catheter's deep cuff in the mid-line linea alba should be avoided.

Patients with autosomal dominant polycystic kidney disease (ADPKD) are at higher risk of developing hernias during PD. The massive cyst burden in many of these patients, combined with a probable underlying collagen defect in the ligamentous structures of the abdominal wall, increases risk of hernia when dialysate is carried in the day dwell. In the ADPKD patient, if the kinetics allow, consideration should be made to PD regimens with APD cycling at night and dry days or reduced volume of dialysate in the day time. Intra-abdominal pressures are highest in the sitting position, compared to standing or lying, so reducing the day dwell may reduce the risk of hernia formation in all patients, but especially in the patient with ADPKD. If adequacy parameters can be maintained, larger, easily reducible hernias may not require repair and the hernia can be treated with a truss and lower dialysate volumes during the day exchange

Management of the PD patient that requires hernia repair can be challenging. The medical team must decide to discontinue PD and temporarily transfer to HD or continue PD throughout the surgical course. It is possible to manage a PD patient through hernia repair surgery without a transfer to temporary HD or exposing the patient to the risk of vascular access catheter placement. Many centers describe successful continuation of PD throughout the pre- and post-operative hernia repair.

Surgical Approach for Hernia Repair

A recommended surgical approach for the PD patient requiring hernia repair is to employ a "tension-free" strategy in which the hernia sac is not opened but inverted back into the peritoneal cavity, an overlying prolene mesh is placed in the extra-peritoneal space to support the musculature and take tension off the wound, allowing for continuation of PD. As the mesh is external to the peritoneum, the risk of any subsequent mesh infection due to peritonitis is averted. The mesh supports the abdominal wall and prevents any direct pressure to be exerted on the prior hernia defect or skin incision - the so called "tension-free" repair. Inguinal hernia tension-free repairs have used the Prolene Hernia System (PHS: Ethicon Inc. Johnson and Johnson, New Jersey, USA). Using this tension-free approach, practitioners have been able to initiate PD within hours to days of hernia repair, and avoid the inconvenience, morbidity, and expense involved with transfer to temporary hemodialysis.

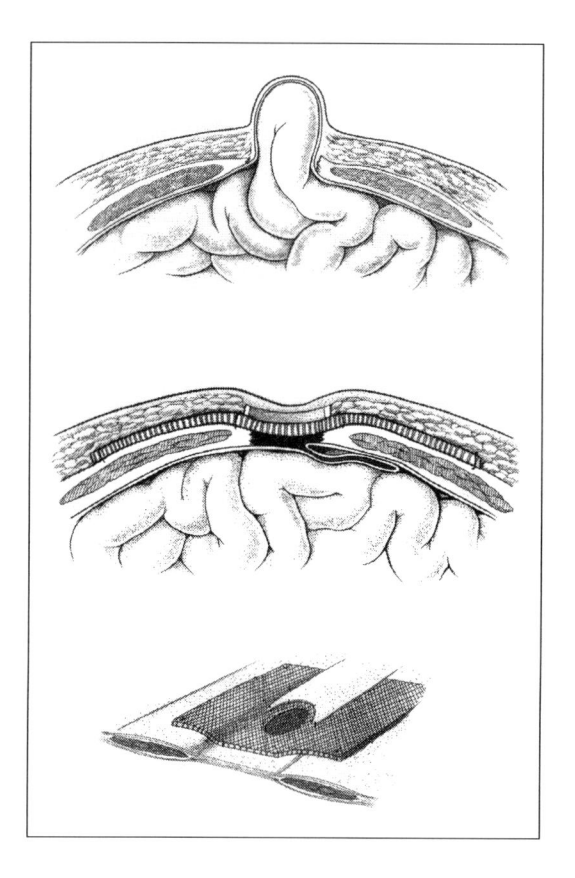

Preoperative hernia presentation

Hernia sack is inverted without damaging peritoneum followed by placement of external mesh

Coronal view showing "butterfly" or "H" mesh in place creating tension-free hernia repair

A reasonable protocol for maintaining the patient on PD throughout the hernia repair period:

1. On the morning of surgery, drain all PD fluid

2. Send for hernia repair, ideally using tension-free techniques described

3. Hold PD for 24 - 48 hours

4. Lower volume, recumbent PD with dry days, for up to 2 weeks

5. Lower volume day exchanges can be added at 2 weeks

6. Resume full dose PD therapy at 4 - 5 weeks.

Adapted from reference Shah, Chu, Bargman.

Hydrothorax

The normal diaphragm is a thin musculo-fibrous membrane formed by the embryological fusion of the septum transversum, abdominal wall, mesogastrium and pleuroperitoneal membranes. Failure to fuse properly leads to diaphragmatic hernias, or vents in the membrane leading to a porous diaphragm syndrome. Defects in the diaphragm can be single or multiple, pinhole to web-like, and are usually due to abnormalities in the tendinous structures within the diaphragm. Acquired defects have been described due to increased abdominal pressure occurring with coughing, trauma, endometrial or malignant implants on the diaphragm, and possibly the increased pressure created during heavy exercise or pregnancy.

A pleural effusion in a PD patient raises concern that the patient may manifest a porous diaphragm syndrome, allowing dialysate to transverse the diaphragm and enter the pleural space. Presenting complaints may be shortness of breath or a dry cough. The prevalence of PD-related hydrothorax is estimated at 1.6 %, is right-sided in up to 88% of cases, and may be more common in females and patients with underlying ADPKD.

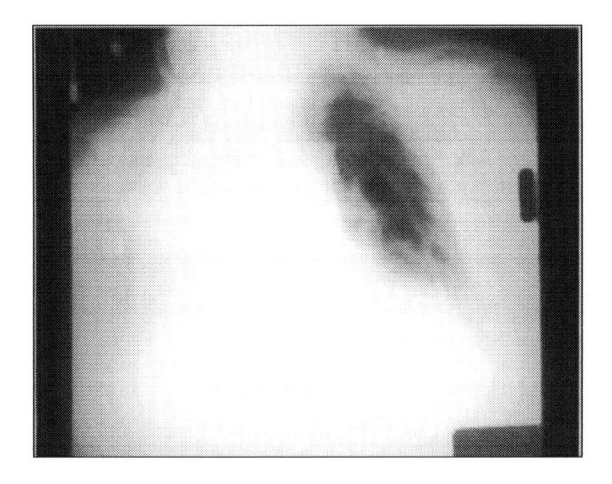

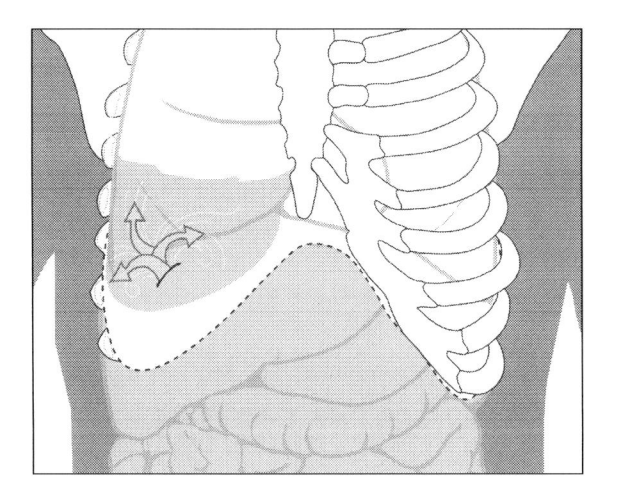

Right-sided hydrothorax in a PD patient with underlying ADPKD

The right-sided predominance is felt to be due to the observation that more embryological diaphragmatic defects are in the right hemidiaphragm. The liver capsule can create a piston effect propelling dialysate across the right-sided diaphragmatic defect. The heart and pericardium, covering a portion of the left diaphragm, may act to tamponade any defects in the left hemidiaphragm.

PD related hydrothorax is typically right-sided due to congenital or acquired diaphragmatic defects

Diagnosing a PD-related hydrothorax

A hydrothorax from PD fluid in the pleural space is typically transudative in nature, demonstrates higher glucose concentration compared to the serum (so called "sweet effusion), has low protein content, and a variable cell count that includes peritoneal mesothelial cells.

Patients using icodextrin can have a sample of the pleural fluid taken with a drop of povidone-iodine added- if the mixture creates a noticeably blue-black color it would confirm the starch-iodine reaction that absorbs visible light. Use of this "black line sign" confirms peritoneal icodextrin has reached the pleural cavity.

To confirm a pleuroperitoneal communication, some authors describe use of radioisotope or CT scanning. With scintigraphy, Technetium 99 tin-colloid, 15 mCi is aseptically injected into the peritoneal cavity via the PD catheter during a long dwell. Anterior and posterior imaging is taken within one hour and then delayed images are obtained at 3 and 6 and 24 hours. Unfortunately, the sensitivity of scintigraphy is low.

Contrast CT imaging is done by aseptically adding 150 ml of contrast media to a 2 L solution bag and infused into the peritoneal cavity. After dwelling for several hours 10mm axial sections are taken from the thorax to abdomen to attempt to locate the communication. Again, sensitivity of this imaging modality is low (<50%).

Attempts to directly visualize the communication during thoracoscopy, guided by discoloration of the PD fluid with methylene blue, indigo carmine, or indocyanine green have been described. In many instances, these dyes have assisted in the identification of diaphragmatic blebs or defects and allowed for surgical intervention. Chemical peritonitis has been reported after dye addition but potential benefits in guiding a surgical intervention would seem to outweigh the risk. Many reports document safe use of injectable dyes to assist in the location of diaphragmatic defects.

Treatment of PD-related hydrothorax

In small case series, a PD-related hydrothorax has occasionally been noted to spontaneously resolve and require no further intervention. In cases of small effusions, lower volume PD could be attempted, especially avoiding higher dwell volumes while the patient is sitting, as the sitting position is associated with highest intra-abdominal pressure.

In patients with persistent effusions, an intervention is required if the patient is to continue long-term PD. Treatment approaches vary from therapeutic thoracentesis, followed by sclerosing therapy, to more invasive thoracoscopic procedures.

Thoracic surgeons or pulmonologists could be consulted to consider pleurodesis with talc, oxytetracycline, autologous blood or fibrin glue. These physicians are well versed in treating recurrent pleural effusions, as pleurodesis was the historic treatment for effusions related to chronic TB or malignancy. More modern approaches to hydrothorax would involve video-assisted thoracoscopic surgery (VATS). VATS procedures use mini-laparoscopic type equipment to enter the pleural space and attempt to directly visualize and allow direct suturing of the site of the diaphragmatic leak. VATS-assisted placement of an overlying mesh to seal the defect has also been described. VATS procedures to guide talc pleurodesis have been successful in cases where a definitive communication could not be visualized. In these cases, the patients are converted to hemodialysis via temporary vascular access catheters and then placed under general anesthesia and intubated with a dual lumen endotracheal tube that allows for separate lung ventilation, and facilitates deflation of the ipsilateral lung. The patient is placed in the decubitus position with the effected lung field positioned up to allow for the thoracoscope to be inserted. Additional ports are created to allow for surgical oversewing or for the talc instillation (typically 10 grams of talc powder). Chronic PD therapy is resumed several weeks post-operatively. Recurrence of hydrothorax is possible but rare.

Lastly, there are reports of diaphragmatic defects being repaired with surgeons being guided by observing injected air bubbles moving from the abdominal compartment into the pleural space. During the VATS procedure, the pleural space is partially filled by sterile water, CO2 is injected into the abdomen using the catheter and any bubble formation is noted at the location of the diaphragmatic defect.

Clinical Approach to Hydrothorax

1. Perform thoracentesis for symptomatic relief and for diagnosis of a "sweet" effusion

2. PD should be temporarily held to allow for absorption of the pleural fluid via pleural lymphatics

3. Lower volume PD could be attempted, in the recumbent position, avoiding the increased intra-abdominal pressure noted in the sitting position with patient observed for possible spontaneous closure

4. If spontaneous closure does not occur PD is again held and a pulmonologist or thoracic surgeon consulted for possible talc or other chemical pleurodesis or VATS procedure

5. If these procedures not available or patient unable, convert to HD

Subcutaneous Leaks

A leak of dialysate into the subcutaneous tissue usually presents with unusual swelling along the abdominal wall, flank area, scrotum, labia or thighs. The overlying skin may take on a boggy appearance with unusual pitting at the belt line. The patient may report weight gain but without pedal edema and a diminished dialysate drain. In the obese patient, a subcutaneous leak may be very insidious and hard to initially detect.

The etiology of the leak is usually due to a disruption in the integrity of the deep cuff. The deep cuff is within the rectus muscle and has had in-growth of muscle tissue around the cuff to prevent a leak of fluid from the peritoneal space. If, however, the deep cuff becomes dislodged temporarily, due to trauma or initial poor placement, the cuff no longer has in-growth of tissue to act as a barrier. The leaking dialysate can track through the subcutaneous tissue into dependent areas such as the genitals.

Leaks usually present within the first few weeks after catheter insertion and imply that the deep cuff has not had sufficient in-growth of tissue. To reduce the incidence of early leaks, catheter placement using laparoscopic rectus sheath tunneling has been advocated. In this procedure the deep cuff is placed within the rectus muscle sheath and then a segment of the catheter is tunneled inferiorly within the sheath before entering the peritoneal space. Other risk factors associated with leaks are hypoalbuminemia and malnutrition, cuff placement in the midline linea alba, and high fluid volumes initially prescribed in new starts.

If an acute leak has been discovered, clinicians can temporarily hold PD for 1-2 days and then employ lower volume, supine PD with dry days for an additional time period. Many acute leaks may spontaneously heal. Leaks occurring over 30 days after starting PD have been attributed to weaker abdominal muscle tone and have been noted more in females, many of whom have mutiparity. Other causes of late leaks include trauma to the catheter with partial dislodgement of the deep cuff or tracking of fluid into the subcutaneous tissues from a hernia.

In many cases temporary cessation of PD followed by lower volume exchanges may allow the peri-catheter leak to heal. If, however, the leak persists after temporary cessation of PD, surgical repair of the deep cuff or replacement of the catheter may be required. In this case, the surgeon should strongly consider simultaneous removal of the old catheter with replacement of a new catheter, without any disruption in PD. Several authors have described simultaneous catheter replacement as a way to avoid conversion to temporary HD. Catheter placement is followed by supine, low volume dialysis until the deep cuff has sealed.

Dialysate leaks can be detected by CT, MRI, or nuclear imaging studies. With CT imaging, contrast can be added to the dialysate and infused with the patient instructed to ambulate for several hours before the imaging occurs. Scintigraphy after the addition of 2 mCi of Tc-99m surfur colloid to 2000 mL dialysate infusion has been described. Alternatively, recent reports demonstrate that the dialysate itself enhances under T2 images with MRI. No gadolinium is required to make the diagnosis as the PD fluid itself acts as the contrasting agent.

Genital Swelling

Scrotal swelling and labial swelling in females is typically attributed to 2 main causes- a patent processus vaginalis (PPV) or subcutaneous tissue leak of dialysate that distributes into the scrotum or labia. The predominant cause of marked, isolated scrotal or labial swelling is the PPV. In these cases, the PPV is small enough to prohibit bowel entry and the formation of a true hernia but, rather, allows for dialysate to descend into the patent processus vaginalis and enter the scotum. The genital swelling can be quite remarkable in this situation.

Patients with subcutaneous leaks will often have signs of leak in the subcutaneous tissue of the lower abdomen with evidence of these changes continuing into the genitalia- changes such as a palpable thickness of the tissue or visible peau d'orange appearance of surrounding skin.

To differentiate between these 2 presentations and to confirm the diagnosis, a CT peritoneogram or nuclear medicine scan can be useful. In CT peritoneography, 100 to 150 mL of contrast material can be added to a 2 L dialysate bag and infused into the patient. The patient is asked to remain ambulatory (active) for 30 to 60 minutes to increase the intra-abdominal pressure and then undergo CT images of the abdomen and processus vaginalis. Similarly, 2 mCi of Tc-99m surfur colloid can be sterilely injected into 2000 mL of dialysate, infused and after similar period of activity the patient can undergo peritoneal scintigraphy.

In patients diagnosed with a PPV, surgical correction will be required to resolve the genital edema. Patients with significant residual kidney function can be attempted with nightly exchanges and dry days if kinetic clearance targets can be achieved.

Hemoperitoneum

Hemoperitoneum refers to blood-tinged PD fluid. Benign causes of hemoperitoneum include retrograde menstruation, ovulation or rupture of an ovarian cyst, endometriosis, pregnancy, trauma from the PD catheter itself, or an acquired coagulopathy.

More malignant causes of hemoperitoneum include malignancy from peritoneal primary tumors or metastatic seeding, ovarian or colon cancer or other intra-abdominal malignancies. Other rare causes of hemoperitoneum include pancreatitis, encapsulating peritoneal sclerosis, rupture of the liver capsule, or spleen. Most sources of bleeding are from the intraperitoneal location but hemoperitoneum may also present from retroperitoneal sources such as a retroperitoneal hematoma, varix, or renal cyst. A careful clinical history of associated pain onset may direct clinicians to the inciting location.

Causes of hemoperitoneum

Ovulation	Peritonitis
Retrograde menstruation	Malignancy - Ovarian, Colon
Complication of pregnancy	Peritoneal metastases
Ruptured ovarian cyst	Encapsulating peritoneal sclerosis
Endometriosis	Pancreatitis
Ectopic pregnancy	Splenic laceration or rupture
Acquired coagulopathy	Cyst rupture- liver, kidney
Catheter trauma	Post-procedure-colonoscopy, radiation
External abdominal trauma	Vascular aneurysms

In the patient presenting with hemoperitoneum, the physical exam should be directed toward rapidly excluding hemodynamic instability or serious underlying abdominal pathology, which would require urgent surgical evaluation. Once the patient is deemed stable, a hemoperitoneum is observed expectantly as most cases are benign and transient and resolve within days. In many cases, the hemoperitoneum will clear with flushing of the peritoneum with several rapid exchanges, preferably of unwarmed, room temperature solutions to induce transient vasoconstriction. Although it would seem counter intuitive, low dose intraperitoneal heparin should be considered to avoid clot formation that could obstruct the catheter. As the administered heparin has not been shown to be systemically absorbed, intraperitoneal heparin may be an important measure to avoid catheter loss due to clots or subsequent fibrin formation.

More persistent or profuse hemoperitoneum may require abdominal imaging and surgical consultation and possibly laparascopic investigation. Temporary cessation of PD may be required post operatively but low volume PD can often be resumed within 48 to 72 hours to avoid transfer to hemodialysis.

> Clinical Approach to Hemoperitoneum
>
> 1. Assess for hemodynamic stability
>
> 2. Abdominal examination to exclude acute abdomen / abdominal catastrophe
>
> 3. If patient stable, consider trial of unwarmed, room temperature dialysate flushes to induce peritoneal vessel vasoconstriction
>
> 4. Consider intraperitoneal heparin 500-1000 units per 2L dwell
>
> 5. Consider desmopressin
>
> 6. If persists, abdominal imaging and surgical consultation should be obtained

Chylous Dialysate

Chyloperitoneum has been described in patients on peritoneal dialysis. The drained dialysate has a milky white, turbid appearance with varying cell count, and contains triglyceride levels that exceed those in the plasma. Turbidity of dialysate can vary depending on the content of recently ingested dietary fat.

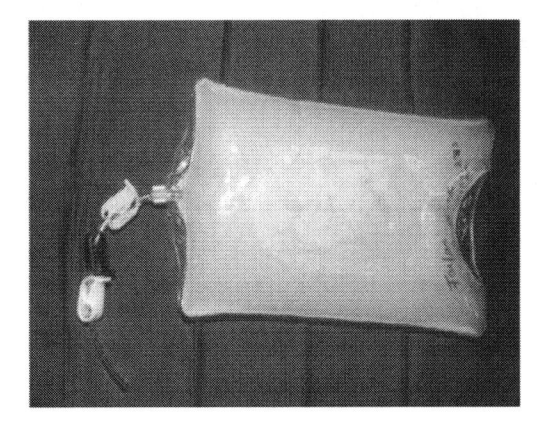

Chylous dialysate in a patient subsequently diagnosed with lymphoma

Dialysate bacterial cultures are negative. Several causes of chylous peritoneum have been described including lymphatic obstruction due to trauma, surgery, an inflammatory process, constrictive pericarditis, or malignancy, particularly lymphoma. In developing countries chylous ascites has been associated with tuberculosis and filariasis.

Causes of Chyloperitoneum

Lymphoma	S/p recent PD catheter placement
Non-lymphoma abdominal malignacy	S/p abdominal aortic aneurysm repair
Lymphatic metastases	S/p cholecystectomy
Infectious peritonitis, especially mycobacterial, filariasis	Pancreatitis
Adenitis in SLE	Cirrhosis
Amyloidosis	Superior vena cava syndrome
Calcium channel blocker medications	Mimicked by calcium-hydroxyphosphate-apatite crystals

Many descriptions of chylous dialysate occurring after percutaneous PD catheter placement suggest that fine lymphatic vessel may be inadvertently injured during the placement procedure. In most of these cases, the chyloperitoneum spontaneously resolves within weeks but may require temporary cessation of PD.

Both dihydropyridine and non-dihydropyridine calcium channel blockers have been described to cause chyloperitoneum. Although the mechanism is unclear many of these agents are lipophilic and able to insert into the lipid bilayer of smooth muscle cells and perhaps cause dilation of the lymphatic vessels, opening up clefts in the vessels that allow for lipid-rich lymphatic fluid to leak into the peritoneal cavity. In these cases, the chylous dialysate was noted to resolve after discontinuation of the medication. A recent report described an additional medication-induced presentation of chyloperitoneum involving aliskiren.

Chylous ascites was also described as occurring after repeated peritonitis episodes suggesting lymphatic obstruction due to subsequent scarring and adhesion formation. Lastly, milky ascites was recently noted in a long-standing PD patient due to calcium-hydroxyphosphate-apatite crystals presenting as calcifying sclerosing peritonitis.

As mentioned, many cases of chyloperitoneum require no treatment and resolve spontaneously. In persistent chyloperitoneum, the turbidity of the fluid, which is attributed to the triglyceride-rich lymphatic fluid, can be lessened by changing the diet to a low fat, low triglyceride diet to reduce lymph flow. Care must be taken, however, to ensure that patients maintain overall good nutrition and can tolerate the ongoing loss of fats in the dialysate. The diet can be supplemented with medium-chain triglycerides which are absorbed directly into the portal system instead of intestinal lymphatics. Resolution of chylous ascites has been described with orlistat (Xenical), a reversible inhibitor of pancreatic and gastric lipases. Orlistat prevents digestion of triglycerides into free fatty acids within the intestines and prevents absorption. Subcutaneous octreotide, a somatostatin analogue capable of reducing gastric, pancreatic and intestinal secretions has successfully treated chylous ascites in a dialysis patient, but the overall clinical experience with these agents is limited.

Clinical Approach to Chylous Dialysate

1. Rule out infectious peritonitis - bacterial, fungal, mycobacterial

2. Abdominal imaging to exclude malignancy or other lymphatic pathology

3. Discontinue calcium channel blocker medications or aliskiren

4. Dietary alteration to reduce long-chain fatty acids and increase medium-chain triglycerides

5. Consider oral orlistat

6. Consider subcutaneous octreotide

7. Consider laparoscopic exploration of source of lymphatic leak after prior ingestion of high fat meal and/or sudan black ingestion

---

Complications Unique to the Female Patient

Vaginal leaking of dialysate is an extremely rare complication and may present early in the initiation of PD or present later in the course of therapy. The main causes of vaginal dialysate leaks include fallopian tube drainage of dialysate into the uterus, a uterine/peritoneal fistula or erosion of the catheter into the uterine or vaginal cavity.

The fallopian tubes contain fimbriae with ciliary hairs that function to sweep ova released from the ovary into the fallopian tube. Rarely, the fimbria capture the distal dialysis catheter allowing infused fluid to overcome the natural resistance to flow within the fallopian tubes and direct dialysate down the fallopian tubes and into the uterus and vagina. Catheters are subsequently freed of the fimbria, during laparotomy, and this procedure combined with tubal ligation has repaired the leak.

Late vaginal leaks have been described, mainly as a post-operative complication after hernia repair or other operative procedure. The vaginal leak has been determined to be a surgical complication of inadvertent damage to the wall of the uterus or catheter erosion into the uterine wall. Surgical repair of the fistula has allowed resumption of PD.

Uterine and uterovaginal prolapse has been described as a complication of PD and can be considered analogous to the hernia presentation. Weakened pelvic supporting structures may not sufficiently support the weight of the instilled dialysate, in the upright position, and create the pelvic prolapse. Women at highest risk are those with multiple vaginal childbirths, advanced age, obesity, and chronic constipation. Often the prolapse appears only during an upright dialysate dwell and is noted to resolve when fluid is drained. Management of this complication can involve surgical interventions to improve pelvic support but more conservative approaches have included use of APD, as opposed to CAPD, and reducing the day dwell volume, especially in patients with significant residual kidney function. Also, use of a vaginal ring pessary has been successful in reducing prolapse symptoms.

Back Pain

A 2 liter bag of PD dialysate in the abdomen represents a 2 kilogram weight that can put mechanical stress on the lumbar spine. The dialysate may increase the tendency of the spine to assume a more lordotic position. This can be exacerbated by weakened anterior abdominal muscles due to de-conditioning or prior surgeries. Treatment of PD-related back pain can involve lower back strengthening exercises that emphasize strengthening of the "internal corset" muscles, a reduction in the ambulatory dwell volume, or a dry day and strictly nightly recumbent cycler regimen, in those with significant residual kidney function.

Drain Pain

As also discussed in Chapter 8, patients on peritoneal dialysis occasionally experience abdominal pain during the phase of the dialysis exchange when fluid is draining from the peritoneal cavity. Commonly referred to as "drain pain", this discomfort is attributed to contact between the lining of the peritoneal membrane and the dialysis catheter.

A variety of general recommendations have been made to reduce or eliminate drain pain. Patients can change body position during the drain phase to determine if discomfort can be minimized in a certain body position. Constipation may contribute to drain pain so laxative therapy may reduce the discomfort. Dietary changes to reduce constipation may also be of benefit.

In the CAPD patient, drain pain can be minimized by manual cessation of the drain at the point of abdominal discomfort or by slowing the dialysate flow rate during the drain by changing the height of the drain bag. Success reducing drain pain has been described with these maneuvers.

An APD prescription change may reduce drain pain. Changing to a tidal modality that allows a small portion of the drain volume to remain in the abdomen to act as a "cushion" and prevent complete drainage of the abdomen may reduce drain discomfort. If drain pain persists, there are several cycler-specific changes that have been described. As drain pain is attributable, in part, to the catheter's suction force created by the fluid draining by gravity and by the cycler-generated negative pressure, raising the cycler relative to the body position (or lowering the patient relative to the cycler) may reduce this suctioning force. Alternatively, if a patient is prescribed a NIPD prescription with a dry day, the initial drain pain may be mitigated by performing a manual fill prior to connecting to the cycler. This manual fill prevents the abdomen from being dry during the cycler's initial drain phase.

In many patients, drain pain may dissipate over time. In those patients that experience continued drain pain, despite the above maneuvers, catheter repositioning or replacement may be required.

Clinical Approach to Drain Pain

1. Institute trial of aggressive laxative therapy

2. Evaluate for body position that reduces or eliminates complaint

3. If persists, abdominal x-ray to evaluate catheter position and check for residual stool

4. Institute tidal PD regimen to allow for reservoir "cushion" of fluid which reduces full drain to final exchange only

5. If on APD therapy, consider raising cycler level up to 12 inches relative to mid-abdomen to reduce cycler machine "pull" of dialysate

6. If drain pain persists question is raised of catheter involvement with adhesions or catheter positioned too deeply within the peritoneum and therefore irritating innervated peritoneal surface- consider surgical intervention to reposition deep catheter segment by use of a purse-string suture to resuspend catheter in different pelvic location

Encapsulating Peritoneal Sclerosis (EPS)

EPS is perhaps the most serious complication of long-term PD characterized by symptoms mimicking an intermittent small bowel ileus such as nausea, vomiting and intestinal obstruction. Inability to take oral nutrition consistently leads to weight loss and need, in some patients, for parenteral nutrition. EPS typically occurs in a patient on longstanding PD with demonstrated ultrafiltration failure and high peritoneal membrane transport status.

Diagnosis is confirmed by radiographic imaging with CT scanning of the abdomen which reveals a markedly thickened peritoneal membrane extending from the visceral peritoneal to parietal peritoneal surface with encasement of small bowel that limits normal motility. Also referred to as abdominal "cocooning", the thickened fibrotic membrane creates cystic fluid collections that establish the diagnosis of EPS.

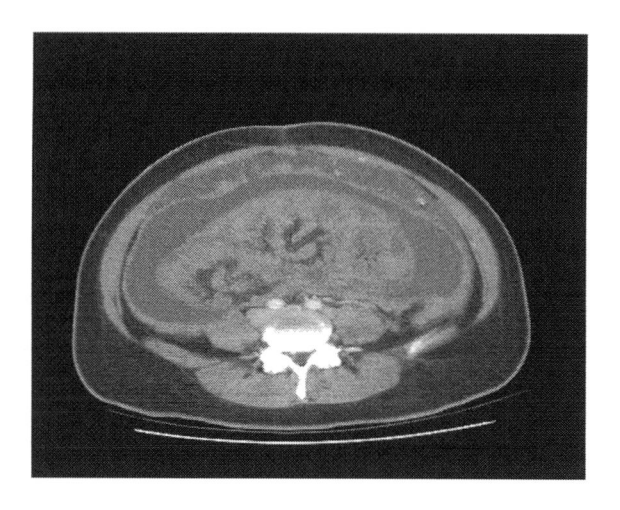

CT scan of encapsulating peritoneal sclerosis showing thickened peritoneal membrane, ascites and cocooning of bowel

EPS has been described worldwide in PD patients both on continuous and intermittent PD regimens. The prevalence estimates vary between 0.5% and 7.3% and risk appears to increase with years on PD. EPS can present after cessation of PD therapy and a recent cluster of publications has reported on EPS occurring in the post-transplant period. Morbidity and mortality rates are high with cause of death being malnutrition and sepsis.

The etiology of EPS is unclear. Peritoneal dialysis solutions are inherently bio-incompatible and expose the peritoneal membrane to glucose, glucose degradation products, advanced glycation end-products, lactate and low pH. As a result, the peritoneal membrane undergoes changes characterized by loss of normal mesothelial cell morphology, expansion of the submesothelial compact zone and neovascularization of the peritoneal membrane. It is unclear if EPS represents a serious final progression, in some patients, of this underlying peritoneal reaction to dialysate or is due to a "second hit" insult to the peritoneum already damaged by the dialysis process. The inflammatory/fibrotic peritoneal capsule that characterizes EPS is likely due, in part, to aberrant fibroblast activity with abnormal fibroblast expression of growth factors such as TGF-*B* which stimulates production of collagen and other extracellular matrix components. Interestingly, mesothelial cells exposed to peritoneal dialysate have been described to undergo a morphometric/functional alteration and change phenotype to become myofibroblasts- a process termed epithelial-to-mesenchymal transition (EMT).

These myofibroblasts migrate into the sub-compact zone and may overproduce TGF-*B* driving thickening of the membrane. Some fibroblasts have also been identified as having estrogen receptors and it is unclear whether estrogen stimulation could be permissive in the development of EPS.

As mentioned, several recent reports suggest that post-transplant patients who have been on long-standing PD may be at increased risk of EPS. With successful transplantation there is cessation of PD and therefore cessation of peritoneal lavage that may allow reactive peritoneum to accumulate fibrin, growth factors, or cytokines and trigger increased fibrosis. Additionally, the recent trends in transplantation medicine of employing prednisone sparing immunosuppressive regimens and the use of pro-fibrotic calcineurin inhibitors, such as cyclosporine and tacrolimus, may contribute to the inflammation and fibrosis that herald the development of EPS in the post-transplant period. Further research is needed to clarify these issues.

Treatments of EPS include cessation of PD and nutritional support with total parenteral nutrition if needed. Medical and surgical approaches have been advocated. Medical approaches involve initiation of general anti-inflammatory and/or anti-fibrotic agents such as glucocorticoids, mycophenolate mofetil, colchicine or tamoxifen.

A tamoxifen precursor was originally developed as a possible contraceptive agent then altered to become the current agent and employed as a selective estrogen receptor modulator as adjuvant therapy for breast cancer. Tamoxifen demonstrated an anti-fibrotic activity and has been a treatment of retroperitoneal fibrosis, fibrosing mediastinitis, idiopathic sclerosing cervicitis and rapidly growing desmoid tumors. Use of tamoxifen in EPS was first described in 1992, with typical doses being 10 to 40 mg a day.

In EPS, experience with tamoxifen is limited to case reports and small case series. These reports document stabilization, improvement, or resolution of EPS, but the number of unpublished non-responders is not known. Tamoxifen has been used as monotherapy or in combination with glucocorticoids.

Tamoxifen therapy is generally well-tolerated and safe. Constitutional side effects include flushing, fatigue, nausea, and tachycardia. Safe use of tamoxifen has been described in patients with recent fungal infections and underlying chronic viral infections such as HIV and hepatitis C. The primary adverse event, in the breast cancer risk trials, was an increase in the hypercoagulable state resulting in increased risk of deep venous thrombosis. Tamoxifen was shown to increase levels of certain coagulation factors while decreasing anticoagulant protein levels. Additionally, a recent report noted platelet activation with exposure to tamoxifen. Platelets of men and women have estrogen receptors on the plasma membrane that may trigger platelet activation, on exposure to tamoxifen. Alternatively, tamoxifen has recently been shown to increase platelet intracellular calcium concentrations leading to platelet activation. If clotting risk is related to enhanced platelet activation it seems prudent to consider co-administration with anti-platelet agents such as aspirin. More work is needed, however, before evidence-based recommendations can be made.

The mechanism of action of tamoxifen in EPS is unclear. Some reports suggest that tamoxifen may down-regulate TGF-*B*, a growth factor implicated in adverse peritoneal membrane changes. Other literature, however, reports that tamoxifen increases TGF-*B* production. Further work is needed to clarify the mechanism of action invoked by tamoxifen to better understand the rationale for use. No randomized controlled trial of tamoxifen, or any other medical therapy in EPS exist, so firm clinical recommendations are difficult to establish.

Intermittent peritoneal lavage, after cessation of long-standing PD, has been recommended by some authors to reduce the likelihood of progressing to EPS. By maintaining the abdominal catheter after converting to HD, once daily to once weekly lavage of the abdomen with dialysate was felt to dilute and remove accumulating inflammatory mediators that may be permissive in the development of EPS. More clinical experience with this lavage strategy to reduce incidence of EPS is needed.

In patients that do not respond to an attempt at empiric medical therapy and present with recurrent obstructive gastrointestinal symptoms, surgical intervention may be indicated. Japanese centers report the largest surgical experience in the world. Kawanishi and colleagues described the surgical approach and results of over 100 operations in 86 patients. The encased bowel is carefully freed from the adhering fibrous capsule by peritonectomy and enterolysis.

Meticulous attempts are made to peel the fibrotic encapsulating membrane off underlying bowel wall, avoiding bowel perforation or bowel resection. Even in the most skilled hands, however, the fibrous peel may be so adhered or calcified that partial bowel resection, combined with diverting colostomy or jejunoscopy may be required. Recurrence of the encapsulation was noted in over 20% of operative cases, often requiring recurrent surgical interventions.

Recently, Kawanishi and colleagues applied an additional procedure in some cases - a Noble plication procedure. In the Noble plication, first describe in 1937 and subsequently modified by others, the small bowel is aligned and kept together with running sutures through the serosal surface and mesentery. By aligning the small bowel loops in an orderly manner, the bowel has less likelihood of developing adhesions between the bowel segments and less chance of descending into the deep pelvis. Initial descriptions of this adjunctive procedure, added to peritonectomy and enterolysis, showed no initial recurrences of EPS in 13 patients. Other rare reports describe various drainage and splinting procedures, with Miller-Abbott or Jones tubes, with some success.

At the time of diagnosis of EPS, discontinuation of PD but continuation of weekly peritoneal lavage, using the catheter, has recently been shown to be effective, in some cases. More research is needed to clarify whether retaining the catheter for intermittent lavage, after cessation of PD, can impact the course of EPS.

Clinical Approach to EPS

1. With confirmation of EPS by CT imaging, conversion to hemodialysis is recommended

2. Consider intermittent peritoneal lavage after PD has been discontinued

3. Maintain adequate nutrition - parenteral nutrition may be necessary

4. Strongly consider medical therapy with anti-inflammatory and/or anti-fibrotic agents

5. If continued obstructive gastrointestinal symptoms, surgical intervention can be considered with emphasis on avoiding bowel resection with priority given to removal of fibrotic capsule only - peritonectomy

6. In post-transplant patients, consider converting pro-fibrotic calcineurin inhibitors to alternate immunosuppressive agent

---

Eosinophilic Peritonitis

Eosinophilic peritonitis typically occurs within the first few weeks of initiating PD. Patients may present with mild abdominal discomfort and cloudy peritoneal fluid, mimicking early bacterial peritonitis. The PD fluid is notable for a predominance of eosinophils and fluid cultures remain sterile. Over half of the patients also demonstrate a peripheral eosinophilia. Estimates of 2 to 4 % of patients may present with eosinophilic peritonitis. The eosinophilic peritonitis usually spontaneously resolves over the ensuing weeks but some reports have shown a smoldering course of up to 6 months. After ruling out bacterial, fungal and mycobacterial infection some authors suggest temporary antihistamines or low dose steroid therapy to quicken the resolution.

The etiology of eosinophilic peritonitis is unclear and many have speculated that it represents a mild allergic reaction to possible plasticizers in the PD bags or catheter or an eosinophilic reaction to the solutions, past antibiotics, insufflation gases used during laparoscopic catheter placement, or inadvertent air injection during the exchanges.

Possible etiologies of non-infectious eosinophilic peritonitis

1. Transient hypersensitivity to plasticizers or siliconized rubber in the catheter
2. Intraperitoneal air
3. Intraperitoneal blood
4. Dialysate additives such as antibiotics, heparin
5. Accidental instillation of minute amounts of the sterilizing povidone-iodine
6. Icodextrin
7. Encapsulating peritoneal sclerosis

The presentation has been described after surgical and percutaneous catheter placements possibly indicating transient reactions to the catheter. Eosinophilic peritonitis rarely recurs but recurrent episodes of have been associated with encapsulating peritoneal sclerosis.

Clinical approach to eosinophilic peritonitis

1. Rule out infectious causes including bacterial, fungal, mycobacterial
2. Watchful waiting- may take weeks to months to resolve
3. Consider abdominal CT imaging to exclude any underlying pathology
4. Consider short trial of anti-histamines or oral steroid therapy to quicken resolution

Pancreatitis

Some reports, but not all, suggest there may be an increased incidence of pancreatitis in PD patients. In one review reporting a positive association, the incidence of acute pancreatitis was 18 per 1000 patient-years in PD patients compared to 6.5 per 1000 patient-years in HD. It is difficult to assess true causality, however, due to the other significant contributors to pancreatitis such as alcohol ingestion, underlying cholelithiasis, medications, etc.

The pancreas is in the retroperitoneal position, covered by a layer of peritoneum, yet dialysate can gain access via the epiploic foramen, to the lesser sac, to be in contact with the peritoneum overlying the anterior head of the pancreas. Several potential triggers of pancreatitis have been proposed, but not proven, including intra-abdominal pressure exerted by dialysate or the higher calcium content of some PD solutions. Hypercalcemia is noted in many dialysis patients due to calcium containing phosphate binders, vitamin D administration or hyperparathyroidism and was noted in up to a third of cases presenting with pancreatitis. The role that hypercalcemia or calcium in the dialysate may play in precipitating pancreatitis is still unclear.

Pancreatitis presents with abdominal pain and can mimic the presentation of peritonitis. PD fluid has been described as clear, cloudy, hemorrhagic, tea or dark colored. Dialysate cell counts have been described as normal or elevated, and, if elevated, can exceed 100 cells/mm^3. Infectious peritonitis should always be excluded. Diagnosis can be made by elevations is serum amylase - greater than 3 fold elevations in most cases but not all. Elevated lipase values are often also noted. Amylase concentrations greater than 100 U/L in the dialysate are suggestive of pancreatitis. The diagnosis can be further confirmed by computerized tomography showing signs of pancreatitis.

In patients treated with icodextrin, serum amylase levels may be falsely lowered, as icodextrin itself competes with the test reagents used in many common assays. The serum lipase level should be considered the main serum diagnostic aid in patients suspected of pancreatitis who are using icodextrin.

Most patients have been managed conservatively with few reports of abscess, pseudo-cyst formation or death.

The Colors of Dialysate

Many non-infectious complications or other clinical scenarios can be notable for a change in color of the dialysate. The red colored dialysate in hemoperitoneum and the milky white chylous peritoneum were previously discussed. A dark greenish dialysate, often with small digested food material, indicates the probable rupture of a posterior duodenal ulcer with fresh bile entering the peritoneal fluid or a ruptured gall bladder. Recognition of this leads to rapid operative intervention, the site of perforation clear to the surgeon due to this bile in the dialysate. Alternately, dark feculent material, without the bilious color, would suggest a large bowel perforation.

In a rare instance the dialysate returned with a bright green, fluorescent color. This can be, obviously, shocking and concerning to the patient and medical staff. The color change occurred due to clearance of dye used for fluorescein angiography done to investigate diabetic retinopathy.

A blue-black colored dialysate bag or tubing can be encountered in patient's using icodextrin. Icodextrin can have an interaction with iodine similar to the Schiff reaction.

In the Schiff reaction iodine interacts with the coils of beta amylase molecules in starch to form a dense complex that absorbs various spectra of visible light. Icodextrin resembles starch, being a soluble glucose polymer, and interacts with the iodine contained in povidone-iodine preparations used to sterilize the injection port or the cap on the transfer set. A dark precipitate in the tubing (dark line sign) has been described due to this icodextrin-iodine interaction.

Additional colors described in the literature are the brownish-black discoloration, so-called "prune juice" dialysate, due to the presence of methemalbumin. Intraperitoneal hemoglobin, separated into heme and globin, can allow the heme to be oxidized to hematin which can complex with albumin to form methemalbumin. This prune juice dialysate has been described in cases of pancreatitis. A darker rusty coloration has occurred after the intravenous administration of iron dextran combined with rifampicin. Brownish, "cola-colored" dialysate has also been attributed to myoglobin during cases of rhabdomyolysis.

Shoulder Pain Secondary to Pneumoperitoneum

Pneumoperitoneum can occur if air from the dialysis tubing has not been properly flushed before infusion of dialysate. During set up of the PD solutions all air from the tubing should be flushed into the drainage bags. Omitting this step can allow air to be infused, with solution, causing abdominal discomfort. Pneumoperitoneum can also be the presenting signs of more serious pathology such as an intestinal perforation such as a perforated peptic ulcer or peritonitis with a gas-producing organism. Diagnosis of pneumoperitoneum is typically made with an upright abdominal xray, where air accumulation under the superior right hemidiaphragm is typical. Air can also be detected by computerized tomography.

In patients determined to have pneumoperitoneum the clinical approach should be a focused history to determine any PD-related cause for the air such as a break in exchange technique, recent transfer set change, catheter manipulation by interventionalist, or error in the set-up of the cycler device. The physical examination should be directed at determining any acute abdominal pathology that could herald an intestinal perforation combined with a careful examination of the drained dialysate to examine for the presence of food, bile, feces, or a cloudy bag suggesting peritonitis. Peritonitis with mixed gram-negative or anaerobic organisms combined with pneumoperitoneum should be considered an intestinal perforation and surgical consultation should be obtained.

If the patient is deemed stable and intestinal perforation has been deemed unlikely, attempts can be made to treat a pneumoperitoneum by placing the patient in the trendelenburg position with gentle manual pressure on the abdomen to attempt to extrude the air during the drain phase. Otherwise, symptoms gradually improve as the intra-abdominal air is absorbed. Several weeks may pass before pneumoperitoneum has been completely resolved.

Increased Intraperitoneal Volume

Increased intraperitoneal volume (IIPV) occurs when the total intraperitoneal volume exceeds the intended target fill volume, increasing risk for patient discomfort or injury. IIPV has been described in patients employing CAPD and APD, and is the result of patient or cycler programming errors in which an infusion of new dialysate occurs before adequate drainage of the previous dwell. Cases of IIPV have been described when a cycler alarm has been over-ridden, or if ultrafiltration is not calculated correctly in the prescription. Patients performing CAPD should be instructed to ensure that the previous dwell has been as fully drained as possible before infusing the subsequent dwell. In patients on APD, the minimum drain volume for night cycles should be programmed to be > 85% of the fill volume.

References:

Hernia

Afthentopoulos IE, Panduranga Rao S, Mathews R, Oreopoulos DG. Hernia development in CAPD patients and the effect of 2.5 L dialysate volume in selected patients. Clin Nephrol 1998;49:251-257.

Bargman JM. Hernia in peritoneal dialysis patients: limiting occurrence and recurrence. Perit Dial Int 2008;28:349-351.

Crabtree JH. Hernia repair without delay in initiating or continuing peritoneal dialysis. Perit Dial Int 2006;26:178-182.

Del Peso G, Bajo MA, Costero O, et al. Risk factors for abdominal wall complications in peritoneal dialysis patients. Perit Dial Int 2003;23:249-254.

Garcia-Urena MA, Rodriguez CR, Ruiz VV, et al. Prevalence and management of hernias in peritoneal dialysis patients. Perit Dial Int 2006;26:198-202.

Gianetta E, Civalleri D, Serventi A, et al. Anterior tension-free repair under local anesthesia of abdominal wall hernias in continuous ambulatory peritoneal dialysis patients. Hernia 2004;8:354-357.

Kantartzi K, Passadakis P, Polychronidis A, et al. Prolene hernia system: an innovative method for hernia repair in patients on peritoneal dialysis. Perit Dial Int 2005;25:295-297.

Lewis DM, Bingham C, Beaman M, et al. Polypropylene mesh hernia repair-an alternative permitting rapid return to peritoneal dialysis. Nephrol Dial Transplant 1998;13:2488-2489.

Lichtenstein IL, Shulman AG, Amid PK, Montllor MM. The tension-free hernioplasty. Am J Surg 1989;157:188-193.

Martinez-Mier G, Garcia-Almazan E, Reyes-Devesa HE, et al. Abdominal wall hernias in end-stage renal disease patients on peritoneal dialysis. Perit Dial Int 2008;28:391-396.

Shah H, Chu M, Bargman JM. Perioperative management of peritoneal dialysis patients undergoing hernia surgery without the use of interim hemodialysis. Perit Dial Int 2006;26:684-687.

Hydrothorax

Camilleri B, Glancey G, Pledger D, Williams P. The icodextrin black line sign to confirm a pleural leak in a patient on peritoneal dialysis. Perit Dial Int 2004;24:197.

Chow KM, Szeto CC, Li PKT. Management options for hydrothorax complicating peritoneal dialysis. Semin Dial 2003;16:389-394.

Fletcher S, Turney JH, Brownjohn AM. Increased incidence of hydrothorax complicating peritoneal dialysis in patients with adult polycystic kidney disease. Nephrol Dial Transplant 1994;9:832-833.

Herbrig K, Reimann D. Reply. Nephrol Dial Transplant 2003;18:2682.

Jagasia MH, Cole FH, Stegman MH, et al. Video-assisted talc pleurodesis in the management of pleural effusion secondary to continuous ambulatory peritoneal dialysis: a report of three cases. Am J Kidney Dis 1996;28:772-774.

Kirschner PA. Porous diaphragm syndromes. Chest Surgery Clinics of North America 1998;8:449-472.

Kumagai H, Watari M, Kuratsune M. Simple surgical treatment for pleuroperitoneal communication without interruption of continuous ambulatory peritoneal dialysis. Gen Thorac Cardiovasc Surg 2007;55:508-511.

Lang CL, Kao TW, Lee CM, et al. Video-assisted thoracoscopic surgery in continuous ambulatory peritoneal dialysis-related hydrothorax. Kidney Int 2008;74:136.

Lew SQ. Hydrothorax: pleural effusion associated with peritoneal dialysis. Perit Dial Int 2010;30:13-18.

Macia M, Gallego E, Garcia-Cobaleda I, et al. Methylene blue as a cause of chemical peritonitis in a patient on peritoneal dialysis. Clin Nephrol 1995;43:136-137.

Mak S, Nyunt K, Wong P, et al. Long-term follow-up of thoracoscopic pleurodesis for hydrothorax complicating peritoneal dialysis. Ann Thorac Surg 2002;74:218-221.

Momenin N, Colletti PM, Kaptein EM. Low pleural fluid-to-serum glucose gradient indicates pleuroperitoneal communication in peritoneal dialysis patients: presentation of two cases and a review of the literature. Nephrol Dial Transplant 2012;27:1212-1219.

Puri V, Orellana FA, Singer GG, Wald MS. Diaphragmatic defect complicating peritoneal dialysis. Ann Thorac Surg 2011;92:1527.

Szeto CC, Chow MC. Pathogenesis and management of hydrothorax complicating peritoneal dialysis. Curr Opin Pulm Med 2004;10:315-319.

Tang S, Chui WH, Tang AWC, et al. Video-assisted thoracoscopic talc pleurodesis is effective for maintenance of peritoneal dialysis in acute hydrothorax complicating peritoneal dialysis. Nephrol Dial Transplant 2003;18:804-808.

Yen HT, Lu HY, Liu HP, Hsieh MJ. Video-assisted thoracoscopic surgery for hydrothorax in peritoneal dialysis patients- check-air-leakage method. Eur J Cardiothorac Surg 2005;28:648-649.

Subcutaneous leaks

Benaroia M, Morton AR, Cheeseman FD, et al. Spontaneous peritoneal membrane rupture with extravasation of peritoneal fluid into the lower limbs and flank in a peritoneal dialysis patient. Perit Dial Int 2008;28:554-557.

Lam MF, Lo WK, Chu FSK, et al. Retroperitoneal leakage as a cause of ultrafiltration failure. Perit Dial Int 2004;24:466-470.

Lam MF, Lo WK, Tse KC, et al. Retroperitoneal leakage as a cause of acute ultrafiltration failure: its associated risk factors in peritoneal dialysis. Perit Dial Int 2009;29:542-547.

LeBlanc M, Ouimet D, Pinchette V. Dialysate leaks in peritoneal dialysis. Semin Dial 2001;14:50-54.

Prischl FC, Muhr T, Seiringer EM, et al. Magnetic resonance imaging of the peritoneal cavity among peritoneal dialysis patients, using the dialysate as "contrast medium". J Am Soc Nephrol 2002;13:197-203.

Prokesch RW, Schima W, Schober E, et al. Complications of continuous ambulatory peritoneal dialysis: findings on MR peritoneography. Am J Roentgenol 2000;174:987-991.

Tun KN, Tulchinkshy M. Pericatheter leak in a peritoneal dialysis patient SPECT/CT diagnosis. Clin Nucl Med 2012;37:625-628.

Yavuz K, Erden A, Ates K, Erden I. MR peritoneography in complications of continuous ambulatory peritoneal dialysis. Abdomin Imaging 2005;30:361-368.

Genital swelling

Hollett MD, Marn CS, Ellis CS, et al. Complications of continuous ambulatory peritoneal dialysis: evaluation with CT peritoneography. AJR 1992;152:983-989.

Hemoperitoneum

Goodkin DA, Benning MG. An outpatient maneuver to treat bloody effluent during continuous ambulatory peritoneal dialysis (CAPD). Perit Dial Int 1990;10:227-229.

Lew SQ. Hemoperitoneum: bloody peritoneal dialysate in ESRD patients receiving peritoneal dialysis. Perit Dial Int 2007;27:226-233.

Lew SQ. Persistent hemoperitoneum in a pregnant patient receiving peritoneal dialysis. Perit Dial Int 2006;26:108-110.

Maaz DE. Troubleshooting non-infectious peritoneal dialysis issues. Nephrol Nurs J 2004;31:521-532.

Tse K, Yip P, Lam M. Recurrent hemoperitoneum complicating continuous ambulatory peritoneal dialysis. Perit Dial Int 2002;22:488-491.

Chylous dialysate

Aalami O, Allen D, Organ C. Chylous ascites: a collective review. Surgery 2000;128:761-778.

Chen J, Lin RK, Hassanein T. Use of orlistat (xenical) to treat chylous ascites. J Clin Gastroenterol 2005;39:831-833.

Cheung CK, Khwaja A. Chylous ascites: an unusual complication of peritoneal dialysis. A case report and literature review. Perit Dial Int 2008;28:229-231.

Geary B, Wade B, Wollmann W, El-Galley R. Laparoscopic repair of chylous ascites. J Urol 2004;171:1231-1232.

Lee PH, Lin CL, Lai PC, Yang CW. Octreotide therapy for chylous ascites in a chronic dialysis patient. Nephrology 2005;10:344-347.

Ram R, Swarnalatha G, Santhosh Pai BH, et al. Cloudy peritoneal fluid attributable to non-dihydropyridine calcium channel blocker. Perit Dial Int 2012;32:110-111.

Ramos R, Gonzalez MT, Moreso F, et al. Chylous ascites: an unusual complication of percutaneous peritoneal catheter implantation. Perit Dial Int 2006;26: 722-723.

Saka Y, Tachi H, Sakurai H, et al. Aliskiren-induced chyloperitoneum in a patient on peritoneal dialysis. Perit Dial Int 2012;32:111-112.

Teitelbaum I. Cloudy peritoneal dialysate: it's not always infection. Contrib Nephrol 2006;150:187-194.

Tsao Y, Chen W. Calcium channel blocker-induced chylous ascites in peritoneal dialysis. Kidney Int 2009;75:868.

Complications unique to the female patient

Bradley AJ, Mamtora H, Pritchard N. Transvaginal leak of peritoneal dialysate demonstrated by CT peritoneography. Br J Radiol 1997;70:652-653.

Caporale N, Perez D, Alegre S. Vaginal leak of peritoneal dialysis liquid. Perit Dial Int 1991;11:284-285.

Coward RA, Gokal R, Wise M, et al. Peritonitis associated with vaginal leakage of dialysis fluid in continuous ambulatory peritoneal dialysis. Br J Med 1982;284:1529.

Dickson MJ, Railton A. Continuous ambulatory peritoneal dialysis and uterovaginal prolapse. Hosp Med 2000;61:283.

Dimitriadis CA, Bargman JM. Gynecologic issues in periotoneal dialysis. Adv Perit Dial 2011;27:101-105.

Liberek T, Lichodziejewska-Niemierko M, Kowalewska J, et al. Uterine-prolapse- a rare or rarely reported complication of CAPD? Perit Dial Int 2002;22:95-96.

Macallister RJ, Morgan SH. Fallopian tube capture of chronic peritoneal dialysis catheters. Perit Dial Int 1993;13:74-76.

Plaza MM. Intrauterine device-related peritonitis in a patient on CAPD. Perit Dial Int 2002;22:538-540.

Back pain

Bargman JM. Complications of peritoneal dialysis related to increased intraabdominal pressure. Kidney Int 1993;43[Suppl 40]:S75-80.

Mahale AS, Katyal A, Khanna R. Complications of peritoneal dialysis related to increased intra-abdominal pressure. Adv Perit Dial 2003;19:130-135.

Drain pain

Juergensen PH, Murphy AL, Pherson KA, et al. Tidal peritoneal dialysis to achieve comfort in chronic peritoneal dialysis patients. Adv Perit Dial 1999;15:125-126.

Fernando SK, Finkelstein FO. Tidal PD: its role in current practice of peritoneal dialysis. Kidney Int 2006;70:S91-S95.

Encapsulating peritoneal sclerosis

Augustine T, Brown PW, Davies SD, et al. Encapsulating peritoneal sclerosis: clinical significance and implications. Nephron Clin Pract 2009;111:c149-c154.

Balasubramaniam G, Brown EA, Davenport A, et al. The Pan-Thames EPS study: treatment and outcomes of encapsulating peritoneal sclerosis. Nephrol Dial Transplant 2009;24:3209-3215.

Brown EA, Van Biesen W, Finkelstein FO, et al. Length of time on peritoneal dialysis and encapsulating peritoneal sclerosis: position paper for ISPD. Perit Dial Int 2009;29:595-600.

Brown MC, Simpson K, Kerssens JJ, Mactier RA. Encapsulating peritoneal sclerosis in the new millennium: a national cohort study. Clin J Am Soc Nephrol 2009;4:1222-1229.

Guest S. Tamoxifen therapy for encapsulating peritoneal sclerosis: mechanism of action and update on clinical experiences. Perit Dial Int 2009;29:252-255.

Johnson DW, Cho Y, Livingston BER, et al. Encapsulating peritoneal sclerosis: incidence, predictors, and outcomes. Kidney Int 2010;77:904-912.

Korte MR, Fieren MW, Sampimon DE, et al. Tamoxifen is associated with lower mortality of encapsulating peritoneal sclerosis: results of the Dutch Multicenter EPS Study. Nephrol Dial Transplant 2011;26:691-697.

Lo WK, Kawanishi H. Encapsulating peritoneal sclerosis- medical and surgical treatment. Perit Dial Int 2009;29[Suppl 2]:S211-214.

Yamamoto T, Nagasue K, Okuno S, Yamakawa T. The role of peritoneal lavage and the prognostic significance of mesothelial cell area in preventing encapsulating peritoneal sclerosis. Perit Dial Int 2010;30:343-352.

Eosinophilic peritonitis

Chan MK, Chow L, Lam SS, Jones B. Peritoneal eosinophilia in patients on continous peritoneal dialysis: a prospective study: a prospective study. Am J Kidney Dis 1988;11:180-183.

Fontan MP, Rodriguez-Carmona A, Galed I, et al. Incidence and significance of peritoneal eosinophilia during peritoneal dialysis-related peritonitis. Perit Dial Int 2003;23:460-464.

Fourtounas C, Dousdampanis P, Hardalias A, et al. Eosinophilic peritonitis following air entrapment during peritoneoscopic insertion of peritoneal dialysis catheters. Semin Dial 2008;21:180-182.

Ikee R, Oka M, Maesato K, et al. Eosinophilic peritonitis and ultrafiltration failure on initiation of CAPD. Perit Dial Int 2008;28:197-199.

Jo YI, Song JO, Park JH, et al. Idiopathic eosinophilic peritonitis in continuous ambulatory peritoneal dialysis: experience with percutaneous catheter placement. Nephrology 2007;12:437-440.

Nakamura Y, Okada H, Yasui A, et al. Sclerosing encapsulating peritonitis associated with recurrent eosinophilic peritonitis. Nephrol Dial Transplant 1999;14:768-770.

Thakur SS, Unikowsky B, Prichard S. Eosinophilic peritonitis in CAPD: treatment with prednisone and diphenhydramine. Perit Dial Int 1997;17:402-403.

Pancreatitits

Bruno MJ, van Westerloo DJ, van Dorp WT, et al. Peritoneal dialysis: an under-appreciated cause of acute pancreatitis. Gut 2000;46:385-389.

Gupta A, Vuan Z, Balaskas E, et al. CAPD and pancreatitis: no connection. Perit Dial Int 1992;12:309-316.

Lankisch PG, Weber-Dany B, Maisonneuve P, Lowenfels AB. Frequency and severity of acute pancreatitis in chronic dialysis patients. Nephrol Dial Transplant 2008;23:1401-1405.

Manga F, Lim CS, Mangena L, Guest M. Acute pancreatitis in peritoneal dialysis: a case report with literature review. Eur J Gastroenterol Hepatol 2012;24:95-101.

Quraishi ER, Goel S, Gupta M, et al. Acute pancreatitis in patients on chronic peritoneal dialysis: an increased risk? Am J Gastroenterol 2005;100:2288-2293.

Shrestha BM, Brown PWG, Wilkie ME, Raftery AT. The anatomy and pathology of the lesser sac: implications for peritoneal dialysis. Perit Dial Int 2010;30:496-501.

Villacorta J, Rivera M, Alvaro SJ, et al. Acute pancreatitis in peritoneal dialysis patients: diagnosis in the icodextrin era. Perit Dial Int 2010;30:374-377.

Colors of dialysate

Carter TB, Garris AG, Ullian ME. Rusty peritoneal dialysis fluid after intravenous administration of iron dextran. Am J Kidney Dis 1996;27:147-150.

Chen YT, Huang CC, Kuo CC, et al. Green dialysate. Kidney Int 2010;77:369.

Connacher AA, Stewart WK. Pancreatitis causes brownish-black peritoneal dialysate due to the presence of methaemalbumin. Nephrol Dial Transplant 1987;2:45-47.

Okada K, Onishi Y, Hagi C, et al. Bloody discoloration of peritoneal dialysate bags. Perit Dial int 1999;19:593-594.

Ramos R, Gonzalez MT, Moreso F, et al. Chylous ascites: an unusual complication of percutaneous peritoneal catheter implantation. Perit Dial Int 2006;26: 722-723.

Robertson S, Huxtable H, Blakemore C, et al. The icodextrin black line sign. Perit Dial Int 2001;21:624-625.

Sekercioglu N, Jassal SV. Early morning blues- a complication of icodextrin. Perit Dial Int 2004;24:197-199.

Shiao CC, Leu SC, Kao JL, et al. "Soybean sauce" peritoneal dialysate. NDT Plus 2011;4:75-76.

Pneumoperitoneum

Cancarini GC, Carli O, Cristinelli MR, et al. Pneumoperitoneum in peritoneal dialysis patients. J Nephrol 1999;12:95-99.

Chang JJ, Yeun JY, Hasbargen JA. Pneumoperitoneum in peritoneal dialysis patients. Am J Kidney Dis 1995;25:297-301.

Chen YC. Peritoneal dialysis-related peritonitis with Klebsiella pneumoperitoneum mimicking viscus perforation. Perit Dial Int 2012;32:575-577.

Huang JW, Peng YS, Wu MS, Tsai TJ. Pneumoperitoneum caused by a perforated peptic ulcer in a peritoneal dialysis patient: difficulty in diagnosis. Am J Kidney Dis1999;33:e6.

Increased intraperitoneal volume (IIPV)

Davis ID, Cizman B, Mundt K, et al. Relationship between drain volume/fill volume ratio and clinical outcomes associated with overfill complaints in peritoneal dialysis patients. Perit Dial Int 2011;31:148-153.

Chapter 13:
Volume Management in PD Therapy

ONE MAJOR GOAL OF PD therapy is the normalization of extracellular volume. Achieving euvolemia is an indicator of the adequacy of dialysis. Three fundamental concepts in volume management must be acknowledged:

-In PD, failure to control the extracellular volume is largely due to dietary non-compliance. Exposing the peritoneal membrane to chronic hypertonic solutions to remove volume, when the primary problem is dietary non-compliance, will not be successful in the long term. Dietary input and reducing salt intake are important management strategies.

-The anuric patient will have a greater difficulty maintaining euvolemia, so preserving residual kidney function (RKF) is important in maintaining volume control.

-Patients with higher (faster) peritoneal membrane transport characteristics will have a more rapid loss of the dialysate osmotic gradient, be more likely to have poor ultrafiltration with longer dwells, and will be at higher risk of dialysate absorption during the long dwell. The long dwells, in these patients, must be separately analyzed and if poor ultrafiltration is present, the long dwell must be shortened or an alternative osmotic agent, such as icodextrin, initiated.

If adhered to, these interventions can help ensure control of the extracellular volume is maintained during long term PD therapy.

Dietary Salt Restriction

Most patients on PD therapy will require a sodium restriction to maintain euvolemia. Early in the history of PD therapy, there was concern that daily PD with daily volume removal would lead to volume depletion and hypotension. A sodium restriction was not commonly reinforced. With experience, it was determined that most patients remained hypertensive and edematous despite daily ultrafiltration and that, indeed, a sodium restriction was indicated. Though still somewhat controversial, salt restrictions of 6 grams a day are recommended (daily intake of 5.8 grams of salt is equivalent to 100 mmol of sodium). Later chapters review many dietary approaches that help achieve this target for salt intake, such as salt substitutes, cooking techniques, avoidance of "fast foods", canned foods, and preservatives such as MSG.

Preservation of Residual Kidney Function (RKF)

RKF contributes to daily loss of salt and water and patients with significant RKF will be less likely to present with signs of volume expansion, such as hypertension and edema. Patients previously euvolemic, who present with new findings of volume expansion, may have lost residual kidney function.

Loop diuretics are recommended to maintain renal sodium excretion. Chapter 5 reviewed the role of diuretics and mechanisms of diuretic refractoriness that should be addressed to ensure adequate renal tubular response to these agents. Higher doses of diuretics are often required to induce a response. Anuric patients will be at greater risk of hypervolemia so active measures to preserve RKF such as ACE/ARB medications, avoiding nephrotoxins such as aminoglycosides, iodinated radiocontrast, and non-steroidal anti-inflammatory agents are important strategies to maintain the residual kidney contribution to volume control.

Ultrafiltration Profile Using Dextrose Exchanges

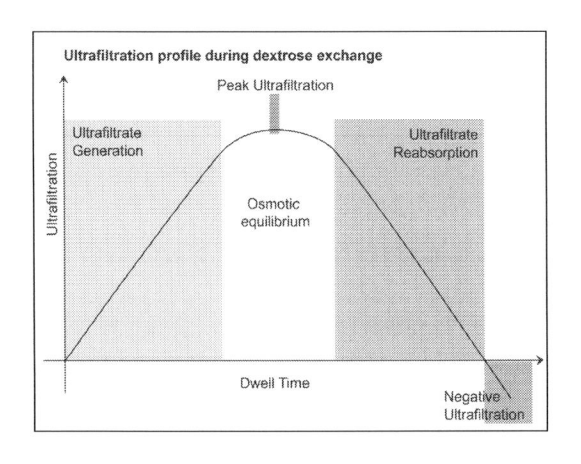

Dextrose as the osmotic agent in standard PD solutions creates a crystalloid osmotic pressure that induces

Three phases of dextrose-mediated ultrafiltration:
A. Brisk initial UF
B. Osmotic equilibrium
C. Reabsorption

ultrafiltration across the peritoneal capillary wall via the small and large pores and the aquaporins. The initial rate of ultrafiltration is brisk due to the hyperosmolality of the solution. However, as dextrose is absorbed into the capillary a point of osmotic equilibrium is reached where the osmotic forces across the capillary are equal and ultrafiltration ceases. As dextrose is further absorbed the osmolality of the capillary plasma will exceed the dialysate and the ultrafiltrate is slowly reabsorbed.

Ultrafiltration and Dialysate Osmolality

The ultrafiltration response to dialysate is determined by the osmotic force generated by various dextrose concentrations. Dextrose solutions containing 1.5%, 2.5% and 4.25% dextrose are commercially available with ultrafiltration profiles as noted below.

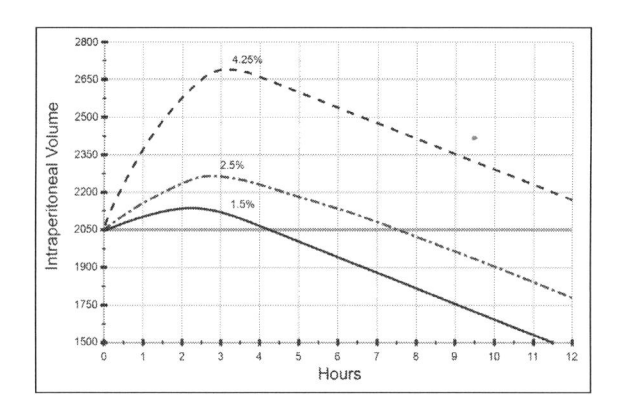

Ultrafiltration profiles of 3 dextrose concentrations

Typical ultrafiltration volumes for 1.5% dextrose solutions are 150 mL, for 2.5% solutions 250 mL and 4.24% solutions can remove in excess of 600 mL. The ultrafiltration response is dependent on the dextrose concentration, dwell volume, dwell time, and peritoneal membrane type (fast, average, slow transporter).

Long dwells risk loss of ultrafiltration and net fluid absorption. Optimization of ultrafiltration can be achieved by dwell times that take advantage of the early peak in ultrafiltration effect before osmotic equilibrium occurs. After osmotic equilibrium, net fluid reabsorption slowly occurs in all patients.

Appropriate PD Prescription

Peritoneal membrane transport characteristics predict the response to an osmotic stimulus. Transport characteristics are determined by the traditional PET. Patient transport types can be described as high, high-average, low-average, or low. Patients with high to high-average (faster) transport properties will be at a greater risk of inadequate peritoneal ultrafiltration due to the more rapid absorption of glucose and dissipation of the osmotic gradient. Patients with lower (slower) transport properties maintain the osmotic gradient longer and have a more sustained ultrafiltration.

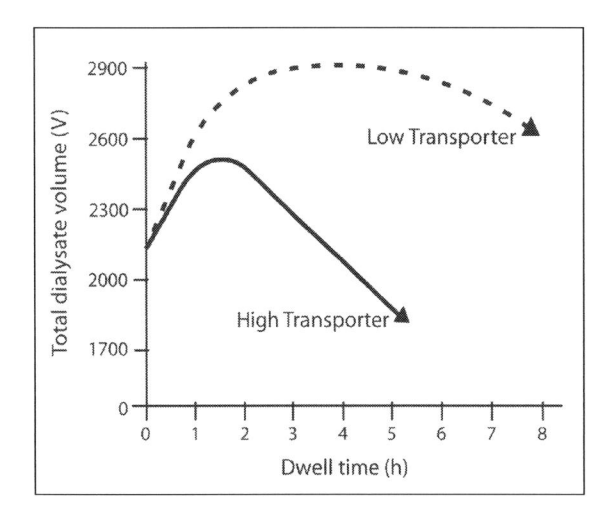

Vast difference in UF profile by peritoneal membrane transport category

An understanding of the underlying peritoneal membrane characteristics allows for optimization of the PD prescription. As shown, patients with high to high-average transport properties will have the greatest initial ultrafiltration in the first hours of the dwell time and then be at risk of ultrafiltrate reabsorption. Patients with lower transport will maintain ultrafiltration for a longer period and require a longer dwell time for therapy optimization.

Patients with high to high-average transport status can be managed well on cycler therapy (APD) that allows for shorter dwell times during the night, but, will be at risk of fluid reabsorption during the long day dwell. Lower transporters are managed well on CAPD regimens with longer dwell times or with longer dwell times and lesser cycles on APD.

It is important to analyze the individual patient's PET characteristics, to predict the optimal dwell time. Many patients on long term PD therapy have been noted to migrate toward higher transport status over time. This suggests that dwell times may need to be shortened in these longer term PD patients. Maintaining euvolemia in longer term patients will be more challenging as these patients have likely lost residual kidney function and be at greater risk of negative ultrafiltration due to membrane changes. In longer term patients who present with loss of volume control, felt due to inadequate ultrafiltration, repeat PET determinations should be considered. New PET information may indicate that changes to the dwell time are needed to enhance ultrafiltration.

Optimization of the Long Dwell

As discussed in Chapter 10, the long day dwell in APD and the night dwell in CAPD provide the least ultrafiltration, due to the long dwell period and subsequent loss of the osmotic gradient seen with dextrose-based solutions. In patients demonstrating evidence of volume excess despite an APD regimen that is felt appropriate for the patient's membrane characteristics, optimization of the long day dwell may be indicated. The long dwell can be interrupted to create 2 dwells of shorter duration- termed a "mid-day exchange". Use of the mid-day exchange will have appreciable impact on quality of life as the patient will be required to perform an additional exchange during the day.

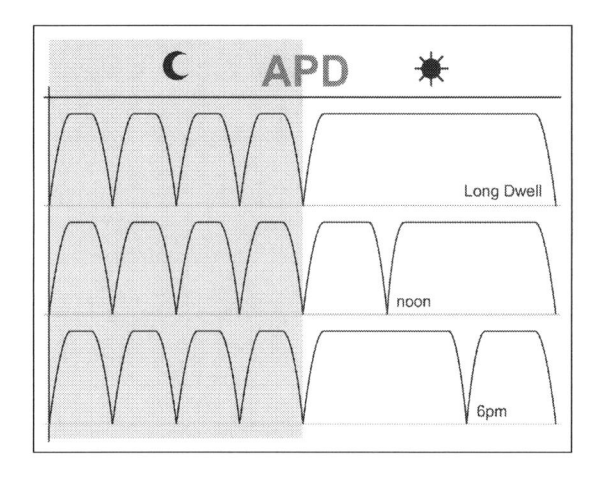

A mid-day exchange shortens the usual day exchange into 2 separate exchanges improving ultrafiltration in each exchange

Clinicians should determine when this additional exchange will be the least intrusive- perhaps during the noon break for some patients or after work, later in the day, for other patients.

Role of Icodextrin

As mentioned, patients with inadequate ultrafiltration during the long dwell will require interruption of the long dwell or a change to an alternative osmotic stimulus.

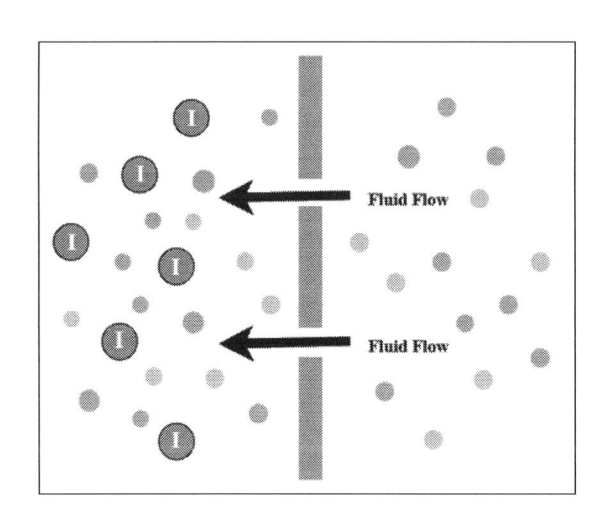

The high reflection coefficient (size) of icodextrin creates a colloidal osmotic effect inducing ultrafiltration

Icodextrin is a non-dextrose solution that exerts a colloidal osmotic pressure to generate ultrafiltration.

Icodextrin is indicated strictly for the long dwell. The ultrafiltration profile of icodextrin reveals a sustained ultrafiltration over 12 to 14 hours. Icodextrin is not indicated for short exchanges as the shorter term ultrafiltration response would be less than that of dextrose solutions.

Icodextrin is useful for the night exchange in CAPD regimens or the long day exchange during APD treatments. Ultrafiltration with icodextrin appears to be independent of peritoneal membrane transport characteristics as similar ultrafiltration volumes were noted in patients of high, average, and low transport properties.

In the randomized controlled MIDAS trial (Multicenter Study of Icodextrin in Continuous Ambulatory Peritoneal Dialysis) 7.5% icodextrin was compared to 1.5% and 4.25% dextrose for ultrafiltration during the long nightly dwell in over 200 CAPD patients. The net mean ultrafiltration with icodextrin was over 500 mL compared to

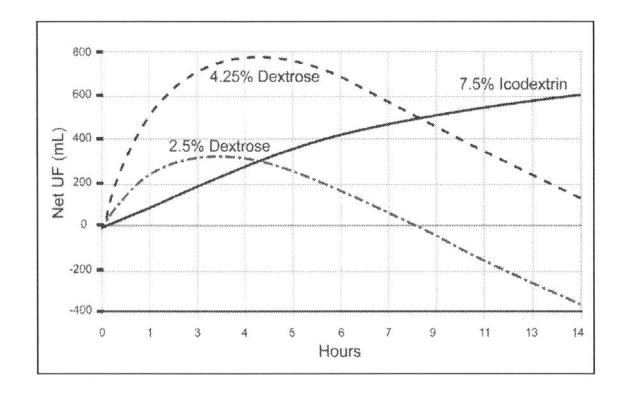

Sustained ultrafiltration profile noted with icodextrin use

155 mL with 1.5% dextrose and 427 mL with 4.25% dextrose solutions.

Finkelstein and colleagues reported on a multicenter, randomized, double-blind trial in 92 patients comparing 4.25% dextrose with icodexrin for the long exchange in APD patients. The patients were all classified as having higher peritoneal membrane permeability. The study demonstrated that icodextrin-mediated ultrafiltration was superior to that observed with hypertonic dextrose in this patient population. Similar observations were published by Paniagua et al, Lin et al, and Davies et al.

Peritoneal aquaporins are activated by the hyperosmolality of standard dextrose solutions. Aquaporins allow for pure water movement from the capillary lumen into the dialysate. During this water movement, sodium is sieved and remains in the capillary lumen. Repeated rapid cycling of dialysate can result in hypernatremia due to sodium sieving. Icodextrin solutions are iso-osmotic and therefore do not activate peritoneal capillary aquaporins. There is no water movement across the aquaporin and no sodium sieving. Fluid movement across the capillary is solely through the small and large pores and therefore more net sodium removal occurs with icodextrin than with dextrose based solutions.

Ultrafiltration Efficiency

Ultrafiltration efficiency refers to the volume of ultrafiltrate created per gram of carbohydrate absorbed. In patients with higher transport status, the ultrafiltration efficiency of icodextrin is over 2-fold greater compared to a 4.25% dextrose solution. Thus, compared to hypertonic dextrose solutions, the use of icodextrin results in lower carbohydrate absorption for the ultrafiltrate achieved. Therefore icodextrin use is a metabolically effective alternative for meeting daily ultrafiltration requirements in patients requiring frequent use of 4.25% dextrose solutions.

Technical Issues Reducing Ultrafiltration

Patients demonstrating poor ultrafiltration should be evaluated for constipation, catheter dysfunction, or subcutaneous dialysate leaks. Careful physical examination can rule out soft tissue induration in the abdomen or genital edema that may suggest a subcutaneous leak. A trial of laxative therapy may be indicated. Catheter flows should be evaluated to rule out omental entrapment, catheter migration, or kinking. If detected, correction of these technical abnormalities can usually restore the normal ultrafiltration response.

Conclusions

Control of the extracellular volume is one of the indicators of "adequacy" of dialysis. Most PD patients will require a significant restriction of dietary salt and water. In those patients with residual kidney function, diuretics should be continued. The patient that reaches anuria will have more difficulty maintaining euvolemia so attempts should be made to preserve residual kidney function with the use of ACE inhibitors or angiotensin receptor blockers. Differing dextrose concentrations are available to assist in adjusting ultrafiltration targets, but long term reliance on hypertonic 4.25% solutions is discouraged. An understanding of baseline peritoneal membrane transport can help estimate the optimal dwell time to achieve maximal ultrafiltration. An overall approach to fluid balance in PD patients is summarized below.

<u>Key Principles in Maintaining Control of Extracellular Volume</u>

1. In patients with evidence of prior hypertension and edema, institution of a low salt diet is required. A 6 gram or less salt diet should be prescribed.

2. In patients with significant residual kidney function, efforts should be made to preserve this excretory function by institution of higher dose diuretic medications and antagonism of the renin-aldosterone axis.

3. Determine the peritoneal membrane characteristics by the PET and estimate appropriate dwell times to achieve peak ultrafiltration.

4. In patients determined to be high to high-average transporters, particular attention is placed on the long exchange which is the exchange with the greatest risk of negative ultrafiltration.

5. If negative ultrafiltration is noted during the long exchange, the osmolality of the long single exchange should be increased, or the single long exchange should be replaced by two exchanges of shorter dwell time or by icodextrin.

6. In diabetics, control of the blood glucose will maximize the osmotic gradient between plasma and dialysate to preserve the osmotic stimulus for fluid removal.

7. Compliance with the prescription should be reviewed with the patient and with a supply inventory.

8. Exclude technical issues such as constipation, catheter dysfunction, or subcutaneous leaks.

9. Patients requiring long term, frequent use of 4.25% dextrose should have an intervention to include dietary and social evaluations, as well as medical interventions to review diuretics, blood glucose control, and possible change to icodextrin. These patients should be informed of the potential need to transfer to HD if there is not clinical improvement. Consideration for placement of an arteriovenous fistula is appropriate. Control of the extracellular volume requires patient compliance and non-compliant patients on home therapies may require transfer to in-center modalities.

References:

Abu-Alfa AK, Burkart J, Piraino B, et al. Approach to fluid management in peritoneal dialysis: a practical algorithm. Kidney Int 2002;62[Suppl 81]:S8-S16.

Asghar RB, Diskin AM, Spanel P, et al. Influence of convection on the diffusive transport and sieving of water and small solutes across the peritoneal membrane. J Am Soc Nephrol 2005;16:437-443.

Ates K, Nergizoglu G, Keven K, et al. Effect of fluid and sodium removal on mortality in peritoneal dialysis patients. Kidney Int 2001;60:767-776.

Davies SJ, Woodrow G, Donovan K, et al. Icodextrin improves the fluid status of peritoneal dialysis patients: results of a double-blind randomized controlled trial. J Am Soc Nephrol 2003;14:2338-2344.

Finkelstein F, Healy H, Abu-Alfa A, et al. Superiority of icodextrin compared with 4.25% dextrose for peritoneal ultrafiltration. J Am Soc Nephrol 2005;16:546-554.

Gunal AI, Duman S, Ozkahya M, et al. Strict volume control normalizes hypertension in peritoneal dialysis patients. Am J Kidney Dis 2001;37:588-593.

Johnson DW, Arndt M, O'Shea A, et al. Icodextrin as salvage therapy in peritoneal dialysis patients with refractory fluid overload. BMC Nephrology 2001;2:2-7.

Jones CH, Newstead CG. The ratio of extracellular fluid to total body water and technique survival in peritoneal dialysis patients. Perit Dial Int 2004;24:353-358.

Konings CJ, Kooman JP, Gladziwa U, et al. A decline in residual glomerular filtration during the use of icodextrin may be due to underhydration. Kidney Int 2005;67:1190-1191.

Konings CJ, Kooman JP, Schonck M, et al. Fluid status in CAPD patients is related to peritoneal transport and residual renal function: evidence from a longitudinal study. Nephrol Dial Transplant 2003;18:797-803.

Konings CJ, Kooman JP, Schonck M, et al. Effect of icodextrin on volume status, blood pressure and echocardiographic parameters: a randomized study. Kidney Int 2003;63:1556-1563.

Lameire N, Van Biesen W. Importance of blood pressure and volume control in peritoneal dialysis patients. Perit Dial Int 2001;21:206-211.

Lin A, Qian J, Li X, et al. Randomized controlled trial of icodextrin versus glucose containing peritoneal dialysis fluid. Clin J Am Soc Nephrol 2009;4:1799-1804.

Lin X, Lin A, Ni Z, et al. Daily peritoneal ultrafiltration predicts patient and technique survival in anuric peritoneal dialysis patients. Nephrol Dial Transplant 2010;25:2322-2327.

Mistry CD, Gokal R, Peers E, MIDAS Study Group. A randomized multicenter clinical trial comparing isosmolar icodextrin with hyperosmolar glucose solutions in CAPD. Kidney Int 1994;46:496-503.

Mujais S, Nolph K, Gokal R, et al. Evaluation and management of ultrafiltration problems in peritoneal dialysis. International Society of Peritoneal Dialysis Ad Hoc Committee on Ultrafiltration Management in Peritoneal Dialysis. Perit Dial Int 2000;20[Suppl 4]:S5-S21.

Paniagua R, Ventura M, Avila-Diaz M, et al. Icodextrin improves metabolic and fluid management in high and high-average transport diabetic patients. Perit Dial Int 2009;29:422-432.

Perl J, Bargman JM. The importance of residual kidney function for patients on dialysis: a critical review. Am J Kidney Dis 2009;53:1068-1081.

Rodriguez-Carmona A, Perez-Fontan M, Garca-Naveiro R, et al. Compared time profiles of ultrafiltration, sodium removal, and renal function in incident CAPD and automated peritoneal dialysis patients. Am J Kidney Dis 2004;44:132-145.

Rodriguez-Carmona A, Perez-Fontan M. Sodium removal in patients undergoing CAPD and automated peritoneal dialysis. Perit Dial Int 2002;22:705-713.

Smit W, Schouten N, Van Der Berg N, et al. Analysis of the prevalence and causes of ultrafiltration failure during long-term peritoneal dialysis: a cross-sectional study. Perit Dial Int 2004;24:562-570.

Vennegoor MA. Salt restriction and practical aspects to improve compliance. J Ren Nutr 2009;19:63-68.

Chapter 14:
PD in the Diabetic Patient

IN MANY COUNTRIES, DIABETIC nephropathy is the most common ESRD-related diagnosis. Compared to non-diabetics, survival is reduced, primarily due to cardiovascular disease and other advanced co-morbidities. Diabetic patients on dialysis often shift their primary care to the nephrologist, who now assumes greater responsibility for managing the disease and its complications.

PD offers the diabetic patient many potential benefits such as lifestyle advantages, avoidance of heparinization, fewer hemodynamic disturbances, the option of intraperitoneal insulin administration, and avoidance of vascular access. Many diabetic patients have had prior medical interventions requiring cannulation of the veins. This reduces the likelihood of successful native fistula creation and results in greater reliance on temporary vascular catheters and grafts with their inherent complications. Therefore, PD may have special advantages yet many unique clinical issues arise in the care of the diabetic patient on PD therapy. This chapter will review management strategies for this population.

Survival of Diabetics on PD

PD has been successfully employed for the management of diabetic ESRD patients but, at present, no randomized controlled trials compare PD to HD outcomes in diabetics. Conclusions about technique success and outcomes are based on retrospective observational data and a newly published propensity-matching cohort study.

In observational studies, the most significant research involves analysis of the United States Renal Data System (USRDS), an annual report prepared by the National

Institutes of Health, National Institute of Diabetes and Digestive and Kidney Diseases, Bethesda, MD. In a 2004 analysis, Vonesh and colleagues compared survival of 398 thousand patients in the USRDS database initiating dialysis between 1995 and 2000. Survival on HD versus PD, in diabetic and non-diabetic patients, different age groups, and in those with and without co-morbidities was reported. Patients were followed for a maximum of three years or until death or transplant. For the entire cohort, there was no significant difference in survival, by any modality. In the sub-group analysis, at three years of follow-up, diabetics less than 45 years of age, with or without co-morbidities, had improved survival on PD. The authors noted this association between diabetes and age and concluded that PD would be the preferred modality in diabetics younger than age 45. Diabetics over age 45 showed improved survival on hemodialysis.

In addition to longer term survival, the researchers then examined outcomes in the first years of dialysis. Diabetics up to age 64 showed a survival benefit in the first year by initiating dialysis with PD. Diabetics 65 years and older showed better early survival on HD. The authors concluded that initiating dialysis with PD, in most diabetics, could offer an early survival advantage.

This observational analysis was followed by a more recent investigation using propensity-matching methodology. By propensity matching, an incident HD patient from the USRDS was matched with an incident PD patient, with careful matching by age, gender, body size, and co-morbidities. Matching of 6337 HD and 6337 PD patients was completed and patients were followed for up to 5 years. Forty six percent of the matched patients, in each group, were diabetic. This study did not report on outcomes of diabetics at different ages but analyzed all diabetics as one group. In an intention-to-treat as well as as-treated analysis, diabetics on PD, followed from day 0, had better survival in the first year of follow-up. Hazard ratios indicated improved survival on HD in subsequent years. Analyzed from day 90, outcomes of diabetics on PD were similar in the first year of dialysis but with higher risk in subsequent years. With this information the authors suggested that their findings were compatible with a dual-modality approach in diabetics, in which dialysis is initiated with PD due to the early survival benefit seen in the day 0 analysis followed by timely transfer to HD.

The apparent early survival advantage of PD, in most patients, may be due to several factors. PD therapy has been demonstrated to preserve residual kidney function in diabetic patients as well as non-diabetics and may convey the initial survival advantage to PD noted in most studies. Avoidance of temporary vascular access in diabetics may also contribute to an early survival advantage. PD therapy should be offered to diabetic patients as part of broad and comprehensive CKD and dialysis options education. Once on PD, the diabetic is best managed with a special clinical action plan to maximize the success rate on the modality.

Glucose Exposure

Reaching ESRD and initiating dialysis does not suggest that control of the blood glucose is any less important. The diabetic initiating PD with dextrose solutions can be expected to have increased medication requirements to maintain glycemic control. Control of the blood glucose level is important not only to reduce diabetic complications but also to maintain the plasma-to- dialysate osmotic gradient necessary to achieve ultrafiltration.

With a 1.5% dextrose PD solution, 15 to 22 grams of glucose are absorbed. With a 2.5% dextrose solution 24 to 40 grams are absorbed and with 4.25% solutions 45 to 60 grams. This additional glucose load adds to daily caloric intake, which can contribute to energy stores, but also to the development of obesity and other metabolic complications such as hyperglycemia, hyperinsulinemia and hyperlipidemia. Control of the blood glucose is of primary importance and strategies should be adopted to reduce unnecessary glucose exposure and control hyperglycemia with oral hypoglycemic agents, subcutaneous or intraperitoneal insulin.

As mentioned, the diabetic on PD must make attempts to avoid the more hypertonic dialysate solutions. To do so, restricted intake of salt is especially important to reduce the ultrafiltration requirements. Repeated interventions may be needed to reinforce a sodium restriction, education on sodium content of processed foods, instruct on use of potassium containing sodium substitutes, and need for ongoing diuretic use. The goal is to have a more educated PD patient, who has a better understanding of how to shop for and prepare food. By limiting the intake of sodium, the patient can avoid higher tonicity solutions and improve glucose control. In the diabetic PD population, the impact of sodium restriction on glucose control must be fully explained so that patients understand the connection between sodium intake, ultrafiltration requirements, and rationale for avoiding the more hypertonic dextrose solutions.

Glucose-Sparing Strategies

As mentioned, use of standard dextrose PD solutions can result in the glucose absorption of 100 to 300 g per day. Icodextrin is an oligosaccharide starch derivative that creates a colloidal osmotic pressure and is indicated for the long dwell, especially in patients with high and high-average transport status. Absorption of icodextrin via the lymphatics is followed by metabolism by serum amylase to maltose and other short chain polysaccharides. They are transported to the intracellular compartment where maltase degrades the compounds to glucose. Therefore icodextrin use does not result in plasma glucose exposure and is, therefore, considered a glucose-sparing solution.

As mentioned, diabetics have been shown to have higher peritoneal membrane permeability and therefore may require hypertonic dextrose solutions to maintain ultrafiltration, especially during the long exchange. The enhanced ultrafiltration achieved with icodextrin can assist in maintaining euvolemia without exposing the diabetic patient to higher dextrose conventional solutions. As the glucose load is reduced with icodextrin use, reductions in insulin dosing may be required. Use of icodextrin for the long dwell reduces glucose exposure to the peritoneal membrane and may result in more stable long term solute transport properties.

In a 2009 randomized controlled trial by Paniagua and colleagues, icodextrin was shown to reduce glucose exposure, fasting serum glucose levels, HbA1c levels, insulin requirements, serum triglycerides, and stabilize body weight in diabetic PD patients with high and high-average transport status.

Several precautions are taken in diabetic patients using icodextrin during the long exchange. The FDA has issued a Drug-Device black box warning for glucose testing devices that are not glucose specific. These devices use the testing reagent glucose dehydrogenase pyrroloquinolinequinone (GDP-PQQ) or glucose-dye-oxidoreductase that is not specific for glucose and detects both maltose and glucose. As icodextrin metabolites are small chain polysaccharides, including maltose, these glucose monitoring devices detect maltose as glucose and record an artifactually elevated reading, indicating hyperglycemia that can lead to excess insulin administration. After reports of deaths due to excess insulin administration, the FDA issued this warning. All diabetic PD patients using icodextrin must use glucose testing devices that are specific for glucose. Patients are also advised to carry wallet warning cards or wrist bracelets to alert medical care givers of this potential for error with certain glucose monitors.

Several common glucose monitoring devices are listed below. The testing reagent used in these devices is given and, again, monitors that contain GDH-PQQ or glucose-dye-oxidoreductase-based reagents should be strictly avoided in patients using icodextrin.

Glucose Monitor Brand	Icodextrin Compatible	Reagent Used	Manufacturer
Most Freestyle models	No	GDH PQQ	Abbott Diabetes Care
Most Precision models	Yes	GDH NAD	Abbott Diabetes Care
Most Advance models	Yes	GOD	Arkray
Most Ascensia models	Yes	GOD or GDH-FAD	Bayer Healthcare
Most One Touch models	Yes	GOD	Lifescan, Inc
Most Accu-check models	No	GDH PQQ	Roche Diagnostics

GOD- glucose oxidase
GDH PQQ- glucose dehydrogenase with pyrroloquinolinequinone
GDH-NAD- glucose dehydrogenase with nicotinamide-adenine dinucleotide
GDH-FAD- glucose dehydrogenase with flavin-adenine dinucleotide

Outside of the USA, several PD solutions are available that are glucose sparing or lower in glucose degradation products. An amino-acid based solution is available, as well as solutions with novel packaging that allows for lower glucose degradation product (GDP) formation during heat sterilization. A popular CAPD regimen in Europe reduces glucose exposure by 50% by using one exchange with icodextrin, one with an amino acid solution, and the remaining with low GDP dextrose solutions.

Monitoring of the HbA1c

Control of the blood sugar in the general diabetic population can reduce microvascular complications and hospitalizations. Monitoring of the glycosylated hemoglobin (HbA1c), which reflects blood glucose control for the prior 3 months, is generally advised. Oganizations such as the American Diabetes Association have established the target HbA1c of less than 7% in the general population. The Kidney Disease Outcomes Quality Initiative (KDOQI) recommends these same targets for patients with CKD and ESRD. However, the HbA1c measurement is less precise in dialysis patients, with the higher rate of RBC turnover (especially in the HD patient) due to increased loss of RBC's and the shorter lifespan of the circulating erythrocyte. Use of erythropoietin, leading to increased numbers of newer, less glycated erythrocytes, leads to reduced levels of HbA1c. The HbA1c was intended to assay the glycation of hemoglobin that occurred over the expected 90 day life span of the erythrocyte. However, as mentioned, if the total erythrocyte lifespan is altered by blood loss in a dialyzer combined with the production of newer cells with erythropoietin, the overall hemoglobin glycation would be less, and the test would result in a falsely reduced value that underestimates true glycemic control. Therefore, the ADA recommendations to maintain the HbA1c below 7% could be considered conservative in the ESRD population.

In ESRD, most long term studies of diabetic control involved hemodialysis patients and these studies have shown conflicting results on the relationship of strict diabetic control and survival. Researchers at the Joslin clinic, analyzing a large diabetic hemodialysis population, were unable to conclusively show an association between the traditional HbA1c ranges and hospitalization or mortality and only noted that the extremes in HbA1c values, of <5% and >11%, were associated with adverse events. The authors could only conclude that the extremely low or high HbA1c values should be avoided in ESRD patients and KDOQI guidelines for HbA1c targets "require more supportive evidence". Simply using HbA1c to try to predict hospitalization or mortality in the diabetic

ESRD population may not be possible, as this patient population has such advanced microvascular and macrovascular disease, of longstanding duration, that diabetic control within a certain range of values may no longer clearly impact on survival outcomes. Just as the so called 4D study could show no benefit of using statins in the hemodialysis patients, this population may have vascular disease that is unique or too advanced to show the survival benefit of any one intervention, such as strict control of the HbA1c level.

Due to these factors, interpretation of HbA1c values in PD patients is controversial. At present, the K/DOQI recommendation to target a HbA1c of <7 % is advised but further research is needed in this important area.

Use of Oral Hypoglycemic Agents

In Type II diabetic patients, oral hypoglycemic agents are often prescribed. Sulfonylurea agents can be used in PD patients but special precautions must be taken to avoid agents with longer half life that may accumulate in ESRD. Glucose based solutions can protect against hypoglycemia but precautions must still be exercised, especially in the anuric patient. Tolbutamide and glipizide are often used, as these agents are shorter acting with largely hepatic clearance. Glyburide should be avoided due to the longer half-life.

Metformin is contraindicated in the patient with advanced kidney disease due to the risk of lactic acidosis. Thiazolidinediones (peroxisome proliferator-activated receptor gamma agonists) have been shown to reduce insulin resistance and insulin requirements and show an anti-inflammatory effect in this population. However, use has been complicated by reports of edema formation and congestive heart failure, resulting in a FDA warning on use of glitazones in patients with cardiac failure. The development of edema in dialysis patients suggests that abnormalities in renal sodium retention may not be the sole mechanism of this fluid retention and further research is needed to evaluate the long term safety of these agents in the PD population.

Subcutaneous and Intraperitoneal Insulin Regimens

During PD therapy, insulin requiring patients can be expected to need adjustment of their insulin dosing due to the improved appetite resulting from corrected uremia and use of dextrose-based dialysis solutions.

Intraperitoneal insulin can free the diabetic patient from painful insulin injections. Intraperitoneal insulin is considered a more physiologic route of administration, as the insulin is absorbed into the portal vein mimicking insulin delivery of the true pancreas. Some, but not all, studies showed a small increase in peritonitis occurrence, presumably from contamination during injection into the dialysate bag.

Recent small reports suggest that diabetics using intraperitoneal insulin develop focal fatty liver deposits under the liver capsule, termed hepatic subcapsular steatosis. The long term clinical implications of intraperitoneal insulin-related steatosis remains unclear, but the steatosis was recently shown to resolve after discontinuation of PD.

Several basic principles guide intraperitoneal insulin use. Only regular insulin is utilized in these protocols and higher doses of insulin are required, compared to the subcutaneous route, due to dilution of the insulin and absorption into the plastic of the bags. Typically 2-3 fold increases in total insulin doses are required if utilizing the intraperitoneal route. Again, only regular insulin is used for the intraperitoneal route of delivery.

To convert the patient presently on subcutaneous insulin to the intraperitoneal route, the clinician determines the total amount of NPH and regular insulin required for the 24 hour period. Multiply this amount by 2 to obtain the initial daily regular insulin units that will be used for intraperitoneal dosing. For patients on CAPD, of the total regular insulin units determined, 85% is divided among day exchanges and 15% is used in the night exchange. For patients on an APD cycler regimen, 50% of the total regular dose is used in the night exchanges and the remaining 50% is used in the day exchange. These doses are then adjusted gradually to determine the final dosing regimen. As mentioned, total regular intraperitoneal insulin requirements are usually 2 to 3 fold higher than the 24 hour subcutaneous insulin requirement.

Regular insulin can be added to icodextrin solutions. Icodextrin is a non-glucose solution and suggests that a reduced amount of insulin should be added to the exchange compared to standard glucose exchanges. Some suggest a 50% reduction in insulin in the icodextrin exchange is reasonable.

Potential advantages of intraperitoneal insulin

>   Avoidance of needle sticks
>   Avoidance of peripheral hyperinsulinemia
>   Insulin delivery into the portal vein mimicking the true pancreas
>   Better metabolic control due to greater insulin sensitivity in the periphery
>   Reduced endogenous hepatic glucose production

Potential disadvantages of intaperitoneal insulin

>   Potential risk of contamination and peritonitis
>   Larger doses are required so less cost effective
>   In high transporters, has been associated with development of hepatic subcapsular steatosis
>   Associated with hypertriglyceridemia

Example: converting a patient from subcutaneous insulin to intraperitoneal insulin

Current subcutaneous insulin regimen:

A.M. - NPH insulin 20 units and Regular insulin 10 units subcutaneously
P.M. - NPH insulin 15 units and Regular insulin 10 units subcutaneously

To convert to intraperitoneal insulin:

First, determine the total daily dose of insulin from above:
20 + 10 + 15 + 10 = 55 units

Due to the dilution of insulin and binding to the plastic bags this calculated dose is doubled:
55 x 2 = 110 units

If patient is on CAPD give 85% in divided doses for day exchange (0.85 x 110 = 93.5) and 15% for the night exchange. The day exchanges can, therefore, contain 31 units of regular insulin in each of the three day exchanges and the night exchange contains 15% of 110 units or 16 units of regular insulin.

If the patient is on an APD regimen, 50% of the total insulin is given in the night exchanges, and 50% is added to the long day exchange - so 55 units of regular insulin are added to the total night dialysate and 55 units of regular insulin are added to the long day exchange when the patient will also be eating breakfast, lunch, and dinner.

If the patient is using icodextrin for the long exchange on CAPD or APD the insulin doses into that exchange would be reduced by half.

With sterile technique and using a one inch needle, the insulin is added to all bags using the medication port. After addition of the insulin in the medication port, the bag is inverted several times to ensure admixture.

After converting to intraperitoneal insulin the patient is advised to use a sliding scale subcutaneous insulin coverage until the intraperitoneal dosing is fully adjusted. Intraperitoneal regular insulin is increased by 2-3 units a day to reach the final dosage which typically, as mentioned, is 2 to 3 fold the initial subcutaneous dose.

Taking all factors into consideration, the decision to convert from subcutaneous insulin to intraperitoneal insulin should be individualized and based on the patient's aversion to skin injections and satisfaction with degree of metabolic control. In patients with acceptable glucose control on a subcutaneous regimen, it may be advisable to continue the regimen and not convert to intraperitoneal dosing, due to the effort required to adjust intraperitoneal dosing, potential risk of peritonitis, larger doses of insulin required with the cost implications, and the potential risk of developing hepatic subcapsular steatosis. Further research is needed to better understand the long term medical benefits, if any, of intraperitoneal insulin with absorption directly into the portal vein.

Residual Kidney Function

Some, but not all, reports suggest that diabetic patients lose residual kidney function (RKF) more rapidly than the non-diabetic. The proposed mechanisms include a diabetic-related chronic inflammatory state with increased levels of pro-inflammatory cytokines such as TGF-B. Strategies to preserve RKF such as the use of ACE inhibitors and avoidance of nephrotoxins may be especially important in this group. Loss of RKF will require fluid removal strictly from peritoneal ultrafiltration and may increase the requirement for hypertonic solutions. Strategies to preserve RKF have been reviewed in Chapter 5.

PD Prescription

The PD prescription in diabetic patients should be guided by the proper understanding of residual kidney function, peritoneal membrane transport type, and sufficient dialysate exposure to meet ultrafiltration and clearance goals. Diabetic patients are more likely to demonstrate higher transport status which can result in an increase in small solute transport and more rapid loss of the osmotic gradient and ultrafiltration. Higher transport status, with ultrafiltration difficulties, contributes to technique failure and mortality.

This suggests that the diabetic patient may be more susceptible to loss of both residual kidney function and ultrafiltration, increasing the risk of chronic fluid overload, hypertension, and left ventricular hypertrophy. Higher transport patients are more suitable to APD therapy with shorter dwell times at night. To prevent inadequate ultrafiltration during the long day exchange, a mid-day exchange or use of an alternative osmotic agent such as icodextrin may be required.

Clearance targets for diabetics are the same as the general PD population. A minimum Kt/V target of 1.7 has been recommended by the K/DOQI working group.

Dietary Interventions

Nutritional parameters should be carefully monitored in diabetic PD patients. As mentioned, many diabetics exhibit higher peritoneal membrane permeability, which has been associated with hypoalbuminemia. Diabetic gastroparesis and a sense of abdominal fullness may be exacerbated by intraperitoneal fluid, affecting the appetite and intake of appropriate nutrition. Visual impairments, problems with manual dexterity, or amputations may impact access to food and food preparation. Patients may have poor understanding of nutrition, have difficulties obtaining groceries, or issues with dentition or swallowing. A detailed and thorough dietary evaluation should be obtained to determine the need for dietary interventions such as protein supplements.

Hypokalemia should be corrected aggressively in diabetics. Peritonitis with enteric organisms has been associated with hypokalemia in this patient population. The presumed mechanism is hypokalemia-induced intestinal motility disorders and bacterial overgrowth that may allow for transmural migration of enteric organisms into the peritoneum.

Diabetes-Related Co-Morbidities

The diabetic patient has an increased risk of cardiovascular (CV) complications, such as myocardial infarction and congestive heart disease, and these complications account for the primary cause of death in this population. At the initiation of dialysis, most patients have advanced vascular disease, as evidenced by the high prevalence of peripheral vascular disease, amputations, cerebral vascular and coronary heart disease. This suggests that aggressive measures should be taken to lower the cardiovascular risk profile in the pre-dialysis period. Once on dialysis, vascular abnormalities may be so advanced that measures intended to lower CV risk may be of limited benefit. The well discussed 4-D study and the recent AURORA study indicate that the use of statin medications in HD patients did not lower the risk of a cardiac event or death and there is no evidence that statin therapy provides a survival benefit to the patient on peritoneal dialysis.

Blood pressure control and control of the extravascular volume status can reduce the risk of new cardiovascular complications. To maintain euvolemia without the need for hypertonic dextrose solutions, patients with residual kidney function should be maintained on diuretic therapy, with strict control of dietary sodium intake. Diabetic patients on CAPD demonstrated a relationship between serum angiotensin converting enzyme (ACE) levels and mortality and treatment with ACE inhibitors or receptor blockers may be of added benefit in this group.

The complicated co-morbidities of the diabetic ESRD patient suggest that renal care givers should consider more frequent follow-up visits, or visits of longer duration. Many nephrologists assume primary care of the diabetic on dialysis, so scheduling of regular eye and foot exams may be needed.

Expanding diabetic education and care management can be of value. A study of intensive diabetic education and care management within a dialysis unit resulted in improved glycemic control, altered patient behavior, and reduced complications. As PD therapy allows for face to face contact between the patient and PD nurse, the opportunities for diabetic case management within the PD unit can be maximized.

Reflux and Gastroparesis

Diabetic PD patients may exhibit a variety of gastrointestinal symptoms due to autonomic neuropathy, uremia, reflux and gastroparesis. Nausea, vomiting, and distension are common complaints. The stomach contains air and therefore can change position as the abdomen is filled with dialysate, thus altering the normal gastric-esophageal angle. This can illicit or exacerbate gastric reflux symptoms in all PD patients but may be worse in the diabetic with pre-existing gastroparesis. Gastroparesis may also be worsened by the pressure-volume effects of dialysate or by the absorbed calories affecting gastric and intestinal motility. Slower gastric emptying was noted with glucose based solutions, compared to icodextrin, suggesting the absorption of glucose calories may contribute to the delay in emptying time. However, gastric emptying times were demonstrated to be prolonged in PD patients, even during periods that the abdomen was dry, implying the delayed gastric emptying was, in part, also due to underlying ESRD. Indeed, other suggested causes of delayed gastric emptying in ESRD patients are uremic toxin retention, bowel mucosal edema, and delayed clearance of intestinal hormones such as cholecystokinin.

Many medical approaches to gastroparesis have been advocated. Use of lower volume exchanges at meal times with larger volumes at night, while recumbent, may be effective. Oral erythromycin regimens such as erythromycin elixir 200 mg given 30 to 60 minutes before meals have been successful. Metoclopramide has been used, but is often associated with extrapyramidal complications. Small feedings, up to 6 times per day, may improve symptoms.

Clinical Action Plan for the Diabetic on PD

This chapter has summarized some unique aspects of care in the diabetic patient on PD. A comprehensive clinical action plan for this population is outlined below:

Check List of Clinical Priorities in Caring for the Diabetic PD Patient

1. Attempt to improve glycemic control as early in CKD as possible with adequate self-monitoring and maintain that control during PD therapy

2. Once on PD, control the blood glucose level to allow for the osmotic gradient to be maintained with lower dialysate dextrose concentrations - avoid use of hypertonic solutions

3. Educate patients to allow for an understanding of the link between sodium intake and the need for hypertonic dextrose solutions

4. Blood pressure control is important, due to the advanced co-morbidities often encountered in this population. Inhibitors of angiotensin II are ideal initial antihypertensive choices due to the potential to also preserve RKF and peritoneal membrane function

5. PD unit should identify which physician will be managing the diabetic care - the nephrologist, endocrinologist, internist, or family physician to facilitate management communication and the forwarding of laboratory testing

6. Evaluate for possible intraperitoneal insulin regimen

7. Carry carbohydrate to avoid hypoglycemia

8. Regularly monitor the HbA1c

9. Take active measures to protect residual kidney function and consider recommendations for using diuretics and medications that inhibit the activity of angiotensin II

10. Ensure special emphasis in this population on avoiding nephrotoxins to preserve RKF

11. Evaluate for neurogenic bladder and need for self catheterization to maintain RKF

12. Analyze the PET carefully, as many diabetics exhibit increased peritoneal permeability and may be better suited for cycler APD therapy, to enable a prescription that contains short dwells at night

13. Carefully monitor the long dwell as higher transport status may result in loss of ultrafiltration in this exchange

14. If ultrafiltration is lost in the long dwell, consider an alternative osmotic agent such as icodextrin or an interruption of the long dwell with an additional exchange

15. For exit site and peritonitis prophlaxis, mupirocin or gentamicin topical antibiotic at the exit site daily is strongly encouraged

16. Correct hypokalemia due to risk of associated peritonitis with enteric organisms

17. Monitor for and treat active periodontal disease

18. Evaluate the patient's glucose monitor to avoid monitors using reagents that are not compatible with icodextrin

19. Monitor nutritional parameters as many diabetics may have high transport status and increased peritoneal protein losses. Consider supplements if indicated

20. Monitor for gastroparesis and if worsening can consider draining abdomen prior to meals, smaller frequent meals, or pro-kinetic therapy such as erythromycin elixir

21. Teach patients how to perform foot checks and have frequent foot examinations in the PD unit. Evaluate for proper shoes and socks. Encourage foot moisturizers to prevent dryness and skin cracking. Evaluate distal pulses

22. PD unit checklist to monitor ophthalmology referrals to maintain recommended yearly dilated eye exams

23. Dietician intervention on meal planning

24. Despite insufficient data to show conclusive benefit, consider dyslipidemia treatment

25. Encourage exercise to maintain steady body weight

26. PD unit staff should consider extending the initial training period for a diabetic patient to allow for these recommendations to be implemented and established as a long term care plan

27. Consider PD unit infrastructure change to allow for more clinical encounters for the diabetic PD patient to address other co-morbidities and expand care management

28. Consider PD unit infrastructure change to allow for RN case management of the diabetic PD population to follow adherence to diabetic specific care protocols

29. Consider continuous education programs on living with diabetes, using support groups consisting of experienced PD nurses, experienced PD patients, dieticians and provide ongoing encouragement and education on community resources

References:

American Diabetes Association. Standards of Medical Care in Diabetes-2006. Diabetes Care 2006;29[Suppl 1]:S4-S42.

Ansari A, Thomas S, Goldsmith D. Assessing glycemic control in patients with diabetes and end-stage renal failure. Am J Kidney Dis 2003;41:523-531.

Babazono T, Nakamoto H, Kasai K, et al. Effects of icodextrin on glycemic and lipid profiles in diabetic patients undergoing peritoneal dialysis. Am J Nephrol 2007;27:409-415.

Beardsworth SF, Ahmad R, Terry E, Karim K. Intraperitoneal insulin: a protocol for administration during CAPD and review of published protocols. Perit Dial Int 1988;8:145-151.

Chung SH, Noh H, Ha H, Lee HB. Optimal use of peritoneal dialysis in patients with diabetes. Perit Dial Int 2009;29(S2):S132-S134.

Chung SH, Han DC, Noh H, et al. Risk factors for mortality in diabetic peritoneal dialysis patients. Nephrol Dial Transplant 2010;25:3742-3748.

Demir S, Torun D, Tokmak N, et al. Resolution of hepatic subcapsular steatosis after discontinuation of CAPD. Nephrol Dial Transplant 2007;22:1247-1249.

Diaz-Buxo JA. Peritoneal dialysis prescriptions for diabetic patients. Adv Perit Dial 1999;15:91-95.

Fang W, Yang X, Kothari J, et al. Patient and technique survival of diabetics on peritoneal dialysis: one-center's experience and review of the literature. Clin Nephrol 2008;69:193-200.

Fine A, Parry D, Ariano R, Dent W. Marked variation in peritoneal insulin absorption in peritoneal dialysis. Perit Dial Int 2000;20:652-655.

Gokal R, Moberly J, Lindholm B, Mujais S. Metabolic and laboratory effects of icodextrin. Kidney Int 2002;62[Suppl 81]:S62-S71.

Holmes CJ, Shockley TR. Strategies to reduce glucose exposure in peritoneal dialysis patients. Perit Dial Int 2000;20[Suppl 2]:S37-S41.

Johnson CA, Amidon G, Reichert JE, Porter WR. Adsorption of insulin to the surface of peritoneal dialysis solution containers. Am J Kidney Dis 1983;3:224-228.

KDOQI clinical practice guidelines and clinical practice recommendations for diabetes and chronic kidney disease. Am J Kidney Dis 2007;49[Suppl 2]:S12-S154.

Kshirsagar AV, Craig RG, Moss KL, et al. Periodontal disease adversely affects the survival of patients with end-stage renal disease. Kidney Int 2009;75:746-751.

Lamb EJ, Worrall J, Buhler R, et al. Effect of diabetes and peritonitis on the peritoneal equilibration test. Kidney Int 1995;47:1760-1767.

Lee JH, Reddy DK, Saran R, et al. Peritoneal accumulation of advanced glycosylation end-products in diabetic rats on dialysis with icodextrin. Perit Dial Int 2000;20[Suppl 5]:S39-47.

Locatelli F, Pozzoni P, Del Vecchio L. Renal replacement therapy in patients with diabetes and end-stage renal disease. J Am Soc Nephrol 2004;15[Suppl 1]:S25-S29.

Marshall J, Jennings P, Scott A, et al. Glycemic control in diabetic CAPD patients assessed by continuous glucose monitoring system (CGMS). Kidney Int 2003;64:1480-1486.

McMurray SD, Johnson G, Davis S, McDougall K. Diabetes education and care management significantly improve patient outcomes in the dialysis unit. Am J Kidney Dis 2002;40:566-575.

Nevalainen PI, Kallio T, Lahtela JT, et al. High peritoneal permeability predisposes to hepatic steatosis in diabetic continuous ambulatory peritoneal patients receiving intraperitoneal insulin. Perit Dial Int 2000;20:637-642.

Nevalainen P, Lahtela JT, Mustonen J, Pasternack A. The influence of peritoneal dialysis and the use of subcutaneous and intraperitoneal insulin on glucose metabolism and serum lipids in type 1 diabetic patients. Nephrol Dial Transplant 1997;12:145-150.

Paniagua R, Ventura M, Avila-Diaz M, et al. Icodextrin improves metabolic and fluid management in high and high-average transport diabetic patients. Perit Dial Int 2009;29:422-432.

Passadakis PS, Oreopoulos DG. Diabetic patients on peritoneal dialysis. Semin Dial 2010;23:191-197.

Quellhorst E. Insulin therapy during peritoneal dialysis: pros and cons of various forms of administration. J Am Soc Nephrol 2002;13[Suppl 1]:S92-S96.

Scarpioni L, Ballocchi S, Castelli A, Scarpioni R. Insulin therapy in uremic diabetic patients on continuous ambulatory peritoneal dialysis; comparison of intraperitoneal and subcutaneous administration. Perit Dial Int 1994;14:127-131.

Scarpioni L, Ballocchi S, Scarpioni R, Cristinelli L. Peritoneal dialysis in diabetics. Optimal insulin therapy on CAPD: intraperitoneal versus subcutaneous treatment. Perit Dial Int 1996;16[Suppl 1]:S275-S278.

Schomig M, Ritz E, Standl E, Allenberg J. The diabetic foot in the dialyzed patient. J Am Soc Nephrol 2000;11:1153-1159.

Shu KH, Chang CS, Chuang YW, et al. Intestinal bacterial overgrowth in CAPD patients with hypokalemia. Nephrol Dial Transplant 2009;24:1289-1292.

Silang R, Regalado M, Cheng TH, Wesson DE. Prokinetic agents increase plasma albumin in hyoalbuminemic chronic dialysis patients with delayed gastric emptying. Am J Kidney Dis 2001;37:287-293.

Smit W, van Esch S, Struijk DG, Krediet RT. Free water transport in patients starting with peritoneal dialysis: a comparison between diabetic and non diabetic patients . Adv Perit Dial 2004;20:13-17.

Szeto CC, Chow KM, Leung CB, et al. Increased subcutaneous insulin requirements in diabetic patients recently commenced on peritoneal dialysis. Nephrol Dial Transplant 2007;22:1697-1702.

Szeto CC, Chow KM. Thiazolidinediones in peritoneal dialysis patients. Perit Dial Int 2009;29:248-251.

Tang W, Cheng L, Wang T. Diabetic patients can do as well on peritoneal dialysis as nondiabetic patients. Blood Purif 2005;23:330-337.

Thorp ML, Wilks TS. Three diabetic peritoneal dialysis patients receiving intraperitoneal insulin with dosage adjustment based on capillary glucose levels during peritoneal equilibration tests. Am J Kidney Dis 2004;43:927-929.

Torun D, Oguzkurt L, Sezer S, et al. Hepatic subcapsular steatosis as a complication associated with intraperitoneal insulin treatment in diabetic peritoneal dialysis patients. Perit Dial Int 2005;25:596-600.

Tzamaloukas AH, Murata GH, Malhotra D. Renal clearances in continuous ambulatory peritoneal dialysis: differences between diabetic and non-diabetic subjects. Int J Artif Organs 2001;24:203-207.

Van Laecke S, Veys N, Verbeke F, et al. The fate of older diabetic patients on peritoneal dialysis: myths and mysteries and suggestions for further research. Perit Dial Int 2007;27:611-618.

Van Vlem BA, Schoonjans RS, Struijk DG, et al. Influence of dialysate on gastric emptying time in peritoneal dialysis patients. Perit Dial Int 2002;22:32-38.

Voges M, Divino-Filho JC, Faict D, et al. Compatibility of insulin over 24 hours in standard and bicarbonate-based peritoneal dialysis solutions contained in bags made of different materials. Perit Dial Int 2006;26:498-502.

Vonesh EF, Snyder JJ, Foley RN, Collins AJ. Mortality studies comparing peritoneal dialysis and hemodialysis: what do they tell us? Kidney Int 2006; 70[Suppl103]:S3-S11.

Wang AY, Wang M, Woo J, et al. Inflammation, residual kidney function, and cardiac hypertrophy are interrelated and combine adversely to enhance mortality and cardiovascular death risk of peritoneal dialysis patients. J Am Soc Nephrol 2004;15:2186-2194.

Williams ME, Lacson E, Teng M, et al. Extremes of glycemic control (HbA1c) increase hospitalization risk in diabetic hemodialysis patients in the USA. Am J Nephrol 2009;29:54-61.

Wong TY, Szeto CC, Chow KM, et al. Rosiglitazone (RSG) reduces insulin requirement and C-reactive protein levels in type 2 diabetic patients on peritoneal dialysis. Am J Kidney Dis 2005;46:713-719.

Wu MS, Yu CC, Wu CH, et al. Pre-dialysis glycemic control is an independent predictor of mortality in type II diabetic patients on continuous ambulatory peritoneal dialysis. Perit Dial Int 1999;19[Suppl 2]:S179-183.

Yao Q, Lindholm B, Heimburger O. Peritoneal dialysis prescription for diabetic patients. Perit Dial Int 2005;25[Suppl 3]:S76-S79.

Chapter 15:
PD in the Obese Patient

REFLECTING THE GENERAL TRENDS in the US population, the proportion of obese patients reaching ESRD is increasing. In this decade, one third of incident dialysis patients are now classified as obese and the prevalence of dialysis patients with a BMI > 35 kg/m² has increased by 63%. Therefore practitioners will need expertise in the management of an obese dialysis patient. Whereas prior nutritional concerns were largely over the malnourished patient with poor appetite, present priorities will need to shift toward development of strategies to manage the more obese patient.

The obese patient on peritoneal dialysis presents many unique concerns and challenges. However, patients who are obese can be successfully managed on peritoneal dialysis and the goals of care in this patient population are similar to those for the general PD population- maximize survival, establish reliable and well planned peritoneal access, preserve residual kidney function, achieve adequate dialysis clearance, and reduce the risk of infectious and non-infectious complications. This chapter will focus on these issues.

Survival Data in the Obese PD Population

In the hemodialysis literature, obesity seems to confer a survival advantage. In peritoneal dialysis, many studies also suggest a survival advantage in the obese patient. This paradoxical "reverse" epidemiology has led to speculation on mechanisms to explain why obesity may confer a survival advantage to patients on dialysis. Dialysis patients have higher energy expenditures and often experience periods of anorexia. Obesity may provide needed energy stores in this population and some speculate that the higher BMI may provide a "nutritional reserve", reducing overall mortality on PD. Others suggest that adipose tissue is not metabolically active and does not contribute to "toxin" production, is not water soluble and, therefore, does not contain urea and other water-bound uremic toxins. Some speculate that adipose cells are a source of stem cells and therefore may play a role in regeneration and mechanisms of tissue repair. These proponents also claim that the obese patient has increased muscle mass. For these reasons, proponents feel the obese dialysis patient would be expected to have a better prognosis than the malnourished patient.

An Australian prospective observational study of outcomes on PD showed that in patients deemed overweight (BMI > 27.5 kg/m^2) twenty-nine percent of patients had died at 3 years compared to 69% of patients in the normal-weight group. The authors concluded that BMI greater than 27.5 was an independent positive predictor of patient survival.

In an analysis of the Medicare population initiating peritoneal dialysis between 1995 and 2000, underweight patients had the highest mortality. Those patients classified as overweight, to frankly obese, had equal or better cumulative survival than normal weight PD patients at 3 years of follow-up.

Similarly, a retrospective analysis of the original USRDS Morbidity and Mortality Wave II Study showed that survival of PD patients with BMI >30 kg/m^2 was equivalent to that of the lower BMI group and concluded that obesity in PD patients did not impact survival on the modality. Similar to the PD patients, obese HD patients showed a survival advantage compared to lower weight patients, and the survival benefit of obesity in HD exceeded that noted in the obese PD population.

Abbott and colleagues performed an analysis of patients initiating dialysis between 1995 and 1997 and again showed that those PD patients at the higher BMI had the best survival. The obese HD patient had superior survival compared to the normal or low weight HD patient. In this study, when a comparison was made in survival of the obese PD patients with the obese HD patients, there was improved survival in obese HD patients.

The preponderance of the information would suggest that the obese PD patient is not at a survival disadvantage compared to the normal or low weight PD patient. However, caution must be used in reaching any conclusion about survival in the obese population, based on dialysis modality. Interpretation of these registry reports is hampered by lack of reporting of residual kidney function (a factor now known to be an independent predictor of survival in PD and HD patients), lack of information about the PD prescription, dialysis adequacy, membrane transport status, medication use, etc. The registry data cannot fully control for potential survival confounders such as cancer, tobacco use, congestive heart failure, etc.

It has been suggested that using the body mass index (BMI) as an indicator of obesity is flawed. For example, a patient with a high BMI may have excellent nutrition and large muscle mass, contributing to the high BMI. Other patients may have a high BMI and low muscle mass, indicating a greater degree of adipose tissue. The degree of adipose tissue may be the true risk factor for survival on PD, not simply the BMI. This would suggest that understanding body *composition* is more important than simply assessing the BMI. An attempt to study the impact of body size and body composition on PD survival was recently reported. Ramkumar and colleagues employed serum creatinine and creatinine clearance determinations to assess the predicted 24-hour urinary creatinine values in over 1000 PD patients from the USRDS database. The urinary creatinine concentrations were used to predict muscle creatine content, as a surrogate estimation of muscle mass. Patients were classified as being high BMI-high muscle mass versus high BMI-low muscle mass. The high BMI-high muscle mass group had better overall survival than a normal BMI control cohort. Death rates were higher in the high BMI-low muscle mass group. They concluded that PD patients with high BMI and larger muscle mass have the best survival of all PD patients and that PD patients should be advised to attempt to gain muscle mass. In addition, gains of further adiposity on PD should be monitored and use of higher tonicity solutions avoided by enforcement of dietary sodium restriction and use of higher dose diuretics.

Attempting to isolate why high BMI-low muscle mass is an independent predictor of survival is difficult, as the low muscle mass group also had a higher prevalence of diabetes, coronary artery disease, peripheral vascular disease, congestive heart failure, and other co-morbidities. Nevertheless, this study raised intriguing questions as to the proper interpretation of a BMI and suggests that further classifications of body size, based on body composition, may help to clarify the association of obesity with survival on dialysis.

At the present level of understanding, obesity should not be considered a contraindication for PD therapy. The obese patient should be offered full dialysis options education and exposure to the home dialysis therapies.

The Obese Patient and Residual Kidney Function

Overall survival on dialysis is determined by the degree of residual kidney function (RKF) and some observational studies have suggested that obese patients have a more rapid loss of RKF, compared to normal or underweight patients. The more rapid decline in RKF in obese patients may be due to the development of diabetes, hypertension, or secondary obesity-related glomerular structural abnormalities. Therefore special emphasis should be placed on protecting RKF in the obese population. As in all PD patients, recommendations are made in the obese population to limit use of aminoglycosides and non-steroidal anti-inflammatory agents or contrast dye. Continuing angiotensin - converting enzyme inhibitors or receptor blockers and diuretics is recommended.

Weight Gain

The effect of PD on weight gain is controversial. Reports have documented weight gain during PD therapy. For example, Jager and colleagues in 2001 reported from 13 Dutch dialysis centers that included consecutive patients starting dialysis from 1993 to 1995 with subsequent nutritional status assessed up to 2 years after initiation of therapy. While in the PD and HD populations overall there was no difference in changes in body mass index over time, an increase in body fat of 3.2 kg was noted in the subgroup of female patients treated with PD compared to HD. However a more recent analysis of a large USA cohort by Lievense and colleagues, using careful 1:1 propensity score-matched cohorts of incident PD and HD patients, found that weight gain was lower in the PD group compared to HD. This decrease in weight gain may be due to the effects of dialysate on appetite, satiety, or due to alterations in gastric motility associated with PD.

Weight gain by modality may be affected by other factors such as co-morbidities, social status and access to higher quality foods, non-fat fluid accumulation, or other residual confounders. Estimates of weight gain during PD are also confounded by baseline weight measurements taken at the initiation of PD but subsequent weight measurements obtained with intraperitoneal dialysate which may overestimate weight changes. Currently, further research is needed to clarify these inconsistencies in the literature and no firm conclusions regarding the effects of dialysis modalities on subsequent weight gain can be made.

Adequacy of Dialysis in the Obese PD Patient

In the past, concern was raised that the obese patient could not achieve adequacy targets for urea and creatinine clearances. This was investigated in a cross sectional study of obese PD patients (BMI >29 kg/m^2), 40% of whom were anuric. In those patients prescribed a mean of 14.6 L of dialysate, 84% achieved a Kt/V of 2.49, well above current adequacy targets. Overall, 96% of all obese patients and 90% of the anuric obese achieved these higher adequacy targets. As this demonstrated, clearance targets are achievable in the obese patient, in part, because adipose tissue is, by definition, anhydrous and does not contribute to total body water and the volume of distribution of urea. Adipose tissue is not particularly active, metabolically, and does not generate significant uremic toxins.

To assure adequacy targets are reached, dwell volumes should be appropriately prescribed to maximize contact of dialysate to peritoneum, to increase the effective surface area of the dialyzing membrane. In a 2003 publication, 17% of solution shipments were for 3 liter exchanges and 26% of exchanges were of 2.5 liters, reflecting on the larger body habitus in more modern times and the trend toward an appropriate increase in the dwell volumes for the obese.

There has been debate over what weight should be used to determine total body water (V) for determination of urea clearance, expressed as the Kt/V. The most accurate formula for determining the volume of total body water (V), in obesity, is the Watson and Watson formula, which was derived from data that included obese patients. However, using isotope dilution techniques, the Watson and Watson formula was shown to overestimate true body water content in obese patients. This suggests that using the Watson and Watson formula to determine V in a Kt/V calculation can underestimate clearance and that actual clearances may be better than indicated by the Kt/V. To overcome this limitation, many practitioners now enter the ideal body weight, not the actual weight, into the Watson calculation. These proponents feel this is appropriate as urea clearance requirements should not increase in relation to anhydrous body fat. Proponents of using the ideal body weight to calculate V, instead of actual weight, state that fat tissue, as mentioned, is anhydrous and does not contain water bound uremic toxins and is metabolically inactive and not generating uremic toxins. At the present time, the weight and formula to use for the determination of V in the obese patient remains controversial. The KDOQI document simply states- "the correct determination of V for overweight patients is unclear".

Catheter Placement in the Obese PD Patient

The obese patient presents technical challenges in catheter insertion. If the catheter exit site is in the lower abdominal quadrants, as with the traditional catheter, there is higher likelihood that the exit site will be difficult to inspect and clean. The exit site may be within a larger pannus and subject to more local movement and trauma. For these reasons, special care should be made in planning the PD catheter placement.

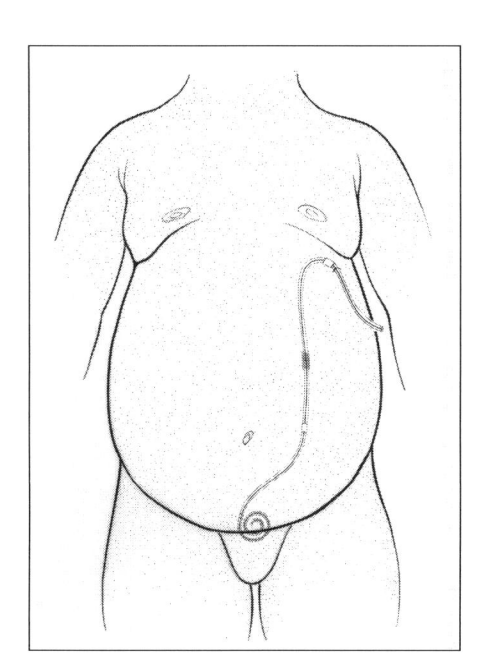

Newer placement techniques should be considered in the obese population. Basic and advanced laparoscopic techniques have led to advancements in catheter placement and the creation of exit site locations that are particularly beneficial to the obese patient. In patients with large dependent abdominal panni,

Obese patients are ideal candidates for upper abdominal exit site locations

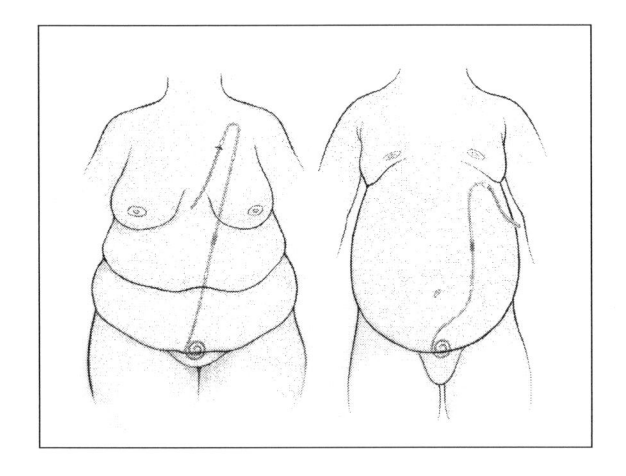

In cases of morbid obesity, the pre-sternal exit site is preferred, to allow for ease of care and reduced tissue movement around the subcutaneous Dacron cuff

consideration should be given to creating an exit site that is located in the upper abdomen or in the pre-sternal location. Catheter extension kits are available that allow for the internal pig-tailed catheter to be connected to a catheter extension, to lengthen the catheter and subcutaneous tunnel to allow for creation of an exit site at a preferred location. Placing the exit site in the upper abdominal wall, or pre-sternal location, allows for better inspection of the exit site, less movement and trauma to the site, easier application of exit site care, and has been shown to reduce catheter complications in the obese patient.

Infection Risk in the Obese PD Patient

Obese patients on PD have been found to have higher rates of peritonitis. An analysis of the ANZDATA Registry found that patients at the extreme of BMI (BMI equal to or greater than 30 kg/m^2) had a shorter time to first episode of peritonitis. The authors had previously noted that obese patients had higher risks of infection with hemodialysis catheters, suggesting that obesity represents a risk factor for all dialysis access infections. Higher peritonitis rates were not seen in those considered just overweight (BMI 25-29.9), and they noted a "vintage" effect, with more infections in the earlier years of observation and lower peritonitis rates noted in more recent years.

Older reports also suggested obese patients had higher rates of exit site infections, but these studies, as well as the Australian study, did not report on the infection rates when recommended strategies to reduce infections, such as prophylactic topical antibiotic administration to the exit site, and advanced catheter placement strategies, were employed. Especially in the obese, it is prudent to determine with the surgeon what the ideal exit site location should be to reduce the chances of chronic exit site infections. Clinicians should reinforce the need for meticulous exit site care and consider ISPD recommendations for daily topical antibiotic placement on the exit site.

Clinical Action Plan for the Obese PD Patient

The obese patient approaching ESRD should be offered PD as a dialysis modality. Special emphasis should be placed on developing a peritoneal access that avoids a lower abdominal exit site if that site cannot be easily visualized and kept clean and be free of abdominal skin folds. Consideration should be given to exit site placement in the upper abdomen or pre-sternal location. Initiating dialysis with PD may preserve residual kidney function and favorably impact survival as well as preserve vascular access for future options. Once on PD therapy use of larger dwell volumes should be considered to maintain adequacy targets. The patient should be encouraged to gain lean body mass and limit further gain in adipose tissue by dietary intervention and avoidance of hypertonic solutions.

References:

Abbott KC, Glanton CW, Trespalacios FC, et al. Body mass index, dialysis modality, and survival: analysis of the United States renal data system dialysis morbidity and mortality wave II study. Kidney Int 2004;65:597-605.

Abbott KC, Oliver DK, Hurst FP, et al. Body mass index and peritoneal dialysis: "exceptions to the exception" in reverse epidemiology? Semin Dial 2007;20:561-565.

Aslam N, Bernardini J, Fried L, Piraino B. Large body mass index does not predict short-term survival in peritoneal dialysis patients. Perit Dial Int 2002;22:191-196.

Crabtree JH. Selected best demonstrated practices in peritoneal dialysis access. Kidney Int 2006;70:S27-S37.

De Mutsert R, Grootendorst DC, Boeschoten EW, et al. Is obesity associated with a survival advantage in patients starting peritoneal dialysis? Contrib Nephrol 2009;163:124-131.

Drechsler C, de Mutsert R, Grootendorst DC, et al. Association of body mass index with decline in residual kidney function after dialysis. Am J Kidney Dis 2009;53:1014-1023.

Fried L, Bernardini J, Piraino B. Neither size nor weight predicts survival in peritoneal dialysis patients. Perit Dial Int 1996;16:357-361.

Ikizler TA. Resolved: being fat is good for dialysis patients: the Godzilla effect. J Am Soc Nephrol 2008;19:1059-1064.

Jager KJ, Merkus MP, Huisman RM, et al. Nutritional status over time in hemodialysis and peritoneal dialysis. J Am Soc Nephrol 2001;12:1272-1279.

Johansson AC, Samuelsson O, Attman PO, et al. Limitations in anthropometric calculations of total body water in patients on peritoneal dialysis. J Am Soc Nephrol 2001;12:568-573.

Johnson DW, Herzig KA, Purdie DM, et al. Is obesity a favorable prognostic factor in peritoneal dialysis patients? Perit Dial Int 2000;20:715-721.

Kramer HJ, Saranathan A. Luke A, et al. Increasing body mass index and obesity in the incident ESRD population. J Am Soc Nephrol 2006;17:1453-1459.

Lievense H, Kalantar-Zadeh K, Lukowsky LR, et al. Relationship of body size and initial dialysis modality on subsequent transplantation, mortality and weight gain of ESRD patients. Nephrol Dial Transplant 2012;27:3631-3638.

McDonald SP, Collins JF, Rumpsfeld M, Johnson DW. Obesity is a risk factor for peritonitis in the Australian and New Zealand peritoneal dialysis populations. Perit Dial Int 2004;24:340-346.

Miller BW. Planning for renal replacement therapy in the patient with obesity. Adv Chronic Kidney Dis 2006;13:418-420.

Piraino B, Bernardini J, Centa PK, et al. The effect of body weight on CAPD related infections and catheter loss. Perit Dial Int 1991;11:64-68.

Ramkumar N, Pappas LM, Beddhu S. Effect of body size and body composition on survival in peritoneal dialysis patients. Perit Dial Int 2005;25:461-469.

Shibagaki Y, Faber MD, Divine G, et al. Feasibility of adequate solute clearance in obese patients on peritoneal dialysis: a cross-sectional study. Am J Kidney Dis 2002;40:1295-1300.

Snyder JJ, Foley RN, Gilbertson DT, et. al. Body size and outcomes on peritoneal dialysis in the United States. Kidney Int 2003:64:1838-1844.

Stack AG, Murthy BVR, Molony DA. Survival differences between peritoneal dialysis and hemodialysis among "large" ESRD patients in the United States. Kidney Int 2004;65:2398-2408.

Chapter 16:
Nutritional and Metabolic Issues in PD

THE PATIENT ON PD therapy has unique nutritional requirements. Dietary recommendations for PD patients are very different than for those on hemodialysis. Daily peritoneal losses of potassium and protein make restrictions of these nutrients unnecessary. The PD patient may develop appetite disturbances due to abdominal fullness and absorption of glucose into the portal circulation leading to lower peak hunger. These and other factors suggest that maintaining adequate nutrition and metabolic control is a clinical challenge in this patient population. This chapter will review the unique dietary concerns and recommendations for the patient on PD therapy.

Sodium Balance in PD Patients

Initially there were concerns that PD patients may develop sodium depletion and hypotension, due to the continuous nature of the therapy. Therefore, no sodium restriction was enforced. Recommendations have come full circle however, as many PD patients were noted to remain hypertensive and edematous. Dietary recommendations were subsequently altered from no restriction to a modest sodium restriction. Present recommendations for salt intake in PD patients are to target 6 grams/day.

In the typical western diet, daily salt intake of 9 or more grams/day is common due to processed foods, "fast-foods", and preservatives such as monosodium glutamate (MSG). To reduce the salt intake in PD patients many recommendations can be made (summarized below). Many salt substitutes use potassium chloride instead of sodium chloride and may be especially useful in PD patients who have ongoing potassium losses.

> Recommendations to reduce salt intake in PD patients
>
> 1. No added salt during food preparation or as seasoning while eating
> 2. Limit processed foods and fast-food franchises
> 3. Read labels and compare sodium content of brands while shopping
> 4. Limit foods that contain MSG as a preservative
> 5. Use of salt substitutes such as AlsoSalt or Morton Salt Substitute
> 6. Avoid salted condiments such as pickles, soy, fish, or teriyaki sauces
> 7. Avoid or reduce portion size of canned, cured meats
> 8. Use spices and herbs to increase tastiness of food without adding salt
>
>   www.alsosalt.com, www.bensonsgourmetseasonings.com

Potassium Balance in PD patients

Potassium disorders are common in PD therapy: 10 to 36% of prevalent patients exhibit hypokalemia with hyperkalemia being less frequent. These disorders are largely due to an imbalance between nutritional intake and the potassium losses in the dialysate.

Hypokalemia in chronic PD therapy may, in part, be attributed to the daily continuous removal of potassium in the dialysate, poor intake of potassium rich foods, the insulin release associated with glucose absorption from the peritoneum, or increased gastrointestinal losses.

Some reports suggest that chronic hypokalemia may precipitate peritonitis by impacting on bowel motility, allowing for bacterial overgrowth and the increased likelihood of transmural migration of enteric organisms into the peritoneum. In the large bowel, hypokalemia may contribute to constipation and treatment with aggressive laxatives has been associated with peritonitis. In addition to the infectious risk, actuarial survival data suggests a higher mortality in those PD patients demonstrating chronic hypokalemia.

Hypokalemia is more common in patients with poor nutritional intake and other markers of malnutrition. These patients may be at greater risk of peritonitis due to their poor nutrition and severe co-morbid diseases. Patients with hypokalemia may also exhibit reduced serum albumin, serum phosphorus, and fasting total cholesterol levels. Hypoalbuminemia may lead to bowel edema increasing the likelihood of intestinal permeability and bacterial translocation.

Hypokalemia should be considered a simple marker for overall nutritional deficits and broad nutritional interventions may be indicated in the hypokalemia patient. Therefore, normalizing the plasma potassium level in PD patients is a clinical priority. Foods rich in potassium but relatively low in phosphorus such as bananas, oranges, tomatoes, potatoes, and spinach should be encouraged.

Due to ongoing potassium losses in the dialysate, the dietary potassium intake should be 70 mmol/day and many patients will require potassium supplementation. Potassium can be replaced orally or with intraperitoneal administration. The typical oral supplementation of potassium chloride (KCl) can vary from 8 to 20 mEq daily or twice a day. Intraperitoneal administration of potassium chloride has been successful, with no associated abdominal complaints or chemical peritonitis. In daily chronic intraperitoneal potassium replacement, typical protocols administer 4 to 8 mEq KCl into each 2 liter dialysate exchange to give a final concentration of 2 to 4 mEq/L in the dialysate. Larger doses of intraperitoneal potassium in the range of 40 to 60 mEqs added to a *once daily* exchange, in short term observations, has been reported but the safety of this regimen in long-term therapy requires further study and introduces the potential risk if misinterpretation by patient or staff as a daily additive to *each* exchange.

Hyperkalemia is rare in PD patients compliant with exchanges. Patients presenting with marked hyperkalemia must be considered to have missed exchanges, have severe dietary non-compliance, or transcellular shift of potassium due to metabolic acidosis, tumor lysis syndrome, rhabdomyolysis, hemolysis, hepatitis, or severe hyperglycemia. Due to the daily removal of potassium with PD therapy, significant hyperkalemia in patients treated with non-steroidal anti-inflammatory agents, angiotensin converting enzyme inhibitors or receptor blockers, spironolactone, or beta blocker agents is rare.

Magnesium Balance in PD patients

Historically, hypermagnesemia in ESRD patients was more common due to the use of magnesium containing antacids, phosphate binders, laxatives, or enemas but restrictions on the use of these products has reduced the incidence of this complication. Hypomagnesemia may be the more frequently encountered magnesium disorder due to malnutrition and losses in the dialysate. Commonly available dialysis solutions contain magnesium concentrations of 0.5 mEq/L and most patients have been demonstrated to maintain serum magnesium levels within normal ranges. Therefore, hypomagnesemia may be most predominantly associated with poor nutritional intake.

Oral magnesium supplementation with magnesium oxide 400 mg tablets twice daily has been reported, which provides 500 mg of elemental magnesium daily. Nutritional recommendations can be made to address hypomagnesemia such as increased intake of magnesium-rich foods such as wheat bran, almonds, and spinach. The administration of intraperitoneal magnesium sulfate was first described by Redrow and colleagues in pregnant patients on PD as a treatment of premature labor. Serum levels were documented to be safe despite administered doses as high as 800 mg per 2-liter exchange. Intraperitoneal administration of magnesium introduces a potential infectious risk and routine dosing regimens are unclear.

Protein Intake in PD Patients

Recommended dietary protein intake for the PD patient is higher than that of the hemodialysis patient or even the general population. These higher recommendations reflect the daily loss of protein and amino acids in the dialysate. Protein losses of 5 - 15 gms/d have been described. Protein losses may be increased in the APD patient compared to CAPD and increase with the number of exchanges and the longer duration of the dwell time.

To maintain neutral nitrogen balance, the dietary protein targets for PD patients are 1.2 to 1.3 grams/kg/day.

In patients being evaluated for malnutrition, the dietary protein intake can be estimated from direct measures such as food diaries, questionnaires, interviews or indirectly by formulae that calculate protein intake derived from urea nitrogen generation. Urea nitrogen generation can be roughly estimated from urea kinetic modeling information. The total urea nitrogen appearing in the residual urine and total dialysate can be used to calculate the urea and protein nitrogen appearance rate (PNA) and these used to estimate dietary protein intake (DPI). To review from earlier chapters, a well dialyzed patient would be expected to have an adequate appetite. Assuming steady state, since urea nitrogen is a breakdown product of protein it is possible to use the daily urea clearance to determine the daily protein intake. Urea generation is proportional to protein breakdown, termed the normalized protein equivalent of nitrogen appearance (nPNA). The nPNA is reflective of dietary protein intake, in stable patients.

Earlier balance studies determined that negative nitrogen balance would occur in a PD patient ingesting less than 1.1 grams of protein/kg/day. Patients ingesting >1.4 grams/kg/day were in definite positive nitrogen balance. A PNA calculation is completed using dialysate urea nitrogen and, if there is significant residual kidney function, 24 hour urine collections. The two results are added to give an estimation of daily protein intake in gms/kg/day. This PNA is normalized to ideal body weight using anthropometric tables to give the nPNA (Frisancho AR. Am J Clin Nutr).

Therefore, using the urea nitrogen values employed in the Kt/V calculation, the clinician can calculate the estimated protein intake as follows:

nPNA (g/24 hrs) = 15.1 + 6.95(urea nitrogen apprearance in g/24 hrs) added to any protein losses, then normalized to ideal body weight

Example:

A 70 kg patient on CAPD with 10 liters of daily dialysate containing 65 mg/dL urea nitrogen would have total urea nitrogen content of 10 x 65 x 10 = 6500 mgs or 6.5 grams of urea nitrogen. The 24 hour urine obtained showed 400 ml of urine containing 640 mg/dL urea nitrogen for 2.56 grams of urea nitrogen. Added together the urea nitrogen appearance in g/24 hrs is 6.5 + 2.5 = 9 grams/24 hr. The dialysate contains 6 grams of protein per day.

The nPNA is 15.1 + 6.95(9) + 6 = 83.65 grams day/ 70 kg (assuming patient is at ideal body weight) = 1.19 g/kg/day

The patient has a borderline estimated dietary protein intake and requires ongoing monitoring and recommendations to increase protein intake.

Patients requiring nutritional supplements can be prescribed a variety of protein-calorie supplements such as Ensure, Nephro, Isocal, Sustacal, or Replete. Pure protein supplements such as Pro-mod powder can be considered.

Hypoalbuminemia in PD Patients

Hypoalbuminemia in PD patients may be due to multiple factors. Inadequate dietary protein intake may play a role as well as extravascular volume expansion, which may dilute the serum albumin concentration. Correction of volume abnormalities has been demonstrated to increase the serum albumin in some studies. The serum albumin level may not entirely be a nutritional marker as chronic inflammation may lower the albumin concentration. The serum albumin is a *negative acute phase reactant* and therefore the serum level is lowered due to hepatic shunting of albumin synthesis toward other proteins involved in the inflammatory response. Sources of chronic inflammation should be investigated including special examination of the feet and possible dental abnormalities such as periodontal disease. Other sources of chronic inflammation should be evaluated including constipation, active co-morbidities, and peripheral vascular disease.

Patients with hypoalbuminemia should be aggressively evaluated, as ongoing protein losses in the dialysate may aggravate the condition. Attention should be directed to the patient's actual protein intake and, if felt to be inadequate, supplements should be considered, as mentioned. In the patient who is both hypertensive and hypoalbuminemic, extravascular volume expansion could contribute to both findings and attempts should be made to contract extracellular volume. In the patient with higher transport status and hypoalbuminemia, the temporary use of a dry day may reduce protein losses into the dialysate. These higher transport patients typically have acceptable clearances due to the more vascular peritoneal membrane so that clearance targets would not be as significantly impacted by use of a temporary dry day. This strategy, combined with the other recommendations above can be considered as interventions in the PD patient with ongoing hypoalbuminemia.

Lipid Abnormalities in PD patients

CKD patients develop many lipoprotein abnormalities characterized by decreased high-density lipoproteins (HDL), low density lipoproteins (LDL) and elevated triglyceride (TG) levels. Patients on PD may have an aggravated dyslipidemia due to the continuous absorption of carbohydrate from the dialysate, leading to increased hepatic lipoprotein and TG synthesis. HDL levels are felt to be lower due the loss of this smaller lipoprotein across the peritoneal membrane and reduced overall synthesis. Compared to HD patients, small cross-sectional studies comparing lipid profiles in HD versus PD patients indicate that PD patients have higher total cholesterol levels, LDL and TG levels and similar HDL levels.

Dialysate protein losses are 5 to 15 grams/d and, in patients who develop hypoalbuminemia, increased hepatic synthesis of lipoproteins, analogous to nephrotic syndrome physiology, could occur. These lipid abnormalities are so common in PD therapy that the patient with normal or low cholesterol values may have malnutrition and chronic inflammation.

K/DOQI clinical practice guidelines for the management of dyslipidemias in CKD have been published and these guidelines suggest that patients with CKD be largely treated as would the patient with coronary heart disease. Therefore, the K/DOQI guidelines recommend following the previously published National Cholesterol Education Program's Adult Treatment Panel III guidelines.

Yet, the evidence supporting these guidelines in dialysis patients is controversial. Whether dyslipidemias in dialysis patients contribute to cardiovascular events is unclear. Several large studies could find no association between lipid profiles and cardiovascular disease. Some studies showed an association and others have shown an inverse relationship between cholesterol levels and death. The atherogenic risk of lipid abnormalities may be confounded by the prevalence of vascular calcifications and pro-inflammatory changes to the vasculature.

The largest intervention trials involving dialysis patients, to date, included only HD patients. These studies examined the impact of statin (HMG-CoA reductase inhibitor) therapy on mortality. The 4-D study (Die Deutsche Diabetic Dialyse Studie) randomized 1,255 German diabetic HD patients to atorvastatin 20 mg/d versus placebo and found no reduction in the primary endpoints of death from cardiac cause, death from stroke, non-fatal myocardial infarction, or non-fatal stroke. Atorvastatin did reduce LDL levels from 121 mg/dl to 75 mg/dl and reduced overall non-lethal cardiac events such as cardiac bypass surgery and percutaneous angioplasty by 18%. Nevertheless, the study was felt to be a negative outcome that did not support the role of statins in reducing cardiac deaths.

The recently published AURORA study randomized 2776 HD patients to rosuvastatin versus placebo for a median of 3.8 years with the primary endpoint being death from cardiovascular event, non-fatal myocardial infarction, or non-fatal cerebrovascular accident. Rosuvastatin lowered LDL levels by 43% yet no effect on the primary endpoints were noted, suggesting the intervention took place too late in the clinical course of these patients or that traditional lipid-related risk factors for cardiovascular disease may not be valid in this population.

An additional statin study, the multinational Study of Heart and Renal Protection (SHARP) was published in 2011. This study examined the effect of simvastatin plus ezetimibe versus placebo in a large group of CKD patients- 3023 patients on dialysis and 6247 patients with non-dialysis CKD. There were 496 patients on PD that were randomized. Outcomes were not reported for the PD patients specifically but for the entire study group there was no significant difference in coronary mortality. There was a reduction in some, but not all, endpoints such as non-hemorrhagic stroke.

Smaller retrospective observational studies suggested lower risk of cardiovascular deaths in those patients taking statin medications, suggesting that PD patients, with generally more atherogenic lipid profiles, may benefit from statin therapy. Lipid disorders in PD are notable for elevated apoB, with or without hypercholesterolemia. ApoB molecules, contained within VLDL and LDL particles, interact with endothelium and trigger the initial growth of an atherosclerotic lesion. Statins reduce apoB levels and these lowering effects may be more important in the PD population. While the 4-D study, AURORA, and SHARP trial found no survival benefit in HD patients, the apoB specific effects may make this class of medication more useful in the PD population.

The conflicting results of these prospective and randomized statin studies may again highlight the fact that cardiovascular disease in dialysis patients is not simply due to atheromatous plaque burden but also a superimposed vascular lesion notable for medial calcifications and evidence of vessel pro-inflammatory changes.

Fibrates (gemfibrozil and fenofibrate) would appear to be ideal medications for PD patients due to their triglyceride lowering properties and ability to increase HDL cholesterol. However, both medications may be contraindicated in the PD patient. Gemfibrozil increases the risk of rhabdomyolysis when added to statin therapy and has reduced excretion in advanced CKD. Fenofibrate is not dialyzable and accumulation in the serum has been noted. The NKF recommends avoiding fenofibrate in the dialysis population and only cautious use of dose adjusted gemfibrozil. The National Lipid Association, due to the concerns over drug accumulation in advanced CKD, recommends that fibrates not be used at all in this population.

Use of bile acid sequestrants such as cholestyramine is problematic in PD patients due to increases in TG levels that occur during therapy. Hypertriglyceridemia is common in PD patients making this agent generally contraindicated. Sevelamer has bile acid sequestrant properties and can lower both total and LDL cholesterol while used as a phosphate binder.

Ezetimibe, which inhibits cholesterol absorption and was combined with a statin in the SHARP trial, has been studied in other small groups of PD patients. Ezetimibe 10 mg/d was used as adjuvant therapy with statin medications and was found to be well tolerated. The combination resulted in significant reductions in LDL in this population. Again, however, the clinical benefits of the LDL reduction are still not clearly demonstrated in large trials.

Fish oil or omega-3 polyunsaturated fatty acids can specifically lower TG levels by decreasing TG synthesis. These agents can also be used in combination with a statin. If fish oils are used, high doses up to 3 to 4 grams/d have been suggested, making intake of many capsules problematic. A commercially available prescription brand of fish oil (Omacor) contains 900 mg of omega-3 fatty acids per pill, substantially reducing the pill burden.

Niacin therapy can increase HDL and reduce TG levels. Use of niacin is limited due to flushing sensations in many patients and, if used, NKF guidelines suggest reducing niacin dosing by 50% in advanced CKD.

Nicotinamide, a metabolite of nicotinic acid, causes less flushing than niacin and has recently been shown to increase HDL levels, lower LDL levels, and lower serum phosphorus levels in most but not all short term studies involving patients with ESRD. Further research is warranted on this potentially useful agent.

Despite the inconclusive evidence discussed above, many leading authorities still recommend treating dyslipidemias in ESRD patients due to the high prevalence of cardiovascular disease. Statins are generally considered the agent of choice and consideration should be given to adding ezetimide, fish oil, or a niacin compound in patients with persistent dsylipidemia.

Weight Gain and PD Therapy

The contribution of glucose absorption during PD therapy to subsequent weight gain has been controversial. Some, but not all, studies have indicated PD patients gain weight during therapy. The most recent study to address the issue of dialysis modality and weight gain in ESRD determined that treatment with PD was less likely to result in significant weight gain. Using 1:1 propensity score-matched cohorts of incident PD and HD patients, Lievense and colleagues determined that the odds of a 2 or 5 or 10%

weight gain were lower for PD patients than HD. The authors were unable to control for the degree of overhydration present in the HD cohort that possibly confounded their result. Yet, the authors applied the most rigorous statistical analysis- propensity matching of PD and HD - and suggested that PD patient weight gain is not greater than that of an HD patient. The authors speculated that delayed gastric emptying or suppression of appetite during instilled dialysate may limit the weight gain in PD patients.

Mineral Bone Disease in PD Therapy

Loss of significant renal function results in abnormalities of bone-mineral metabolism hallmarked by a rise in serum phosphorus levels, vitamin D deficiency with hypocalcemia that triggers secondary hyperparathyroidism. These disorders must be managed with dietary and medical interventions to maintain target levels.

K/DOQI recommendations for calcium, phosphorus and PTH levels are:

Calcium	8.4 – 9.5 mg/dL
Phosphorus	3.5 – 5.5 mg/dL
PTH	150 – 300 pg/mL

Patients with ESRD, HD and PD, are typically prescribed phosphorus restricted diets, phosphorus binding agents to be administered with food, and vitamin D supplementation. A variety of phosphate binders are available that are typically aluminum, calcium, sevelemar, or lanthanum based. Use of these agents in PD patients is similar to those of the general ESRD population with oral dosing being titrated to achieve serum phosphorus control. All binders have been useful in the PD population but use of aluminum based binders has been discouraged due to toxic aluminum accumulation in bone and neural tissue.

As mentioned, nicotinamide has recently been demonstrated to lower serum phosphorus levels in patients with ESRD. Nicotinamide inhibits a sodium-dependent phosphate co-transporter located in the intestine and proximal tubule brush border, reducing intestinal phosphorus absorption and proximal tubule reabsorption. Nicotinamide has the added benefit of raising HDL levels and lowering LDL levels in many, but not all, studies.

Nicotinamide is a promising agent for patients with ESRD due to the phosphorus lowering properties and favorable lipid response but the studies have many limitations- most were not blinded and contain small sample size, are of short-term duration, and cannot establish the longer term safety of the compound. While better tolerated than niacin, high dose nicotinamide is associated with diarrhea.

A phosphorus-lowering chewing gum is expected to be released soon (Fostrap, Nestle SA). The chewing gum is not replace traditional phosphate binders but may serve as an additive mechanism to lower serum phosphorus levels. The active ingredient is derived from crustacean exoskeletons which bind to salivary phosphate. A small clinical trial was conducted in Italy followed by larger double-blind, placebo-controlled studies in Japan and the USA. Results of these studies are expected soon. The chewing gum is considered a "medical food" and therefore does not require FDA approval for use.

Phosphorus Removal with PD

Phosphorus removal with PD has not been extensively studied and undoubtedly varies by underlying peritoneal membrane transport status. Phosphorus is not felt to be freely diffusible across the small capillary pores due to the negative charge, protein binding, and complexing to other cations. Based on size comparisons, phosphate clearance is more closely compared to that of creatinine, and is reported to be approximately 36L/wk/1.73m^2. Weekly creatinine clearance has been used as a surrogate for weekly phosphate clearance. In general, weekly phosphate removal by CAPD has been estimated to be between 2170 to 2790 mg. Clearance by APD is less clear and appears more affected by underlying membrane type. A more extensive review of the topic was published in 2010 by Kuhlmann.

Glucose Exposure in PD

Use of traditional dialysis solutions result in the absorption of 100 to 300 gms of glucose daily. This absorption contributes to the recommended daily caloric intake of 2500 kcal/day (35kcal/kg/day). For example, the CAPD patient using four 2.5% dextrose exchanges will absorb 110 grams of glucose or 440 kcal a day. In patients receiving adequate nutritional intake, with sedentary lifestyles, the calories derived from the dialysate can contribute to weight gain in many patients. Use of dialysate with the lowest osmotic concentration to achieve euvolemia is recommended and usually requires that patients be maintained on a sodium restriction and continued on diuretics, in those with significant RKF. Clinicians should repeatedly counsel patients requiring the need to avoid higher osmotically active glucose concentrations by addressing dietary compliance and strive to not depend on higher glucose exposure as a long term strategy. Icodextrin is used as a glucose sparing agent in those patients requiring enhanced ultrafiltration.

Acid-Base Balance in PD

Chronic metabolic acidosis results in breakdown of lean body mass. Acidosis triggers activation of an ATP-dependent ubiquitin-proteasome proteolytic pathway. Acidosis also triggers the enzyme branched-chain keto-acid dehydrogenase to catabolize valine, leucine, and isoleucine. Proteolysis from these mechanisms can contribute to loss of muscle mass in dialysis patients. Additionally, chronic metabolic acidosis has adverse effects on bone mineralization. Acidosis stimulates osteoclast activity in a futile attempt to release bone buffers (calcium carbonate). For these reasons, full correction of the acid-base status is important in patients with advanced kidney disease.

Despite dialysis, many patients with ESRD develop chronic metabolic acidosis, especially those on intermittent therapies such as in-center HD. PD therapy, being a more continuous dialysis modality, better controls chronic acidosis by adding daily base to the body stores. Standard PD solutions contain lactate as the buffer in concentrations of 35 mmol/L or 40 mmol/L. Novel PD solutions contain bicarbonate as the base or bicarbonate/lactate combinations.

A goal of PD therapy is to fully correct the acid-base status. In patients treated with 35 mmol/L lactate solutions and persistent serum bicarbonate values < 22 mEq/L, consideration should be given to use of 40 mmol/L lactate solutions. Oral bicarbonate therapy can be added and K/DOQI recommendations suggest bicarbonate supplements are indicated in patients with persistent plasma bicarbonate values < 22 mEq/L. The adverse effects of the sodium content of these supplements should be considered and use of the lowest effective dose of oral alkalinization is prudent. Higher dose oral bicarbonate treatment was shown to increase hospitalizations for congestive heart failure and fluid overload.

Patients with unexplained persistent chronic metabolic acidosis, despite use of higher lactate solutions, should be evaluated for excessive protein intake. Many dietary proteins contain methionine and cysteine, that are metabolized to sulfuric and phosphoric acid, creating an acid load that worsens the acid-base status.

Micronutrients and the Requirement for Multi-Vitamins in PD patients

Water soluble vitamins and minerals can be lost during ultrafiltration and therefore should be replaced as a multivitamin supplement. Hemodialysis multivitamins are often restricted in potassium but this is not necessary in the patient on PD therapy. A recent study from Mexico, using careful dietary logs, suggested that PD patients may have significant deficiencies in micronutrient intake suggesting supplementation may be of value.

Subjective Global Assessment (SGA)

Due to difficulties interpreting the patient's true nutritional status based on dietary histories or blood tests, the SGA has become a popular tool. The SGA represents a composite assessment of 8 parameters obtained during a medical history and examination that give an indication of a patient's nutritional status. These parameters are easily scored to give an estimation of the nutritional status as being either normal nutrition, mild to moderate malnutrition, or severe malnutrition. The SGA, as an indicator of nutritional status, has been validated in a large Canadian-USA study (CANUSA) and predicted hospitalization rate and mortality.

Clinical parameters included in a SGA include weight change, dietary intake, gastrointestinal symptoms, functional capacity, disease state and co-morbidities, and physical exam. The SGA can be included in the assessment of PD patients to help predict which patients require nutritional intervention and may be at risk for poor outcomes.

Anthropometric Measures of Nutritional Status

Anthropometric measurements include weight, mid-arm circumference, skinfold thickness, and calculated body mass index (BMI). These measurements can be used as crude determinants of nutritional status when compared to published normative values.

Bioelectrical Impedance to Assess Nutritional Status

Assessing body composition is difficult, clinically, so use of bioelectric impedance (BIA) to determine hydration status and fatty mass composition has gained popularity. This simple bedside technique can differentiate between hydration status, bone mineral content and body fat stores. In patients losing body weight, BIA determinations showing a stable hydration status would imply that the loss in body weight is due to loss of fat tissue.

Star Fruit

Precautions against ingesting star fruit should be made in all dialysis patients and patients with advanced chronic kidney disease. Star fruit, commonly available in supermarkets, contains a potent neurotoxin that has yet to be fully elucidated. Peritoneal dialysis patients that ingest star fruit can experience hiccups, weakness, confusion, agitation, and seizure activity. Deaths from status epilepticus have occurred.

Summary of general nutritional recommendations for PD patients:

1. Salt restriction of 6 gms/d and continued enforcement as a strategy to avoid the metabolic complications of hypertonic dialysate solutions

2. Avoid hypokalemia - potassium rich diet with oral supplements if needed

3. Phosphorus restriction and phosphate binders to achieve a serum phosphorous level of 3.5 to 5.5 mg/dL

4. Vitamin D supplementation

5. Protein intake of 1.2-1.3 grams/kg/d

6. Monitor serum albumin levels and initiate protein supplements if Alb < 3.4 g/dL

7. Replace the losses of water soluble vitamins and minerals by administering a daily multivitamin

8. Consider statins, fish oil, and niacin

References:

General

Burkart J. Metabolic consequences of peritoneal dialysis. Semin Dial 2004;17:498-504.

Wright M, Woodrow G, O'Brien S, et al. Disturbed appetite patterns and nutrient intake in peritoneal dialysis patients. Perit Dial Int 2003;23:550-556.

Sodium balance in PD patients

Aanen MC, Venturoli D, Davies SJ. A detailed analysis of sodium removal by peritoneal dialysis: comparison with predictions from the three-pore model of membrane function. Nephrol Dial Transplant 2005;20:1192-1200.

Fouque D, Kalantar-Zadeh K, Kopple J, et al. A proposed nomenclature and diagnostic criteria for protein-energy wasting in acute and chronic kidney disease. Kidney Int 2008;73:391-398.

McLean R. Cooking a low-salt meal: the ultimate culinary challenge. Kidney Int 2008;74:1105-1106.

Rodriguez-Carmona A, Perez-Fontan M, Garcia-Naveiro R, et al. Compared time profiles of ultrafiltration, sodium removal, and renal function in incident CAPD and automated peritoneal dialysis patients. Am J Kidney Dis 2004;44:132-145.

Vennegoor MA. Salt restriction and practical aspects to improve compliance. J Ren Nutr 2009;19:63-68.

Potassium balance in PD patients

Amirmokri P, Morgan P, Bastani B. Intra-peritoneal administration of potassium and magnesium: a practical method to supplement these electrolytes in peritoneal dialysis patients. Renal Failure 2007;29:603-605.

Chuang YW, Shu KH, Yu TM, et al. Hypokalaemia: an independent risk factor of Enterobacteriaceae peritonitis in CAPD patients. Nephrol Dial Transplant 2009;24:1603-1608.

Lu XH, Su CY, Sun LH, et al. Implementing continuous quality improvement process in potassium management in peritoneal dialysis patients. J Ren Nutr 2009;19:469-474.

Shu KH, Chang CS, Chuang YW, et al. Intestinal bacterial overgrowth in CAPD patients with hypokalaemia. Nephrol Dial Transplant 2009;24:1289-1292.

Szeto CC, Chow KM, Kwan BC, et al. Hypokalemia in Chinese peritoneal dialysis patients: prevalence and prognostic implication. Am J Kidney Dis 2005;46:128-135.

Magnesium balance

Redrow M, Cherem L, Elliott J, et al. Dialysis in the management of pregnant patients with renal insufficiency. Medicine 1988;67:199-208.

Ejaz AA, McShane AP, Gandhi VC, et al. Hypomagnesemia in continuous ambulatory peritoneal dialysis patients dialyzed with a low-magnesium peritoneal dialysis solution. Perit Dial Int 1995;15:61-64.

Protein intake in PD patients and Protein Energy Malnutrition (PEM)

Bergstrom J, Furst P, Alvestrand A, Lindholm B. Protein and energy intake, nitrogen balance and nitrogen losses in patients treated with continuous ambulatory peritoneal dialysis. Kidney Int 1993;44:1048-1057.

Boudville N, Rangan A, Moody H. Oral nutritional supplementation increases caloric and protein intake in peritoneal dialysis patients. Am J Kidney Dis 2003;41:658-663.

De Mutsert R, Grootendorst DC, Indemans F, et al. Association between serum albumin and mortality in dialysis patients is partly explained by inflammation, and not by malnutrition. J Ren Nutr 2009;19:127-135.

Frisancho AR. New standards of weight and body composition by frame size and height for assessment of nutritional status of adults and elderly. Am J Clin Nutr 1984;40:808-819.

Gonzalez-Espinoza L, Gutierrez-Chavez J, Del Campo FM, et al. Randomized, open label, controlled clinical trial of oral administration of an egg albumin-based protein supplement to patients on continuous ambulatory peritoneal dialysis. Perit Dial Int 2005;25:173-180.

Heaf JG, Honore K, Valeur D, Randlov A. The effect of oral protein supplements on the nutritional status of malnourished CAPD patients. Perit Dial Int 1999;19:78-81.

Jones CH, Wells L, Stoves J, et al. Can a reduction in extracellular fluid volume result in increased serum albumin in peritoneal dialysis patients? Am J Kidney Dis 2002;39:872-875.

Kaysen GA. Biological basis of hypoalbuminemia in ESRD. J Am Soc Nephrol 1998;9:2368-2376.

K/DOQI, National Kidney Foundation. Clinical practice guidelines for nutrition in chronic renal failure. Am J Kidney Dis 2000;35[Suppl 2]:S1-S140.

Ray C. Protein supplementation in patients using peritoneal dialysis. J Ren Nutr 2005;15:260-264.

Wang AY, Sea MM, Ip R, et al. Independent effects of residual renal function and dialysis adequacy on actual dietary protein, calorie, and other nutrient intake in patients on continuous ambulatory peritoneal dialysis. J Am Soc Nephrol 2001;12:2450-2457.

Westra WM, Kopple JD, Krediet RT, et al. Dietary protein requirements and dialysate protein losses in chronic peritoneal dialysis patients. Perit Dial Int 2007;27:192-195.

Wolfson M. Management of protein and energy intake in dialysis patients. J Am Soc Nephrol 1999;10:2244-2247.

Lipid abnormalities in PD patients

Babazono T, Nakamoto H, Kasai K, et al. Effects of icodextrin on glycemic and lipid profiles in diabetic patients undergoing peritoneal dialysis. Am J Nephrol 2007;27:409-415.

Baigent C, Landray MJ, Reith C, et al. The effects of lowering LDL cholesterol with simvastatin plus ezetimibe in patients with chronic kidney disease (Study of Heart and Renal Protection): a randomised placebo-controlled trial. Lancet 2011;377:2181-2192.

Bredie SJ, Bosch FH, Demacker PN, et al. Effects of peritoneal dialysis with an overnight icodextrin dwell on parameters of glucose and lipid metabolism. Perit Dial Int 2001;21:275-281.

Fellstrom BC, Jardine AG, Schmieder RE, et al. Rosuvastatin and cardiovascular events in patients undergoing hemodialysis. N Engl J Med 2009;360:1395-1407.

Freidman AN, Fadem SZ. Reassessment of albumin as a nutritional marker in kidney disease. J Am Soc Nephrol 2010;21:223-230.

Goldfarb-Rumyantzev AS, Habib AN, Baird BC, et al. The association of lipid-modifying medications with mortality in patients on long-term peritoneal dialysis. Am J Kidney Dis 2007;50:791-802.

Habib AN, Baird BC, Leypoldt JK, et al. The association of lipid levels with mortality in patients of chronic peritoneal dialysis. Nephrol Dial Int 2006;21:2881-2892.

Harper CR, Jacobson TA. Managing dyslipidemia in chronic kidney disease. J Am Coll Cardiol 2008;51:2375-2384.

National Kidney Foundation. K/DOQI clinical practice guidelines for managing dyslipidemias in chronic kidney disease. Am K Kidney Dis 2003;41[Suppl 3]:S1-S91.

Nutescu EA, Shapiro NL. Ezetimibe: a selective cholesterol absorption inhibitor. Pharmacotherapy 2003;23:1463-1474.

Paniagua R, Ventura MD, Avila-Diaz M, et al. Icodextrin improves metabolic and fluid management in high and high-average transport diabetic patients. Perit Dial Int 2009;29:422-32.

Reiche I, Westphal S, Martens-Lobenhoffer J, et al. Pharmacokinetics and dose recommendations of Niaspan in chronic kidney disease and dialysis patients. Nephrol Dial Transplant 2011;26:276-282.

Rennick A, Kalakeche R, Seel L, Shepler B. Nicotinic acid and nicotinamide: a review of their use for hyperphosphatemia in dialysis patients. Pharmacotherapy 2013;33:683-690.

Ritz E, Wanner C. Lipid abnormalities and cardiovascular risk in renal disease. J Am Soc Nephrol 2008;19:1065-1070.

Scarpioni R. Therapeutic tools for dyslipidemia in peritoneal dialysis patients. J Nephrol 2009;22:46-58.

Shurraw S, Tonelli M. Statins for treatment of dyslipidemia in chronic kidney disease. Perit Dial Int 2006;26:523-539.

Shurraw S, Tonelli M. AURORA: is there a role for statin therapy in dialysis patients? Am J Kidney Dis 2010;55:237-240.

Sniderman AD, Solhpour A, Alam A, et al. Cardiovascular death in dialysis patients: lessons we can learn from AURORA. Clin J Am Soc Nephrol 2010;5:335-340.

Vaziri ND. Causes of dysregulation of lipid metabolism in chronic renal failure. Semin Dial 2009;22:644-651.

Weight gain during PD therapy

Lievense H, Kalantar-Zadeh K, Lukowsky LR, et al. Relationship of body size and initial dialysis modality on subsequent transplantation, mortality and weight gain of ESRD patients. Nephrol Dial Transplant 2012;27:3631-3638.

Mineral bone disease in PD therapy

Bernardo AP, Contesse SA, Bajo MA, et al. Peritoneal membrane phosphate transport status: a cornerstone in phosphate handling in peritoneal dialysis. Clin J Am Soc Nephrol 2011;6:591-597.

Fukagawa M, Komaba H, Miyamoto K. Source matters: from phosphorus load to bioavailability. Clin J Am Soc Nephrol 2011;6:239-240.

Hutchison AJ. Oral phosphate binders. Kidney Int 2009;75:906-914.

Kuhlmann MK. Phosphate elimination in modalities of hemodialysis and peritoneal dialysis. Blood Purif 2010;29:137-144.

Moe SM. Management of renal osteodystrophy in peritoneal dialysis patients. Perit Dial Int 2004;24:209-216.

Moe SM, Zidehsarai MP, Chambers MA, et al. Vegetarian compared with meat dietary protein source and phosphorus homeostasis in chronic kidney disease. Clin J Am Soc Nephrol 2011;6:257-264.

Noordzij M, Voormolen NM, Boeschoten EW, et al. Disordered mineral metabolism is not a risk factor for loss of residual renal function in dialysis patients. Nephrol Dial Transplant 2009;24:1580-1587.

Sahin G, Kirli I, Sirmagul B, et al. Loss via peritoneal fluid as a factor for low 25(OH)D3 level in peritoneal dialysis patients. Int Urol Nephrol 2009; 41:989-996.

Sedlacek M, Dimaano F, Uribarri J. Relationship between phosphorus and creatinine clearance in peritoneal dialysis: clinical implications. Am J Kidney Dis 2000;36:1020-1024.

Schmitt CP, Borzych D, Nau B, et al. Dialytic phosphate removal: a modifiable measure of dialysis efficiency in automated peritoneal dialysis. Perit Dial Int 2009;29:465-471.

Shah N, Bernardini J, Piraino B. Prevalence and correction of 25(OH) vitamin D deficiency in peritoneal dialysis patients. Perit Dial Int 2005;25:362-366.

Tonelli M, Pannu N, Manns B. Oral phosphate binders in patients with kidney failure. N Engl J Med 2010;362:1312-1324.

Uribarri J. Phosphorus additives in food and their effect in dialysis patients. Clin J Am Soc Nephrol 2009;4:1290-1292.

Wang AY, Lam CW, Wang M, et al. Is valvular calcification a part of the missing link between residual kidney function and cardiac hypertrophy in peritoneal dialysis patients? Clin J Am Soc Nephrol 2009;4:1629-1636.

Young DO, Cheng SC, Delmez JA, Coyne DW. The effect of oral niacinamide on plasma phosphorus levels in peritoneal dialysis patients. Perit Dial Int 2009;29:562-567.

Glucose exposure in PD

Holmes CJ, Shockley TR. Strategies to reduce glucose exposure in peritoneal dialysis patients. Perit Dial Int 2000;20[Suppl 2]:S37-S41.

Fortes PC, De Moraes TP, Mendes JG, et al. Insulin resistance and glucose homeostasis in peritoneal dialysis. Perit Dial Int 2009;29[Suppl 2]:S145-S148.

Acid-base

Graham KA, Reaich D, Channon SM, et al. Correction of acidosis in CAPD decreases whole body protein degradation. Kidney Int 1996;49:1396-1400.

Lefebvre A, de Vernejoul MC, Gueris J, et al. Optimal correction of acidosis changes progression of dialysis osteodystrophy. Kidney Int 1989;36:1112-1118.

Mujais S. Acid-base profile in patients on PD. Kidney Int 2003;64[Suppl 88]:S26-S36.

Szeto CC, Wong TY, Chow KM, et al. Oral sodium bicarbonate for the treatment of metabolic acidosis in peritoneal dialysis patients: a randomized placebo-control trial. J Am Soc Nephrol 2003;14:2119-2126.

Micronutrients

Clase CM, Ki V, Holden RM. Water-soluble vitamins in people with low glomerular filtration rate or on dialysis: a review. Semin Dial 2013;26:546-567.

Martin-del-Campo F, Batis-Ruvalcaba C, Gonzalez-Espinoza L, et al. Dietary micronutrient intake in peritoneal dialysis patients: relationship with nutrition and inflammatory status. Perit Dial Int 2012;32:183-191.

SGA, anthropometric measures, and bioelecric impedence

Enia G, Sicuso C, Alati G, Zoccali C. Subjective global assessment of nutrition in dialysis patients. Nephrol Dial Transplant 1993;8:1094-1098.

Woodrow G, Devine Y, Cullen M, Lindley E. Application of bioelectrical impedance to clinical assessment of body composition in peritoneal dialysis. Perit Dial Int 2007;27:496-502.

Star fruit

Chang JM, Hwng SJ, Kuo HT, et al. Fatal outcome after ingestion of star fruit (*Averrhoa carambola*) in uremic patients. Am J Kidney Dis 2000;35:189-193.

Neto MM, Cardeal da Costa JA, Garcia-Cairasco N, et al. Intoxication by star fruit (*averrhoa carambola*) in 32 uremic patients: treatment and outcome. Nephrol Dial Transplant 2003;18:120-125.

Chapter 17:
Survival in the PD Population

THE IMPACT OF PD vs. HD on patient survival has been debated for decades. Publications have reported that PD survival was superior to HD, inferior to HD, or equivalent-making conclusions difficult to reach. What has become apparent, however, is that simple comparisons of large groups of PD patients vs. large groups of HD patients is too simplistic as a variety of confounders such as selection bias, residual kidney function, and type of vascular access have independent effects on outcome. This chapter will review these issues.

Survival on PD vs. HD: Poor Outcomes Overall

In general, patients with ESRD have poorer outcomes compared to the general population. To illustrate, according to life expectancy tables used by the insurance industry, a 40 year old Caucasian male in 2002, with no known medical problems, could be expected to live an additional 37 years. That same individual with ESRD, on dialysis, would be expected to live only 7 years. Survival of ESRD patients in the USA is reduced compared to that of many other countries, often attributed to the higher prevalence of diabetes, advanced age and co-morbidities. For decades, attempts have been made to determine if one dialysis modality, HD or PD, could confer a survival advantage. The gold standard test would be a large, multi-center randomized controlled trial assigning consecutive patients to either HD or PD and following outcomes in subsequent years. An attempt at such a trial was initiated in the Netherlands but largely failed due to patient reluctance to be randomized and their strong preferences for one modality over the other. Of 773 patients eligible for recruitment, the researchers were able to randomize only 38 patients, and showed a survival advantage to PD. No firm conclusions can be made due to the limited sample size.

Observational Survival Comparisons

From the USRDS, retrospective observational survival data is available. Limitations of using USRDS data are that data is censured at 90 days, meaning that a dialysis patient must survive 90 days to be entered into the database. Another limitation is that co-morbidity data is based on data entry on the Center for Medicare and Medicaid Services (CMS) Medical Evidence Form (2728 form). Data entry on this short form often fails to capture all pertinent clinical parameters.

Despite these limitations, recent analyses of the entire ESRD population in USRDS has shown no statistically significant differences in adjusted 5-year survival rates, comparing incident PD and HD. Older studies attempted to understand the effects of co-morbidities on survival. Vonesh and colleagues grouped patients by presence or absence of diabetic nephropathy, age groups and a co-morbidity index. In this analysis, they noted equal survival or a survival benefit to PD in the non-diabetic and in younger diabetics with or without co-morbidities. A survival benefit to HD was noted in patients with diabetic nephropathy and other co-morbidities who were over the age of 45 years.

Vonesh and colleagues also analyzed survival in the first years of treatment, to determine if one modality conferred an early survival advantage. They noted a consistent early survival advantage for PD, in all patient groups, except diabetics over age 65. This observation, that PD may confer an early survival advantage, confirmed observations made in other countries. In the Canada-USA (CANUSA) study, an early survival advantage to PD was noted for the first 36 months of therapy and a Dutch registry of 16 thousand patients showed a clear early survival advantage to PD.

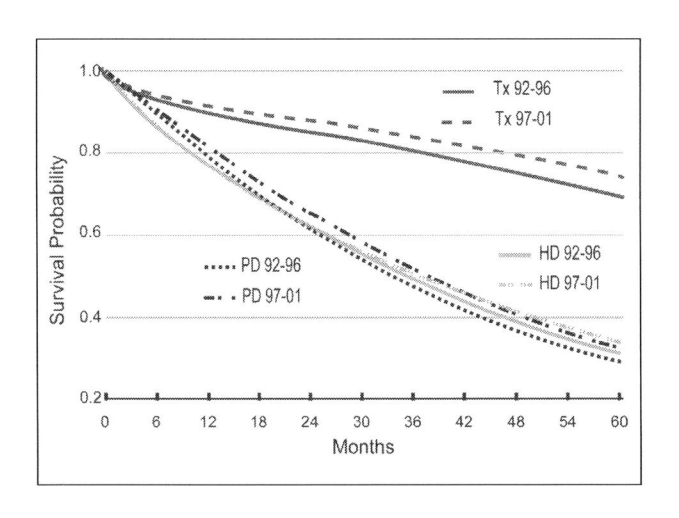

In 2012, an updated analysis of the Canadian Organ Replacement Register determined outcomes of HD and PD. Yeates and colleagues conducted

Similar 5-year survival by dialysis modality. From the U.S. Renal Data System Annual Report, Bethesda MD, National Institutes of Health, National Institute of Diabetes and Digestive and Kidney Diseases

intent-to-treat analyses of survival outcomes of PD v HD as well as outcomes in patients initiating dialysis in three time periods covering 1991 to 2004. The researchers noted improved PD survivals on the most recent time period and due to this concluded that, in their analysis, survival favored PD for the first 2 years and thereafter PD and HD were similar. In a sub-analysis of females over age 65 whom were diabetic, PD showed a significantly higher mortality rate.

Propensity Matching

The above studies are based on observational data and the gold standard comparison would be a randomized controlled trial. As mentioned above, attempts at such studies have failed due to patient reluctance to be randomized. Short of a randomized controlled trial, the next highest level of evidence is termed "propensity matching". A recent study analyzed over 6300 matched pairs of incident HD and PD patients from the U.S. Renal Data System (USRDS). Patients were matched based on age, gender, body size, available co-morbidities and laboratory parameters. Patients were followed from day 0 to 5 years. The cumulative mortality in the matched pairs was 42% at a mean follow-up of 2.3 year. In the primary, intention-to-treat analysis, cumulative survival from day 0 onward was higher for PD than for HD. In a secondary analysis that eliminated deaths before day 90, overall survival was similar. In analyzing specific patient groups by intention-to-treat, survival from 90 days favored PD for patients less than 65 years of age and for patients without diabetes or cardiovascular disease. Patients with diabetes had similar risk on PD in the first year, then higher risk in subsequent years.

Vascular Access Modifies Modality Comparisons

A separate analysis has revealed a possible mechanism for the early survival advantage of PD noted in many studies. A significant number of HD patients initiate dialysis with a temporary dialysis catheter, and these patients had a subsequent higher rate of bacteremia and sepsis. Analysis of longer-term outcomes, after an episode of sepsis, revealed a subsequent 3-fold greater cardiovascular event rate. Over 70% of incident HD patients start dialysis with a temporary vascular access catheter. A single episode of sepsis in HD predicts a higher subsequent cardiovascular event rate and may partially explain the early survival advantage to PD therapy.

In a recent analysis of the Canadian Organ Replacement Registry, Perl and colleagues used sophisticated non-proportional and proportional hazards models to evaluate 1-year survival and overall survival using an intent-to-treat methodology. Outcomes of incident patients on PD were compared to HD patients who initiated dialysis with a temporary vascular access catheter and those that initiated dialysis with a functional fistula or graft. Compared to the PD cohort, 1-year survival was equivalent in the HD population with a functional arm access but mortality was 80% higher in the HD group initiating dialysis with a temporary vascular access catheter. This suggested that the early survival advantage to PD, noted on some registries, may largely be accounted for by the poor outcomes in the HD population initiating dialysis with a temporary catheter. These studies detailing the infectious complications of temporary catheters and cardiovascular risk as well as the impact on survival have led to wider discussions of the use of PD in the incident population that does not have established vascular access. Having a capability to initiate PD more urgently, to avoid temporary vascular access, has been a quality control strategy to reduce the use of temporary catheters.

Selection Bias

PD patients are often younger, have less co-morbidities, and have more sustained residual kidney function. These factors also introduce selection biases into any large analysis of mortality across the dialysis modalities. It is clear that the most impactful future comparisons of dialysis modality survival should control for all the potential selection biases.

A recent publication demonstrated that the perceived survival advantage of initiating dialysis with peritoneal dialysis may, indeed, reflect selection bias. By restricting their analysis to the most ideal situation where patients received 4 or more months of pre-dialysis care and who started dialysis electively as outpatients, Quinn and colleagues could demonstrate no early survival advantage to PD- the survival was equivocal between HD and PD. This study appears to confirm that the higher relative risk of death in those patients who start with HD is likely due, not to the modality itself, but to the selection bias introduced by co-morbidities and the presence of temporary vascular catheters.

Improving PD Outcomes in Recent Cohorts

USRDS and Canadian observational studies have demonstrated improved outcomes in more recent cohorts of patients. Both a USA analysis by Mehrotra et al and Canadian analysis by Yeates et al. have demonstrated improved PD outcomes in the more modern cohorts. In the former analysis, improved PD outcomes in the current cohort remained after adjusting for demographics, case-mix, and laboratory data. Improving outcomes in more modern cohorts may be due to a variety of factors such as physician practice, improvement in management of medical co-morbidities, improved selection of patients suitable for PD, or improved management of PD-related complications such as peritonitis. It is also possible that the recent introduction of continuous quality improvement programs have impacted the more recent cohorts.

Effects of Residual Kidney Function

Many hypotheses have been proposed to explain why PD may confer an early survival advantage for most patients. Survival has been linked to underlying residual kidney function (RKF) in both HD and PD patients- those with significant RKF show a survival advantage. PD has been noted to better preserve RKF, and by this mechanism may confer the early survival advantage. Wang and colleagues noted that RKF in PD patients was predictive of the degree of left ventricular hypertrophy (LVH) and hypothesized that patients with the more constant loss of salt and water by the native kidneys may have less cardiac stress and speculated that RKF gives a survival advantage by a relative reduction in LVH. The myriad of effects of RKF on PD outcomes and technique success are reviewed in Chapter 5.

What factors, impact survival in the anuric PD population? Outcomes in anuric patients were analyzed and survival was related to net daily ultrafiltration and the achieved Kt/V. Markers of better survival were a Kt/V maintained above 1.5 and a daily ultrafiltration volume of 750 mL. This suggests that preservation of RKF should be attempted in early PD but at any point that RKF is lost the peritoneal ultrafiltration should be at least 750 mL/day in the stable patient ingesting their usual daily nutritional intake. Some studies suggest that high transport status may be a marker for increased mortality and technique success. High transport status on the PET has been associated with elevated markers of inflammation and may be one additional manifestation of the malnutrition, inflammation, atherosclerosis (MIA) syndrome. However, increased mortality in the high transport population has not been a consistent finding. High transporters were recently found to have superior survival when treated with APD versus CAPD. Finally, PD patients treated with ACE inhibitors or angiotensin- receptor blockers were found to have better overall survival, suggesting that these agents may play an important role in reducing mortality, independent of their effects on RKF.

Modality Effect on Survival after Failed Kidney Transplant

Patients with failed kidney transplants return to dialysis and have been identified as having a higher mortality than the transplant naïve ESRD population. The effect of dialysis modality on survival in these previously transplanted patients is of concern when educating on dialysis options. A recent study analyzed survival of failed transplant patients to determine the impact of dialysis modality. The authors determined that post-transplant HD and PD patients had similar death rates in all analyses performed, including early deaths, later deaths, and overall deaths. The original postulation was that allograft function may be better preserved in PD and therefore survival rates improved on PD. This was not found, however, and the authors speculated that preservation of transplant residual function may be different from that in native kidneys, or that transplant patients are started back on dialysis at lower GFR values that may reduce the early survival benefit usually associated with PD. Indeed, some studies have shown a more rapid loss of RKF in the transplanted kidneys after resuming dialysis. Further research on modality effects of the previously transplanted patient is needed.

Conclusions

Outcomes on PD have improved in recent cohorts and may reflect on improved management of PD complications and greater understanding of which patients are suitable to PD. The superior early survival of incident patients started on PD may, in part, reflect survival biases and the relatively poorer survival of the HD group that starts dialysis with a temporary vascular access catheter. Longer term survival in the PD population is felt to be equivalent to HD, but certain patient populations may slightly favor one modality over the other. The elderly diabetic population shows improved survival on HD with the non-diabetic populations showing equal to better survival on PD. Survival in ESRD patients, in general, could be improved by considering PD as the initial dialysis therapy taking advantage of the early survival advantage, by wider use of AV fistula's as the initial vascular access if HD is elected, attempts to preserve intrinsic kidney function after initiating dialysis, as well as attempts to control other markers of survival such as adequate nutrition, inflammation, control of extracellular volume, and overall mineral balance.

References:

Brown EA, Davies SJ, Rutherford P, et al. Survival of functionally anuric patients on automated peritoneal dialysis: the European APD Outcome Study. J Am Soc Nephrol 2003;14:2948-2957.

Brimble KS, Walker M, Margetts PJ, et al. Meta-analysis: peritoneal membrane transport, mortality, and technique failure in peritoneal dialysis. J Am Soc Nephrol 2006;17:2591-2598.

Collins AJ, Foley RN, Herzog C, et al. Excerpts from the United States Renal Data System 2009 annual data report. Am J Kidney Dis 2010;55[Suppl 1]:S1-S420.

Collins AJ, Hao W, Xia H, et al. Mortality risks of peritoneal dialysis and hemodialysis. Am J Kidney Dis 1999;34:1065-1074.

Fang W, Oreopoulos DG, Bargman J. Use of ACE inhibitors or angiotensin receptor blockers and survival in patients on peritoneal dialysis. Nephrol Dial Transplant 2008;23:3704-3710.

Fenton SS, Schaubel DE, Desmeules M, et al. Hemodialysis versus peritoneal dialysis: a comparison of adjusted mortality rates. Am J Kidney Dis 1997;30:334-342.

Heaf JG, Lokkegaard H, Madsen M. Initial survival advantage of peritoneal dialysis relative to hemodialysis. Nephrol Dial Transplant 2002;17:112-117.

Jaar BG, Coresh J, Plantinga LC, et al. Comparing the risk for death with peritoneal dialysis and hemodialysis in a national cohort of patients with chronic kidney disease. Ann Intern Med 2005;143:174-183.

Jansen MAM, Termorshuizen F, Korevaar JC, et al. Predictors of survival in anuric peritoneal dialysis patients. Kidney Int 2005;68:1199-1205.

Johnson DW, Hawley CM, McDonald SP, et al. Superior survival of high transporters treated with automated versus continuous ambulatory peritoneal dialysis. Nephrol Dial Transplant 2010;25:1973-1979.

Korevaar JC, Feith GW, Dekker FW, et al. Effect of starting with hemodialysis compared with peritoneal dialysis in patients new on dialysis treatment: a randomized controlled trial. Kidney Int 2003;64:2222-2228.

Liem YS, Wong JB, Hunink MGM, et al. Comparison of hemodialysis and peritoneal dialysis survival in the Netherlands. Kidney Int 2007;71:153-158.

McDonald SP, Marshall MR, Johnson DW, Polkinghorne KR. Relationship between dialysis modality and mortality. J Am Soc Nephrol 2009;20:155-163.

Mehrotra R, Kermah D, Fried L, et al. Chronic peritoneal dialysis in the United States: declining utilization despite improving outcomes. J Am Soc Nephrol 2007;18:2781-2788.

Mehrotra R, Chiu Y, Kalantar-Zadeh K, Vonesh E. The outcomes of continuous ambulatory and automated peritoneal dialysis are similar. Kidney Int 2009;76:97-107.

Murphy SW, Foley RN, Barrett BJ, et al. Comparative mortality of hemodialysis and peritoneal dialysis in Canada. Kidney Int 2000;57:1720-1726.

Perl J, Wald R, McFarlane, et al. Hemodialysis vascular access modifies the association between dialysis modality and survival. J Am Soc Nephrol 2011;22:1113-1121.

Perl J, Hasan O, Bargman JM, et al. Impact of dialysis modality on survival after kidney transplant failure. Clin J Am Soc Nephrol 2011;6:582-590.

Quinn RR, Hux JE, Oliver MJ, et al. Selection bias explains apparent differential mortality between dialysis modalities. J Am Soc Nephrol 2011;22:1534-1542.

Stack AG, Molony DA, Rahman NS, et al. Impact of dialysis modality on survival of new ESRD patients with congestive heart failure in the United States. Kidney Int 2003;64:1071-1079.

Stack AG, Martin DR. Association of patient autonomy with increased transplantation and survival among new dialysis patients in the United States. Am J Kidney Dis 2005;45:730-742.

Vonesh EF, Snyder JJ, Foley RN, Collins AJ. The differential impact of risk factors on mortality in hemodialysis and peritoneal dialysis. Kidney Int 2004;66:2389-2401.

Vonesh EF, Snyder JJ, Foley RN, Collins AJ. Mortality studies comparing peritoneal dialysis and hemodialysis: what do they tell us? Kidney Int 2006;70[Suppl 103]:S3-11.

Weinhandl ED, Foley RN, Gilbertson DT, et al. Propensity-matched mortality comparison of incident hemodialysis and peritoneal dialysis patients. J Am Soc Nephrol 2010;21:499-506.

Wiggins KJ, McDonald SP, Brown FG, et al. High membrane transport status on peritoneal dialysis is not associated with reduced survival following transfer to haemodialysis. Nephrol Dial Transplant 2007;22:3005-3012.

Winkelmayer WC, Liu J, Brookhart MA. Altitude and all-cause mortality in incident dialysis patients. JAMA 2009;301:508-512.

Yang X, Fang W, Bargman JM, Oreopoulos DG. High peritoneal permeability is not associated with higher mortality or technique failure in patients on automated peritoneal dialysis. Perit Dial Int 2008;28:82-92.

Yeates K, Zhu N, Vonesh E, et al. Hemodialysis and peritoneal dialysis are associated with similar outcomes for end-stage renal disease treatment in Canada. Nephrol Dial Transplant 2012;27:3568-3575.

Chapter 18:
Setting Up a PD Program / Infrastructure

PERITONEAL DIALYSIS UNITS CAN be either free-standing units or units attached to physician offices or hemodialysis units. Key components of successful units include adequate staffing, adequate physical structure for patient care, administration, and storage space for supplies, and protocols that allow for certain standardization of care processes. These components will be reviewed in this chapter.

In the USA, a PD program providing dialysis services must operate under the Center for Medicare and Medicaid Services (CMS) mandated regulations if the unit is to participate in the Medicare program. These regulations are termed the Conditions for Coverage and are explained in detail at the www.cms.gov/center/esrd.asp website.

The PD unit must ensure that services provided to the home patient are equivalent to those offered within an in-center dialysis unit, such as dietician and ongoing medical social work evaluations (Section 494.100). The PD unit must retrieve and review the home records of the patient at least every 2 months and keep an active chart that maintains this information for members of the interdisciplinary team to review with the patient. The PD unit must also ensure that a physician or nurse practitioner, clinical nurse specialist, or physician's assistant documents a visit at least once a month. Inspections can be done to ensure that facilities and providers are adhering to these CMS requirements.

The core team that is required to medically supervise a peritoneal dialysis program is the medical director, the nursing staff, medical social worker and dietician.

Medical Director

The medical director must be a board certified physician in internal medicine or pediatrics whom has completed a nephrology training program and has at least 12 months of relevant experience caring for dialysis patients.

The medical director is responsible for the overall medical care provided in the unit. The Conditions for Coverage detail the specific responsibilities of the medical director and state:

The dialysis facility must have a medical director who meets the personnel qualifications to be responsible for the delivery of patient care and outcomes in the facility. The medical director is accountable to the governing body for the quality of medical care provided to patients. Medical director responsibilities include, but are not limited to, the following:

-Quality assessment and performance improvement program
-Staff education, training, and performance
-Policies and performance

The medical director must:(1) Participate in the development, periodic review and approval of a "patient care policies and procedures manual" for the facility; (2) ensure that all policies and procedures relative to patient admissions, patient care, infection control, and safety are adhered to by all individuals who treat patients in the facility, including attending physicians and non-physician providers; and (3) ensure that the interdisciplinary team adheres to the discharge and transfer policies and procedures specified by the facility's governing body.

The medical director provides leadership to the unit and assures that the unit monitors clinical outcomes, has good record keeping, and establishes processes that address suboptimal trends.

The web site www.kidneypatientsafety.org contains useful material to advise medical directors on how to implement the new CMS Conditions for Coverage and provides tools, resources, and educational material on how to improve safety of ESRD patients by reducing the risk of falls, medication errors, and issues of hand hygiene.

PD Nursing Staff

Under the Conditions for Coverage, the dialysis unit must have a nurse manager whom oversees the nursing issues in the unit and must be a full time employee of the facility, a registered nurse, and must have at least 12 months experience in general nursing and an additional 6 months of experience providing care to patients on dialysis. Functions of the nurse manager can include scheduling of the unit nurses, monitoring quality control measures, coordinating with hospitals if patients are hospitalized, organizing the billing and supply ordering/inventory process and communicating to the medical director any clinical concerns.

In addition to the nurse manager, additional home dialysis training nurses must be registered nurses with at least 12 months experience providing nursing care and at least 3 months of experience in the specific dialysis modality that the nurse will be providing care.

In the USA, the nursing-to-patient ratio varies from 1:15 to 1:25, with many units considering a ratio of 1:20 the current standard. A medical assistant can support the nursing staff by performing the scheduling of patient visits, answering phones, assisting with the charts and filing, rooming the patients and checking vital signs. The nursing staff can be further supported by the use of established protocols. Protocols for sampling of dialysate during suspected peritonitis episodes, empiric antibiotic protocols, protocols for exit-site care, erythropoietin administration, PET, and adequacy dialysate collections help maintain standardization and efficiency of nursing care.

Many programs establish a nursing on-call schedule to address patient calls on nights and weekends. The on-call nurse would address patient questions, decide if referral to a physician or emergency room is required and, in some programs, present to the emergency room during a peritonitis episode to expeditiously collect dialysate samples for laboratory testing and then initiation of antibiotics.

Key characteristics of successful PD nurses are those nurses that strongly believe in patient empowerment and the importance of allowing patients to perform self-care at home. PD nurses act as physician extenders and should be confident, efficient, organized and dedicated adult learners who become experts in PD therapy.

Dietician

The PD unit should have a dietician with a usual staffing ratio of 1:75 patients. The PD renal diet is different than HD or CKD so considerable effort is required of the dietician to instruct new patients. The dietician follows nutritional trends and designs interventions to address common PD dietary abnormalities such as hypokalemia, hypoalbuminemia, and hyperphosphatemia. As the dialysate contains carbohydrates, the dietician may need additional time to instruct on caloric restriction.

Medical Social Worker

Dialysis patients have many social needs and a social worker is a vital team member. The staffing ratio for a PD social worker varies, but is typically 1:100 patients, depending on the acuity of the patient population. The social worker can perform home visits to assess whether a prospective patient has the necessary home environment to support PD.

Social workers can assess family dynamics that may affect technique success. Social workers can assist the patient in establishing transportation to the unit, address billing and insurance questions, and educate on community resources such as the National Kidney Foundation or American Association of Kidney Patients. Medical social workers in the PD unit are invaluable for providing emotional support during the initiation of dialysis or during unexpected transitions in care.

Surgeons

The surgeon placing catheters should, ideally, be considered part of the PD team. Establishing an active working relationship with a surgeon for communication regarding catheter outcomes is important. Surgeons can be part of PD unit quality assurance meeting or be informed of the results of such meetings. Getting feedback from surgeons regarding the PD unit's scheduling of catheters and post-operative care is important. For new patients, coordination with the surgeon regarding pre-operative skin marking for the exit site should be established. It is important that the unit give feedback to the surgeon regarding catheter function and complications.

Attitude

Besides these individual members of the PD team, an additional component is important - attitude. Attitude is everything - a PD unit needs to adopt an attitude and mission statement that establishes a spirit of optimism, successful outcomes, team camaraderie, and compassion. This will establish an atmosphere that is welcomed by the patients and other caregivers. If a patient understands that they have the liberating option of home therapy and can be supported by a PD unit of excellence that is nurturing and a special place to visit, the entire medical enterprise - from doctors to nurses to staff to patients and families can have some of the most special relationships in their lives.

In building the infrastructure of a PD unit it is important to build not only the physical plant but to establish the attitude, morale, and philosophy that will promote health and the richness of life's possibilities. The PD unit allows for home therapy- and, compared to in-center HD, dialysis at home can be liberating. The unit can take great pride in enabling patients to have the knowledge and confidence to provide self-care at home. This empowers patients, gives them back a sense of control that perhaps was lost in the pre-dialysis period, and when done well is rewarding for all staff involved.

Patient Training

New patients-in-training will require dedicated nursing time and can put a strain on nursing resources. Adequate nursing staffing, therefore, must consider that the available nurses must not only manage the PD patient's monthly routine visit, be available to address unscheduled visits such as a peritonitis presentation, but may be required to spend significant time in the training of a single patient. Training times for new patients vary between 3 to 10 days, but approximately 7 days is average. Unit administrators must understand the impact that new patient training has on nursing time and assure that proper nursing staffing allows for safe and thorough training which will reduce subsequent complications.

Physical Space

There are certain minimal space requirements that are recommended. One room is needed for patient training and an additional room is recommended per every 20 patients. The rooms should be large enough to allow for at least 3 chairs- for the nurse, patient, and a relative. The patient chair should be able to be reclined to facilitate abdominal examinations and dressing changes. The rooms should contain supply cabinets and a hand washing sink. Many centers discourage phones being placed in the rooms which may distract the nurses and be a source of hand contamination. Besides the patient rooms, a separate administrative room for nursing staff is recommended to allow for charting, managing schedules, and phone access for contact with patients or other clinical staff.

Significant storage space is recommended for solutions, cycler devices, and other supplies. Separate from the patient rooms is a space considered a "dirty utility room" used for discarding dialysate or other body fluids. A conference room to facilitate team meetings is recommended. If possible, the PD unit should have a reception area for waiting patients and families as well as a break room for staff. Two restrooms are recommended - one for patients and one separate for staff.

CKD Education

To assure growth of the PD census, new patients must enter the unit from the general CKD population. CKD education is critical to expose patients to the home dialysis option. Dialysis options education should be done carefully, with time allotted to allow patients and family members to thoroughly learn about PD, have the time to ask questions and discuss among themselves, and have the option of meeting actual PD patients to hear directly about the home dialysis experience. Some centers provide up to three options education sessions before asking a patient to make a decision on the dialysis modality. Some centers allow CKD patients to walk into HD units and spend considerable time sitting in a hemodialysis chair to better understand the lifestyle on hemodialysis. This is followed by visits to the PD unit where manual exchanges are performed by the patient on an abdominal simulation model to demonstrate the PD process.

Each PD unit should adopt a unique approach to dialysis options education to assure that an informed decision is made by the patient. Literature has suggested that when full and complete options education is given, up to 40% of patients elect to initiate PD.

Infrastructure Requirements for Urgent-Start PD

Outpatient PD centers that are capable of performing urgent PD soon after catheter placement will have several unique infrastructure requirements. Initiating urgent PD will require staff-assisted PD to occur in the unit as many patients have presented late in the course of their disease, had a catheter placed expeditiously, and need to initiate PD more urgently to avoid temporary vascular access and urgent HD. Patients initiating PD urgently may be at increased risk of leak, as the catheter may not have had the customary 2-week break-in period. Therefore, the unit should have the capability of performing staff assisted low-volume, recumbent PD in a reclining chair, bed, or stretcher. As this will impact nursing staffing requirements and urgent start PD capability is better suited for larger units with more than a single PD nurse. The unit would need to control supply inventory to assure that supplies are readily on hand should an urgent PD patient be referred to the center. These requirements have been fully elucidated in a recent article by Ghaffari et al.

Quality Assessment and Performance Improvement (QAPI)

The PD unit should develop and sustain a culture of quality with frequent assessment of quality goals. Quality management activity can include regular meetings to review clinical targets such as peritonitis rates, anemia, mineral bone disease, and nutritional parameters. Deaths and hospitalizations should be reviewed to determine if PD therapy contributed to the event, and if so, determine the need for a change in monitoring, training, or policy and procedures. It is important for the PD unit to have this formal continuous quality initiative. A QAPI meeting agenda could address the following:

Current census for the month
Causes of transfers out during the month
Deaths and whether there was any PD attribution to the death
Hospitalizations and whether there was any PD attribution
Peritonitis episodes and re-calculation of the unit's peritonitis rate
Exit site infections and calculation of exit site rate

Clearance measurements performed in the month are reviewed to insure that any inadequate result has been addressed with a prescription change
Anemia Management
Review of outliers in calcium, phosphorus, and PTH protocols
Nutritional review of patients with low serum albumin or hypokalemia and discussion of needed intervention
Any active social issues the MSW feels should be addressed by the group

By performing this QAPI on a frequent basis (monthly to quarterly) the staff are assured that there is better understanding of the functioning of the unit and its outcomes. Without this QAPI effort the unit is like a ship adrift at sea, directionless- aware of neither successes nor failures. Only with the vigorous tracking of outcomes can the QAPI process discover deficiencies and take corrective actions.

The QAPI process should attempt to perform a root cause analysis of infectious episodes and catheter problems. It is important to understand why a catheter did not get placed as desired or did not function to the team's satisfaction. Is there an issue with the surgeon that has become recurrent? Is there a problem with a particular insurance company or barriers that cause delay in obtaining surgical consultation and operating room scheduling? Does the peritonitis or exit site infection rate suggest a need to change the training manual?

Members of the QAPI team can apply Business Management theories such as 6S and Lean techniques to improve workplace efficiency and reduce waste. The team should ask of themselves- are the patient training manuals excessively wordy and unfriendly, are the staff charting mechanisms redundant and wasting time, should paper records move to an electronic format, is the unit using computer-based adequacy programs and peritonitis tracking programs, reporting to upper management on successes and emphasizing the cost-effectiveness of the delivery of dialysis services, instituting employee recognition pathways to encourage a high quality workplace performance, is the physical plant clean and inviting and fostering a sense of professionalism, is the work place dress code professional, is there a mechanism to allow patients to make suggestions and give feedback on the unit's performance? Should there be a PD unit web site, a quarterly newsletter to the patients highlighting events surrounding the lives of fellow patients and the staff, is the unit building relationships among the staff and patients, celebrating birthdays, the birth of a grandchild, graduations, making the unit a shining star of excellence to counter the many negative perceptions of dialysis that exist? In many important ways, these infrastructure issues determine whether a PD unit succeeds or fails.

Several recent publications have suggested that PD census is related to clinical outcomes. Larger PD units were noted to have reduced peritonitis rates, hospitalizations, catheter complications, and improved survival. This suggests that in larger units there is more experience generated in managing the patients. Units of 20 patients or greater were noted to have better outcomes than smaller units. Therefore, small PD units may consider consolidating to allow for full-time nurse staffing in the unit and greater accumulated experience in managing the therapy and any complications.

Hospital and Extended Care Facility Interactions

The PD unit should have access to hospitals capable of caring for the patient with minimal disruption to the therapy. Communication channels should be established to allow unit nurses to assist hospital staff for questions and patient information. A PD patient requiring temporary or permanent nursing home placement should, ideally, not have to be converted to HD but allowed to continue PD therapy in a facility licensed and trained to perform PD. PD unit staff can lobby for the continued development of PD expertise within the inpatient and nursing home setting.

Conclusions

The development of a successful PD program requires adequate staffing, physical space, and processes of care that allow for the efficient delivery of the therapy. Policies and procedures should be established that allow for consistency in patient management and a reduction in ineffective use of time and resources. Establishing a quality control mechanism can allow for an understanding of the unit's successes and weaknesses and allow for continuous improvement.

References:

Bernardini J, Price V, Figueiredo A. Peritoneal dialysis patient training, 2006. Perit Dial Int 2006;26:625-632.

Finkelstein FO. Structural requirements for a successful chronic peritoneal dialysis am. Kidney Int 2006;70:S118-S121.

Finkelstein FO, Ezekiel O, Raducu R. Development of a peritoneal dialysis program. Blood Purif 2011;31:121-124.

Gadallah MF, Ramdeen G, Torres-Rivera C, et al. Changing the trend: a prospective study on factors contributing to the growth rate of peritoneal dialysis programs. Adv Perit Dial 2001;17:122-126.

Ghaffari A, Kumar V, Guest S. Infrastructure requirements for an urgent-start peritoneal dialysis program. Perit Dial Int 2013;33:611-617.

Golper TA, Saxena AB, Piraino B, et al. Systematic barriers to the effective delivery of home dialysis in the United States: a report from the public policy/advocacy committee of the North American chapter of the international society for peritoneal dialysis. Am J Kidney Dis 2011;58:879-885.

Goovaerts T, Jadoul M, Goffin E. Influence of a pre-dialysis education programme (PDEP) on the mode of renal replacement therapy. Nephrol Dial Transplant 2005;20:1842-1847.

Li PK, Chow KM. How to have a successful peritoneal dialysis program. Perit Dial Int 2003:23[Suppl 2]:S183-S187.

Maddux FW, Maddux DW, Hakim RM. The role of the medical director: changing with the times. Semin Dial 2008;21:54-57.

Neil F, Guest S, Wong L, et al. The financial implications for Medicare of greater use of peritoneal dialysis. Clin Ther 2009;31:880-888.

Piraino B, Minev E, Bernadini J, Bender FH. Does experience with PD matter? Perit Dial Int 2009;29:256-261.

Plantinga LC, Fink NE, Finkelstein FO, et al. Association of peritoneal dialysis clinic size with clinical outcomes. Perit Dial Int 2009;29:285-291.

Wish JB. What is expected of a medical director in the Centers for Medicare and Medicaid Services conditions for coverage? Blood Purif 2011;31:61-65.

Chapter 19:
PD in Special Situations

THE PRACTICE OF **PD** therapy can be complicated by special clinical situations such as the need for colonoscopy, an ostomy, percutaneous gastric feeding tube, or the patient who wishes to swim. These and other special situations will be discussed in this chapter.

Patients with Ostomies

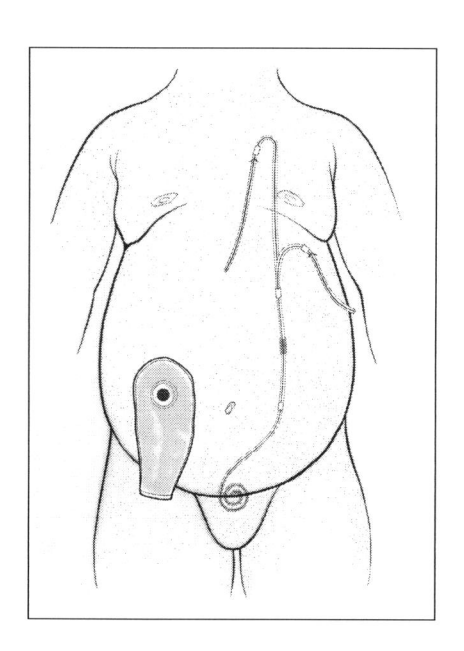

Patients with pre-existing abdominal stomas are candidates for peritoneal dialysis. Initial fear of peritonitis, due to cross contamination, was not found to be warranted. Anecdotal experiences with these patients have shown successful PD therapy with low peritonitis rates. In those cases with peritonitis, staphylococcal infections, not enteric organisms, were most common, as in the general PD population.

However, precautions can be taken in patients with pre-existing stomas to minimize the

Extended catheter options for exit site location in patients with ostomies

chance of cross contamination and include (1) placement of the catheter exit site a significant distance from the stoma on the abdomen (2) placement of a pre-sternal catheter to avoid an abdominal exit site altogether.

Patients with stomas have had prior abdominal surgery and may have adhesions complicating catheter placement and dialysate flow. During catheter placement, advanced laparoscopic techniques using adhesiolysis should be considered, along with repair of any noted incisional hernias.

PD after a Failed Kidney Transplant

The impact of dialysis modality on survival after failed kidney transplant was discussed in Chapter 17. PD can be initiated after failed kidney transplant as the transplanted organ typically resides in the extraperitoneal soft tissue. Management of these patients is unique in regards to the transplant immunosuppression. As discussed in Chapter 5, PD can often be associated with preservation of residual kidney function and therefore continuation of lower level immunosuppression may be indicated to attempt to preserve residual allograft function.

PD Patients Undergoing Transplant - Catheter Removal Recommendations

Management of PD patients subsequently undergoing transplant will require a decision to be made on whether the PD catheter should be removed at the time of transplantation or left in place as an access should there be delayed graft function. Transplant centers may have individual protocols addressing this issue but a recent report in the Canadian Urological Association journal provides additional insight. Warren and colleagues followed 137 PD patients who underwent kidney transplantation. Nineteen patients had their catheters removed at the time of surgery and 118 patients had the catheters left in place. Eighty-nine percent of these latter patients had immediate graft function and had no requirement for use of the catheter. Despite not being used, the authors felt the catheter itself was associated with peritonitis in 5 patients, catheter-related infection in 2 patients and one catheter patient required an exploratory laparotomy for presumed peritonitis. Overall, of the 15 patients requiring post-transplant PD there was a high rate of peritonitis in the post-operative period (33%) and high rate of dialysate leak necessitating HD (20%). The authors concluded that maintaining the PD catheter post-transplant was associated with a 7% rate of peritonitis versus 0% if removed and subjected the patients to a second surgery for catheter removal. This experience is from a single center and may not reflect the experience in other centers. Further research in this important area of patient management is needed.

Patients with Percutaneous Endoscopic Gastrostomy (PEG) or other Gastric Feeding Tubes

Initiating PD in the patient with a pre-existing gastrostomy is generally safe and without risk of dialysate leak or peritonitis. The gastrostomy, in these cases, is well-healed and the peritoneum is intact and isolated from the percutaneous sinus tract. However, placing a new gastrostomy tube in the patient on PD represents a different level of complexity, with greater peri-operative morbidity. Increased rates of bacterial and fungal peritonitis have been described post-operatively. Special precautions are, therefore, warranted and include the cessation of PD for several months after gastrostomy placement, combined with both bacterial and fungal prophylaxis. In this population, surgical gastrostomy placement, as opposed to percutaneous placement, may be associated with less risk of subsequent leakage.

A recently described higher percutaneous esophageal tube, that enters the cervical esophagus under ultrasound guidance and then is passed from the upper esophagus into the stomach, has been employed in PD patients in Japan. This tube has been termed a percutaneous transesophageal gastro-tube (PTEG) and had low rates of post-procedure complications.

Patients with Suprapubic Bladder Catheters

PD therapy has been described in patients with indwelling suprapubic bladder catheters. These catheters are extra-peritoneal and do not come into contact with the open peritoneum or dialysate. The bladder catheter skin entrance site may represent a source of potential cross-contamination. These patients would be ideal candidates for exit site placement in more remote locations such as an upper abdominal or pre-sternal site.

PD in the HIV Patient

Patients with underlying human immunodeficiency virus (HIV) have been treated with PD. Highly active antiretroviral therapy has improved the long term prognosis of infected patients and many patients have been managed with dialysis and transplantation. Spent dialysate, tubing, and bags should be disposed of as biohazard waste material as per general Centers of Disease Control recommendations.

Pregnancy and the PD Patient

Becoming pregnant while on dialysis is rare. In patients with ESRD, the incidence of pregnancy in women of childbearing age is 1 to 7%, with those pregnancies often notable for higher rates of complications such as premature labor, intrauterine growth retardation, and infant death. In 1999, estimates suggested that less than 50% of pregnancies resulted in delivery of a surviving infant. More current information, however, suggests successful pregnancies are described in up to two thirds of patients. The overall incidence of pregnancy may be lower in PD patients, compared to HD patients, due to the intraperitoneal fluid presenting a possible barrier to ovum movement after ovulation and subsequent ovum implantation. Once pregnant, the diagnosis is often delayed due to a pre-existing irregular menstrual pattern.

Some literature suggests that managing the pregnant dialysis patient on PD is advantageous, due to the more continuous nature of the process, without the more dramatic shifts in electrolytes and volume status associated with intermittent HD. Rapid shifts in volume and solute may affect uteroplacental circulation and fetal homeostasis. Other advantages to PD, in the management of the pregnant patient, are higher hematocrits maintained with less erythropoietin requirement, less hypotensive episodes, and lack of the need for systemic heparinization.

Though unproven, it is believed that increasing the dose of dialysis delivered could be beneficial to the mother and developing fetus. The patient prescription can be empirically increased, preferentially by increasing the number of cycles, as opposed to increasing the dwell volume. Daily total volumes up to 12 liters have been described. In the patient on CAPD, successful pregnancies have been describe with reducing the dwell volume to 1.5 liters and increasing the exchange frequency to 5 times a day, beginning in the 4th month of the pregnancy.

Tidal PD may be of particular benefit to the pregnant patient. In this regimen a small residual volume is left in place to prevent uterine obstruction of the catheter and a dwell volume is exchanged over more frequent cycles. The total intraperitoneal volume can be reduced to less than 2 liters, if required. Care must be made to instruct the patient not to bypass a slow drain alarm and re-fill the abdomen without assuring that the expected drain volume had occurred.

PD complications during pregnancy may raise unique concerns. Peritonitis during pregnancy has been described and was successfully treated during the gestation. In one report, peritonitis was described to trigger premature labor.

Hemoperitoneum, due to retrograde flow of blood from the uterus to the open fallopian tube fimbrae, should be promptly reported as it could herald a complication such as placental detachment or spontaneous abortion.

Pregnant patients delivering by caesarian section have resumed PD several days after surgery. In these cases the caesarian approach was termed "low abdominal" or "transverse abdominal" and was felt to be an extraperitoneal incision.

Patients with an Intrauterine Device

Female patients with an intrauterine device (IUD) are candidates for PD. The intrauterine location of the device is extraperitoneal and has not adversely affected dialysate administration. Only rare case reports describe IUD perforation of the uterus and subsequent peritonitis. Uterine perforation may present with polymicrobial peritonitis and/or fungal peritonitis. Broad spectrum antibiotics and antifungal agents, combined with transvaginal or laparoscopic removal of the IUD resulted in resolution of infection. A recent report by Wu and colleagues demonstrated the value of prophylactic antibiotics prior to IUD placement.

PD for the Management of Severe Congestive Heart Failure

Patients with severe underlying cardiomyopathy may poorly tolerate the aggressive ultrafiltration associated with intermittent hemodialysis. PD has been proposed as a suitable treatment, as fluid removal is gentle and better tolerated. Clinical experience with PD in the management of severe congestive heart failure (CHF) is limited to case reports and small case series but document improvement, in many patients, in New York Heart Association functional class. Use of once-daily icodextrin, to enhance fluid removal in patients not at end-stage renal disease, has been described but no large experience with this management strategy exists. Patients with severe cardiomyopathy have increased operative risk during access surgery so percutaneous catheter placement may be preferred.

PD in the Patient with Underlying Liver Disease and Ascites

Patients with cirrhosis and ascites have been successfully managed on peritoneal dialysis and some centers consider PD the preferred dialytic option for this patient population. The cirrhotic often poorly tolerates the more aggressive ultrafiltration on HD, due to lower baseline blood pressures and hepatorenal physiology. The increased bleeding risk in cirrhosis makes HD heparinization difficult.

PD offers several advantages - a more gentle hemodynamic profile, the ability to drain accumulated ascites, making subsequent paracentesis unnecessary, and avoidance of heparinization.

At the time of initial PD catheter placement, some reports describe an initial large volume paracentesis to decompress the ascites, and allow for catheter placement with reduced chance of early leak. This initial large volume paracentesis is often combined with infusions of intravenous albumin to provide hemodynamic support. The catheter is allowed to heal for several weeks, but if used sooner, the patients are initiated with lower volume, supine cycler therapy to reduce the chance of leak. The initial PD regimen is termed a "controlled paracentesis" as the dialysate drain will contain a mixture of residual ascites and the dialysate. The drain volume is restricted to allow for only the slow eventual decompression of all remaining ascites. The largest published series of cirrhotics on PD showed similar or reduced peritonitis rates. Infection rates may be reduced by avoiding hypokalemia and, possibly, by the use of lactulose as a laxative. A recent report described a reduced peritonitis rate in cirrhotics taking lactulose. Lactulose increases intestinal transit time, thus reducing likelihood of bacterial overgrowth, and is metabolized to lactate and pyruvic acid, thus acidifying the stool. The authors speculated that these factors may reduce the likelihood of enteric peritonitis. Further investigation is warranted.

Maintaining adequate nutrition is a significant concern in the cirrhotic PD patient. Ongoing protein losses in the dialysate can allow for the development of malnutrition and serum albumin levels, and other nutritional parameters must be closely monitored. Early interventions to increase the nutritional intake may be necessary to counter the protein losses in dialysate.

PD in Autosomal Dominant Polycystic Kidney Disease (ADPKD)

Patients with underlying ADPKD can be managed on PD but are at higher risk of certain complications - associated with the cyst burden and perhaps the underlying collagen defect that is the hallmark of the disease. Patients with ADPKD on PD are at increased risk of hernia formation, leaks, and possibly hydrothorax. Initial concerns that ADPKD patients may have increased enteric peritonitis rates, due to underlying diverticulosis, have not be substantiated in more recent reports.

A recent report by Kumar and associates determined that ADPKD patients on PD, compared to matched non-affected patients, had similar baseline peritoneal membrane function, clearances, ultrafiltration volumes, PET results, dialysate inflow or outflow times, and residual dialysate volumes. Technique survival and peritonitis rates, including enteric peritonitis, were similar. In the 56 patients studied 5 required subsequent umbilical hernia repair and 3 patients

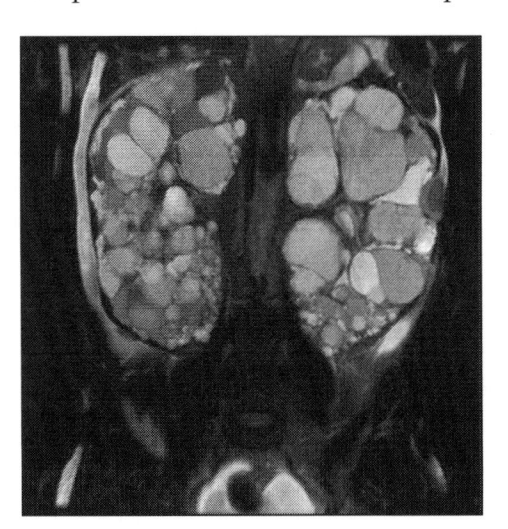

MRI of a PD patient with underlying ADPKD, showing massive cyst burden in the intra-abdominal cavity

had early leaks, within one week of starting PD. Hernias appear to be the main complication associated with PD therapy in the ADPKD population and detection of pre-existing hernias with simultaneous repair at the time of initial catheter placement is recommended.

PD in Swimmers

Patients on PD therapy can swim despite the presence of an abdominal catheter. Ocean water and pool water are generally less contaminated with bacteria yet even fresh water swimming has been described.

Attempts to protect the catheter and exit site from contact with water is prudent. Protection from water has been described by applying a clear semi-occlusive adhesive dressing or overlying ostomy bag. Thorough cleaning and drying of the exit site after swimming is recommended.

PD in the Visually Impaired or Blind Patient

Patients with severe visual impairment or complete blindness have been successfully trained to perform CAPD. To assist the patients, talking watches, weight scales, blood pressure monitors, and glucometers are available. To perform the PD connection, a variety of training approaches have been described. In one approach, the patient secures the dialysate tubing on the edge of a table by using a specially designed clip. The cap is removed in sterile fashion while the tubing is held in the clip. The patient then removes the cap of their transfer set and holds the transfer set in one hand, reaches back to the work table to remove the dialysate tubing from the clip, and using a "three finger approach" the connection is completed in sterile fashion.

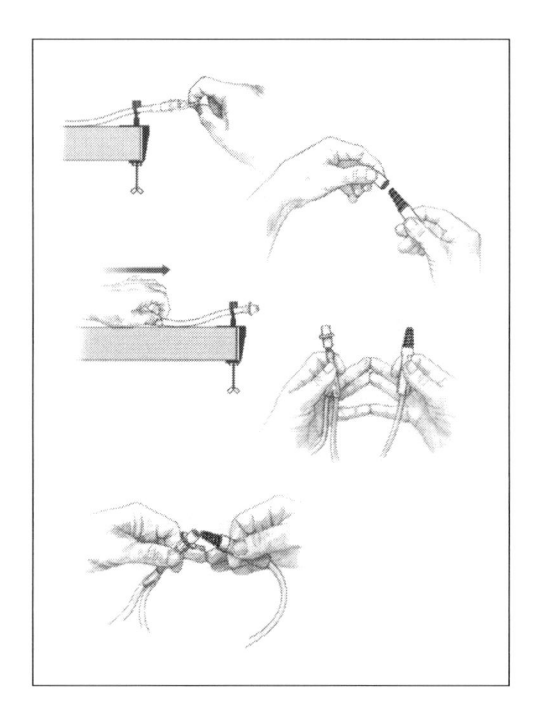

To assist in the training, audio tapes can be made to reinforce the instructions for reviewing at home. During the delivery of supply boxes, the solution boxes should be placed in a consistent order, from 1.5% to 2.5% to 4.25% to allow the patient to reliably locate the correct solution. If there is some limited vision, magnifying glasses and large print laminated cards can assist in the training.

Patients with Pets at Home

Patients with pets in the home are candidates for PD but special precautions should be taken to reduce the possibility of a pet contaminating the PD home supplies or adding infectious risk during the set-up and initiation of the exchanges. Pet-related peritonitis with Pasteurella multocida has been described in patients with cats, dogs, hamsters and other animals in the home. Cats are notorious for their attraction to the dialysate tubing as a source of entertainment and challenge and most cats may indeed prefer to nap on the warm surface of the cycler heater tray. Pets should be kept out of the room used for performing the exchanges, if at all possible, and should not be present during the set-up and connection to the dialysate bags. In patients with pets it may be prudent to increase the hand hygiene regimen prior to making an exchange to include more prolonged hand washing and use of alcohol-based hand products after the hand wash. Careful wipe down of the cycler device and other support devices may be needed if a pet has had access to the treatment room.

Patients with a Ventriculoperitoneal Shunt (VP Shunt)

The presence of a VP shunt is considered a relative, but not absolute, contraindication to PD therapy. Many case reports describe successful experiences with PD, even in patients in which subsequent peritonitis occurs. In cases of peritonitis, ascending infection via the shunt, to the ventricles, can occur but appears rare as current shunt designs allow flow in one direction only, to prevent reflux flow. Most reports of PD in patients with VP shunts are in the pediatric population and the time course of PD is relatively shorted by earlier transplantation. A recent report in pediatric patients by Dolan and colleagues from the International Pediatric Peritoneal Dialysis Network stated in 18 PD patients with VP shunts there were no instances of ascending shunt infection, descending peritonitis from meningitis, or other complications such as catheter dysfunction. These authors concluded that the presence of a VP shunt in an anticipated patient or the subsequent need for a shunt in a pre-existing patient on PD can be considered safe.

CSF secretion is approximately 750 mL per day and therefore adds to the volume of fluid in the abdomen, yet reports describe no increased abdominal discomfort or hydrostatic pressure increases of significance. Encapsulating peritoneal sclerosis has been described in patients with VP shunts not on PD as well as on PD therapy and longer term follow-up for this complication is prudent.

PD in the Patients with an Abdominal Aortic Graft

PD has been performed chronically in patients with abdominal vascular prosthesis as treatment for an abdominal aortic aneurysm. The aorta resides in the retroperitoneal space and peritonitis leading to subsequent infection of an established retroperitoneal aortic mesh graft or stent has not been described. Maccario and colleagues reported on 8 patients with intra-abdominal prosthetic grafts who were maintained on PD. Patients were followed for a total of 208 months and there were 6 episodes of peritonitis with no evidence of abdominal aortic graft infection. Peritonitis episodes infrequently lead to bacteremia, further reducing the risk of hematogenous spread of peritoneal infection to a vascular prosthesis. Additionally, aortic prostheses develop a neo-intimal endothelial surface which further protects against bacterial seeding of the prosthesis during bacteremia.

Stent-grafts to repair iliac or aortic aneurysms can be placed from extraperitoneal insertion sites and the peritoneal cavity is not entered, so PD has been continued post-procedure. Patients requiring an open repair of a AAA have been typically converted to HD, after PD catheter removal, and then re-evaluated for PD candidacy after full recovery of the larger abdominal wound.

Gastric Banding or Gastric Bypass Surgery in PD

Currently there is insufficient information to make recommendations about the safety of adjustable gastric banding procedures on patients maintained on peritoneal dialysis. Theoretically, laparoscopic gastric bands and the connection leading to the subcutaneous port may be at risk of seeding during PD-related peritonitis necessitating removal but no reports, to date, have appeared in the literature to document this complication. Chen and colleagues reported on a non-uremic patient with an adjustable gastric band who developed peritonitis requiring laparotomy and removal of the device.

Gastric bypass surgery in obese patients on dialysis has not been widespread due to the complexity of co-morbid conditions often present and the perceived risk of the surgery. Yet some experience with gastric bypass surgery in dialysis patients is available. Alexander et al. described 19 dialysis patients that underwent gastric bypass procedures. The dialysis modality was not reported. PD patients undergoing gastric bypass would presumably require temporary conversion to HD until complete wound healing. The dialysis patients described above had been on dialysis for a mean of 2.6 years prior to surgery and the reduction in excess BMI was 66 % at 12 months. Patients with gastric bypass procedures before initiating dialysis have been placed on PD uneventfully with only minor upper abdominal adhesions noted during catheter placement surgery.

References:

Ostomies

Korzets Z, Golan E, Naftali T, Bernheim J. Peritoneal dialysis in the presence of a stoma. Perit Dial Int 1992;12:258-260.

Kidney transplantation

Bakir N, Surachno S, Sluiter WJ, et al. Peritonitis in peritoneal dialysis patients after renal transplantation. Nephrol Dial Transplant 1998;13:178-183.

Warren J, Jones E, Sener A, et al. Should peritoneal dialysis catheters be removed at the time of kidney transplantation? Can Urol Assoc J 2012;6:376-378.

PD in patients with percutaneous feeding tubes (PEGs)

Fein PA. Safety of PEG tubes in peritoneal dialysis patients. Semin Dial 2002;15:213-214.

Fein PA, Madane SJ, Jorden A, et al. Outcome of percutaneous endoscopic gastrostomy feeding in patients on peritoneal dialysis. Adv Perit Dial 2001;17;148-152.

Lew SQ, Gruia A, Hakki F. Adult peritoneal dialysis patient with Tenckhoff and percutaneous endoscopic gastrostomy catheters. Perit Dial Int 2011;31:360-361.

Von Schnakenburg C, Feneberg R, Plank C, et al. Percutaneous endoscopic gastrostomy in children on peritoneal dialysis. Perit Dial Int 2006;26:69-77.

PD in patients with suprapubic bladder catheters

Twardowski ZJ, Prowant BF, Pickett B, et al. Four-year experience with swan neck presternal peritoneal dialysis catheter. Am J Kidney Dis 1996;27:99-105.

PD in the HIV patient

Novak JE, Szczech LA. Management of HIV-infected patients with ESRD. Adv Chronic Kidney Dis 2010;17:102-110.

Ahuja TS, Collinge N, Grady J, Khan S. Is dialysis modality a factor in survival of patients with ESRD and HIV-associated nephropathy? Am J Kidney Dis 2003;41:1060-1064.

Soleymanian T, Raman S, Shannaq FN, et al. Survival and morbidity of HIV patients on hemodialysis and peritoneal dialysis: one center's experience and review of the literature. Int Urol Nephrol 2006;38:331-338.

Pregnancy

Chang H, Miller MA, Bruns FJ. Tidal peritoneal dialysis during pregnancy improves clearance and abdominal symptoms. Perit Dial Int 2002;22:272-274.

Chou CY, Ting IW, Lin TH, Lee CN. Pregnancy in patients on chronic dialysis: a single center experience and combined analysis of reported results. Eur J Obstet Gynecol Reprod Biol 2008;136:165-170.

Gadallah MF, Ahmad B, Karubian F, Campese VM. Pregnancy in patients on chronic ambulatory peritoneal dialysis. Am J Kidney Dis 1992;20:407-410.

Gomez Vazquez JA, Martinez Calva IE, Mendiola Fernandez R, et al. Pregnancy in end-stage renal disease patients and treatment with peritoneal dialysis: report of two cases. Perit Dial Int 2007;27:353-358.

Hou S. Conception and pregnancy in peritoneal dialysis patients. Perit Dial Int 2001;21[Suppl 3]:S290-S294.

Jakobi P, Ohel G, Szylman P, et al. Continuous ambulatory peritoneal dialysis as the primary approach in the management of severe renal insufficiency in pregnancy. Obstet Gynecol 1992;79:808-810.

Jefferys A, Wyburn K, Chow J, et al. Peritoneal dialysis in pregnancy: a case series. Nephrology 2008;13:380-383.

Lew SQ. Persistent hemoperitoneum in a pregnant patient receiving peritoneal dialysis. Perit Dial Int 2006;26:108-111.

Reddy S, Holley JL. Management of the pregnant chronic dialysis patient. Adv Chronic Kidney Dis 2007;14:146-155.

Shemin D. Dialysis in pregnant women with chronic kidney disease. Semin Dial 2003;16:379-383.

Smith WT, Darbari S, Kwan M, et al. Pregnancy in peritoneal dialysis: a case report and review of adequacy and outcomes. Int Urol Nephrol 2005;37:145-151.

PD in patients with an intrauterine device (IUD)

Bieber SD, Jefferson JA, Anderson AE. Migration of an intrauterine device and peritonitis in a peritoneal dialysis patient. Clin Nephrol 2013;80:146-150.

Plaza MM. Intrauterine device-related peritonitis in a patient on CAPD. Perit Dial Int 2002;22:538-539.

Wu HH, Li IJ, Weng CH, et al. Prophylactic antibiotics for endoscopy-associated peritonitis in peritoneal dialysis patients. PLos One 2013;8:e71532.

Congestive heart failure

Hebert MJ, Falardeau M, Pichette V, et al. Continuous ambulatory peritoneal dialysis for patients with severe left ventricular systolic dysfunction and end-stage renal disease. Am J Kidney Dis 1995;25:761-768.

Khalifeh N, Vychytil A, Horl WH. The role of peritoneal dialysis in the management of treatment-resistant congestive heart failure: a European perspective. Kidney Int 2006;70[Suppl 103]:S72-S75.

Mehrotra R, Khanna R. Peritoneal ultrafiltration for chronic congestive heart failure: rationale, evidence and future. Cardiology 2001;96:177-182.

Mehrotra R, Kathuria P. Place of peritoneal dialysis in the management of treatment-resistant congestive heart failure. Kidney Int 2006;70[suppl 103]:S67-S71.

Sanchez JE, Ortega T, Rodriguez C, et al. Efficacy of peritoneal ultrafiltration in the treatment of refractory congestive heart failure. Nephrol Dial Transplant 2010;25:605-610.

Sheppard R, Panyon J, Pohwani AL, et al. Intermittent outpatient ultrafiltration for the treatment of severe refractory congestive heart failure. J Card Failure 2004;10:380-383.

PD in the patient with liver disease and ascites

Afsar B, Elsurer R, Bilgic A, et al. Regular lactulose use is associated with lower peritonitis rates: an observational study. Perit Dial Int 2010;30:243-245.

Chaudhary K, Khanna R. Renal replacement therapy in end-stage renal disease patients with chronic liver disease and ascites: role of peritoneal dialysis. Perit Dial Int 2008;28:113-117.

Chow KM, Szeto CC, Wu A, et al. Continuous ambulatory peritoneal dialysis in patients with hepatitis B liver disease. Perit Dial Int 2006;26:213-217.

De Vecchi AF, Colucci P, Salerno F, et al. Outcome of peritoneal dialysis in cirrhotic patients with chronic renal failure. Am J Kidney Dis 2002;40:161-168.

Guest S. Peritoneal dialysis in patients with cirrhosis and ascites. Adv Perit Dial 2010;26:82-87.

Howard CS, Teitelbaum I. Renal replacement therapy in patients with chronic liver disease. Semin Dial 2005;18:212-216.

Selgas R, Bajo MA, Del Peso G, et al. Peritoneal dialysis in the comprehensive management of end-stage renal disease patients with liver cirrhosis and ascites: practical aspects and review of the literature. Perit Dial Int 2008;28:118-122.

PD in ADPKD

Alam A, Perrone RD. Management of ESRD in patients with autosomal dominant polycystic kidney disease. Adv Chronic Kid Dis 2010;17:164-172.

Fletcher S, Turney JH, Brownjohn AM. Increased incidence of hydrothorax complicating peritoneal dialysis in patients with adult polycystic kidney disease. Nephrol Dial Transplant 1994;9:832-833.

Goffin E, Pirson Y. Is peritoneal dialysis a suitable renal replacement therapy in autosomal dominant polycystic kidney disease? Nat Clin Pract Nephrol 2009;5:122-123.

Kumar S, Fan SL, Raftery MJ, Yaqoob MM. Long term outcome of patients with autosomal dominant polycystic kidney diseases receiving peritoneal dialysis. Kidney Int 2008;74:946-951.

PD in swimmers

Cugelman A. Steps to safe swimming for patients on peritoneal dialysis. CANNT J 2011;21:53-54.

Sandahl L, Owens E. Use of an ostomy pouch for pediatric CAPD swimmers. ANNA J 1989;16:274-277.

Plante B, Amadei M, Herbert E, O'Regan S. Tegaderm dressings for peritoneal dialysis and gastrojejunostomy catheters in children. Adv Perit Dial 1990;6:279-280.

Visual-impairment and PD

Bentley ML. Keep it simple! A touch technique peritoneal dialysis procedure for the blind and visually impaired. CAANT 2001;11:32-34.

Boyer M, Lepage-Sabourin L, Poirier F, Smith C. Teaching CAPD to the visually impaired. CAANT 1998;8:28-29.

Chandran PKG, Lane T, Flynn CT. Patient and technique survival for blind and sighted diabetics on continuous ambulatory peritoneal dialysis: a ten-year analysis. Int J Artif Organs 1991:14:262-268.

Shokar S. Keep it simple: teaching totally blind patients using Baxter's twin bag peritoneal dialysis system. CAANT 2001;11:8.

Wright LS. Training a patient with visual impairment on continous ambulatory peritoneal dialysis. Nephrol Nurs J 2005;32:675-677.

Pets

Sol PM, van de Kar NC, Schreuder MF. Cat induced pasteurella multocida peritonitis in peritoneal dialysis: a case report and review of the literature. Int J Hyg Environ Health 2013;216:211-213.

PD in the patient with a ventriculoperitoneal shunt

Dolan NM, Borzych-Duzalka D, Suarez A, et al. Ventriculoperitoneal shunts in children on peritoneal dialysis: a survey of the International Pediatric Peritoneal Dialysis Network. Pediatr Nephrol 2013:28:315-319.

Grunberg J, Rebori A, Verocay MC. Peritoneal dialysis in children with spina bifida and ventriculoperitoneal shunt: one center's experience and review of the literature. Perit Dial Int 2003;23:481-486.

Kazee MR, Jackson EC, Jenkins RD. Management of a child on CAPD with a ventriculoperitoneal shunt. Adv Perit Dial 1990;6:281-282.

Ram Prabahar MR, Sivakumar M, Chandrasekaran V, et al. Peritoneal dialysis in a patient with neurogenic bladder and chronic kidney disease with ventriculoperitoneal shunt. Blood Purif 2008;26:274-278.

Warady BA, Hellerstein S, Alon U. Advisability of initiating chronic peritoneal dialysis in the presence of a ventriculoperitoneal shunt. Pediatr Nephrol 1990;4:96.

Abdominal aortic aneurysms

Maccario M, De Vecchi A, Scalamogna A, et al. Continuous ambulatory peritoneal dialysis in patients after intra-abdominal prosthetic vascular graft surgery. Nephron 1997;77:159-163.

Misra M, Goel S, Khanna R. Peritoneal dialysis in patients with abdominal vascular prostheses. Adv Perit Dial 1998;14:95-97.

Norwood MGA, Polimenovi NM, Sutton AJ, et al. Abdominal aortic aneurysm repair in patients with chronic renal disease. Eur J Vasc Endovasc Surg 2004;27:287-291.

Polner K, Gosi G, Vas SI, et al. Management of abdominal aortic and iliac artery aneurysms by stent-graft implantation in a patient on CAPD. Clin Nephrol 2009;71:359-362.

Gastric banding and gastric bypass

Alexander JW, Goodman HR, Gersin K, et al. Gastric bypass in morbidly obese patients with chronic renal failure and kidney transplant. Transplantation 2004;78:469-474.

Chen CC, Huang MT, Wie PL, et al. Severe peritonitis due to streptococcus viridans following adjustable gastric banding. Obes Surg 2010;20:1603-1605.

Appendix 1.
Useful web addresses

American Association of Kidney Patients	www.aakp.org	National non-profit organization started by CKD patients for the education of other patients, has links for patient questions.
AMA's Practice Management Center	www.ama-assn.org/go/pmc	Site provides physicians and their staff with practice management tools and resources.
American Society of Diagnostic and Interventional Nephrology	www.asdin.org	Society for interventional nephrologists with core curriculum for peritoneal dialysis catheter procedures
American Society of Nephrology	www.asn-online.org	Society that provides education through an annual meeting, smaller satellite meetings, and annual board review programs. Has self assessment programs termed NephSAP that are free to ASN members and awards CME credits.

Baxter Healthcare	www.baxter.com	Home site for Baxter with associated site renalinfo.com has information about kidney disease and dialysis with information on Baxter products, information on solutions such as Extraneal and recipes.
Baxter PD Site	www.glucosesafety.com	Web site lists the glucose monitors that use GDH-PQQ reagents that may read icodextrin related serum maltose as glucose and therefore report falsely elevated glucose readings
Center for Medicare and Medicaid Services	www.cms.hhs.gov	Home site for Medicare information related to ESRD with links to ESRD networks, clinical performance measures (CPM's), quality improvement initiatives, and dialysis facility information.
Covidian (formally Kendall brands)	www.kendallhq.com	Web site lists ordering information for a variety of PD catheters and accessories including the Quinton, Missouri, Toronto-Western, Moncrief-Popovich in swan neck and presternal designs. Also has abdominal stencils for pre-operative skin marking.
Dialysis Patient Citizens	www.dialysispatients.org	Organization of over 20 thousand dialysis patients with a mission to improve kidney care by state and federal advocacy and education. Has a Facebook page that encourages dialysis patients to network and exchange ideas and experiences.
Fresenius Medical Care	www.fmc-ag.com	Home site for world's largest provider of dialysis services and products, with PDF's for dialysis overview and the history of PD.
Home Dialysis Central	www.homedialysis.org	Central clearing house for useful information and web links relevant to home dialysis

Hypertension, Dialysis, and Clinical Nephrology	www.hdcn.com	Considered perhaps the single most extensive website in nephrology education with slide presentations, streaming audio from major renal meetings, and relevant publications.
International Society of Peritoneal Dialysis	www.ispd.org	Home site for the ISPD- meetings, guidelines, scholarship information and teaching materials.
Internet School of Nephrology	www.ukidney.com	Site with video presentations on PD, blogs and discussion forums.
iTunes	www.itunes.com/podcasts/nephrozone	PD related podcasts by leading authorities in the field.
Kidney Care Partners	www.kidney-carepartners.org	Coalition of patient representatives, dialysis professionals, providers, and manufacturers that broadly advocates on behalf of CKD and dialysis patients.
Kidney School, Life Options	www.lifeoptions.org	Web site started with support from Amgen with free booklets that discuss employment, exercise and encouragement while on dialysis. The Kidney School link contains interactive teaching modules such as coping, living with kidney disease, how kidneys work and how they fail, lab test interpretation, nutrition, and sexuality issues.
Medcomp	www.medcompnet.com	A provider of various PD catheters with recently introduced extended catheter kits and stencils
Merit Medical Systems	www.merit.com	Recently acquired Medigoup- provides Flex-Neck PD catheters and placement kits.
National Kidney Disease Education Program	www.nkdep.nih.gov	Teaching materials for the public and physicians with standardized MDRD equation.

National Kidney Foundation	www.kidney.org	Site is for patients as well as professionals. Has educational material for nephrologists to use when communicating with primary care physicians, tools to help implement K/DOQI guidelines.
National Renal Administrators Association	www.nraa.org	Nonprofit organization representing dialysis facilities in USA that includes medical directors, nurse managers, technicians, and financial/billing managers for dialysis clinics.
Nephron Information Center	www.nephron.com	Web site that aggregates renal publications, news events, lists all dialysis units approved by Medicare with maps to location, etc.
Patient's Pride	www.patientspride.com	Company started by PD patient Shiela Shaw who ultimately received a living related transplant. Sheila designed and produced a soft cotton waist band that more comfortably holds the external catheter assembly. The web site also contains motivational material for patients and caregivers.
Renal Physicians Association	www.renalmd.org	Association of nephrologists active in promoting excellence in care which advocates for public policy initiatives that affect the practice of nephrology and it's fair renumeration.
RenalWeb	www.renalweb.com	Clearing house of dialysis related resources, products, discussion groups, etc.

Buettner K, Fadem SZ. The internet as a tool for the renal community. Adv Chronic Kid Dis 2008;15:73-82.

Index

3 pore model 15

A

AAA 257
Abdominal aortic aneurysm 257
ACE inhibitors 46
ACE inhibitors and RRF 46
Acid-base 220
Acute PD 93
Adapters, catheters 68
ADEMEX 35
Adequacy of dialysis 33, 206
Adhesiolysis 75
ADPKD 148, 254
Advanced laparoscopic placement techniques 75
Air, intraperitoneal 165
Albumin level 215
Alcavis 119
Alcohol-based hand products 125
Amino acid solutions 58
Aminoglycosides 45
Amylase, icodextrin metabolism 58
Angiotensin receptor blockers 46
APD 105
Aquaporins 16, 20

B

Back pain 157
Bacterial peritonitis 122
Balance 54
BALANZ study 60
Bicarbonate, infusion pain 88
BicaVera 54
Bile 164
Bile acid sequestrants 218
Bilious dialysate 164
Bio-electric impedence 222
Black line sign 165
Bladder catheters 251
Blind patient 255
BMI 203
Body composition 205
Body mass index 203
Bone disease 219
Buried catheters 76

C

Caesarian section, pregnancy 252
Calcium channel blockers, chylous ascites 155
Caloric absorption 220
CANUSA 34
CAPD 105
Carbohydrate absorption 187, 220
Catheter migration 84
Catheter placement, acute PD 94
Catheter repositioning 85
Catheters 65
Cats 135
Cell count, peritoneal fluid 127, 139
Chewing gum, phosphate removal 220
Chlorhexidine 120
Cholesterol 216
Chylous dialysate 154
Cirrhosis 253
Colloidal osmotic pressure 56
Colonoscopy, antibiotic prophylaxis 124
Colostomy 249

Conditions for coverage 239
Congestive heart failure 253
Constipation 83, 182
Contrast agents 45
Convection 17
C-section 252
Cuff erosion 87
Cuff placement 68
Culture techniques 127
Cycler PD 106

D

DATT 28
Dental prophylaxis 124
Diabetic patient 185
Dialysis Adequacy and Transport Test (DATT) 28
Dianeal 53
Dianeal – N 54
Dietician 241
Diffusion 16
Distributed model 15
Diuretics 46
Diverticulosis 133
Dogs 135
DPI 214
Drain pain 88, 157

E

EDEN study 60
Education, dialysis options 243
Embedded catheters 76
EMT 20
Encapsulating peritoneal sclerosis 159
Enterococcal peritonitis 134
Eosinophilic peritonitis 138, 162
Epithelial-to-mesenchymal transition 20
EPS 159
Exit site infections 118, 120
Exit site, location 69, 118
Extended care facilities and PD 246
Extended catheters 70
Extraneal 55

Ezetimibe 218
F
Fast PET 27
Feeding tubes 251
Fibrates 217
Fibrin 86
Fluid status 175
Fluoroscopically-guided catheter placement 72
Fogarty catheter manipulation 85
Fungal exit site infections 121
Fungal peritonitis 137
G
Gastric banding 257
Gastric bypass 257
Gastric feeding tube 251
Gastroparesis 195
Gastrostomy 251
Genital swelling 152
Gentamicin cream 119
Glucose degradation products (GDPs) 54
Glucose exposure 187, 220
Glucose meters 57
Glucose-sparing strategies 187
Gram-negative peritonitis 133
Gynecology procedures 125, 138
H
Hand washing 125
HbA1c 189
Hemoperitoneum 152
Heparin 129
Hernia 145
Historical perspective 1
HIV patient on PD 251
HMG-CoA reductase inhibitors 216
Hot tubs 70
Household pets 135
Hydrothorax 148
Hyperkalemia 212
Hyperphosphatemia 219
Hypertonic saline soaks 120

Hypoalbuminemia 125, 215
Hypokalemia 125, 212
Hypomagnesemia 213
Hypophatemia 219

I

Icodextrin 55, 111, 187
IIPV 166
Ileostomy 249
IMPENDIA study 60
Increased intraperitoneal volume 166
Incremental PD 112
Infrastructure of a PD unit 239
Infusion pain 88
Insulin 190
Insulin, intraperitoneal 190
Intermittent PD 113
International Society of PD 10, 117, 129
Interventional radiology 73, 85
Interventionalists 72, 89
Intra-abdominal pressure 71, 95

Intraperitoneal antibiotics 130
Intraperitoneal insulin 190
Intraperitoneal volume, increased 166
Intrauterine device 253
IPD 113
ISPD 10, 117, 129
IUD 253

J

Jacuzzi, use in the PD patient 70

K

Kidney transplant 250
Kinetic modeling 33
Kt/V 34

L

Lactulose 126
Laparoscopic catheter placement 75
Laparotomy, catheter placement 74
Large pores 15
Late-referred patient 93

Laxatives 84, 88, 126
Leaks 151
Lipase 58
Lipids 216
Liver disease 253
Long dwell 110, 178
Lymphatics, fluid reabsorption 19
Lymphatics, icodextrin absorption 57

M
Magnesium 213
Magnesium deficiency 213
Maltose 57, 187
Medical director 240
Membrane transport characterisics 24
Mesh, for hernia repair 146
Methemalbumin 165
Middle molecule, clearance 17
Migration, catheter 84
Mineral bone disease 219
Mini-PET 28
Modified PET 27
Moncrief-Popovich technique 76
Morbid obesity, technique success 203
Multivitamins 221
Mupirocin 118
MVI 221
Mycobacterial peritonitis 136

N
Nasal carriage 118
Neurogenic bladder 251
Neutral pH solutions 54
Nicotinamide 218
NIPD 106
NKF-DOQI 34
nPNA 39
Nursing homes 246
Nursing staff 240
Nutrineal 58
Nutrition 211

O

Obesity 70, 203
Obesity, catheter placement 70, 207
Obesity, peritonitis 208
Obesity, survival 203
Octreotide 156
Omental wrap 87
Omentopexy 76, 87
Open laparotomy 74
Orlistat 156
Osmotic conductance 19
Osmotic properties 18, 177
Ostomies 249

P

Pain on draining 88, 157
Pain on filling 88
Pancreatitis 163
Pasteurella peritonitis 135
Patent processus vaginalis 152
PDC 28
PEG 251
Percutaneous catheter placement 72
Percutaneous gastrostomy 251
Peritoneoscopic catheter placement 73
Peritonitis 122
Peritonitis, diagnosis 126
Peritonitis, eosinophilic 138, 162
Peritonitis, fungal 132
Peritonitis, mycobacterial 136
Peritonitis, recurrent 136
Peritonitis, relapsing 136
Peritonitis, treatment 128
Personal Dialysis Capacity Test (PDC) 28
PET 23
PET, fast 27
PET, modified 27
Pets, in the home 135, 256
Phosphorus restriction 219
Phospho-soda bowel preparations 84

Phosphorus removal 220
Physioneal 54
Pleurodesis 149
PNA 39, 214
Pneumoperitoneum 165
Polycystic disease 148, 254
Polymicrobial peritonitis 133
Polysporin ointment 119
Polyurethane 65
Potassium disorders 125, 212
Povidone-iodine/icodextrin complex 165
Pregnancy 148, 153, 251
Prescription management, acute 95
Prescription management, chronic 105
Pre-sternal catheters 70, 208
Processus vaginalis 152
Protein intake 39, 214
Protein nitrogen appearance 214
Pseudomonal peritonitis 133
QAPI 244

Q-R

Quality control 244
Rash, icodextrin 58
Rectus sheath tunneling 75
Recurrent peritonitis 136
Reflection coefficient 56
Relapsing peritonitis 136
Renin-angiotensin system 46
Residual kidney function 43, 176, 193, 205, 235
Rhabdomyolysis 165

S

Salt intake 176, 211
Salt substitutes 211
Scrotal leak 152
Scrotal swelling 152
Seldinger technique 72
Sevelamer 219
SGA 221
Silicon catheters 6, 65
Small pores 15

Social worker 241
Sodium balance 211
Sodium hypochlorite 120
Sodium sieving 19
Solutions 53
SPA 28
Standard peritoneal permeability analysis 28
Staphylococcal peritonitis 132
Star fruit 222
Statins 216
Stiff wire manipulation 85
Stomas 249
Suprapubic bladder catheters 251
Surgeons 242
Survival 43, 185, 203, 231
Swan neck catheters 67
Swimming 255

T

Tamoxifen 160
Tenckhoff catheters 5, 67
TGF-beta 20, 160
Thorascopic surgery, video assisted 150
Three pore model 15
Thrombolytics, intraperitoneal 89
Tidal PD 88, 112
Tissue Plasminogen Activator 89
TPA 86, 89
Training, patient 242
Transplant immunosuppression 48
Transplant outcomes 235, 250
Transport characteristics 24
Treatment of peritonitis 128
Triglycerides 154, 216
Triple antibiotic cream 119
Tunnel infections 122

U

Ultrafiltration 17, 96, 110, 175
Ultrafiltration efficiency 19, 180
Ultrasound guidance 72
Urgent-start PD 98, 244

USRDS 11, 232
Uterine prolapse 157
V
Vaginal leaks 156
Vancomycin-resistant enterococcus peritonitis 134
VATS procedure 150
VEGF 21
Ventriculo-peritoneal shunt 256
Video-assisted thoroscopic surgery 150
Visually-impaired patient 255
Vitamin D 219
Vitamins 221
Volume status 175
V-P shunt 256
VRE 134
W
Water channels 16, 20
Water soluble vitamins 221
Watson formula 38
Weight gain 206, 218
X-Z
Y-Tec 73

About the Author:

STEVEN GUEST **MD** ATTENDED medical school at Vanderbilt University School of Medicine and completed his nephrology fellowship at the Massachusetts General Hospital. For twelve years Dr. Guest served as the PD program director at the Santa Clara Valley Medical Center which functioned as the primary PD training site for the Stanford University School of Medicine nephrology training program. As a Stanford Adjunct Clinical Associate Professor of Medicine he was awarded many prestigious teaching awards including the Henry J. Kaiser award for excellence in clinical education.

Dr. Guest also served as the PD program director at Kaiser Permanente Santa Clara. He received sub-specialist of the year teaching awards and was named a Consumer's Checkbook Top Doctor. In 2008, Dr. Guest joined Baxter Healthcare Corporation and speaks on various PD topics throughout the USA. He has published many articles focusing on the clinical aspects of PD therapy.

Printed in Great Britain
by Amazon